Pneumonia: Diagnosis, Prognosis and Treatment

Pneumonia: Diagnosis, Prognosis and Treatment

Edited by Natalia Fitzgerald

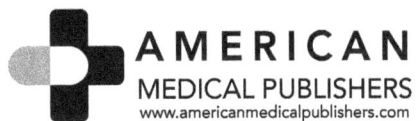

AMERICAN
MEDICAL PUBLISHERS
www.americanmedicalpublishers.com

American Medical Publishers,
41 Flatbush Avenue,
1st Floor, New York,
NY 11217, USA

Visit us on the World Wide Web at:
www.americanmedicalpublishers.com

ISBN: 978-1-63927-231-0

Cataloging-in-Publication Data

Pneumonia : diagnosis, prognosis and treatment / edited by Natalia Fitzgerald.
     p. cm.
Includes bibliographical references and index.
ISBN 978-1-63927-231-0
1. Pneumonia. 2. Pneumonia--Diagnosis. 3. Pneumonia--Treatment.
4. Lungs--Diseases. I. Fitzgerald, Natalia.
RC771 .P543 2022
616.241--dc23

Table of Contents

Preface

The purpose of the book is to provide a glimpse into the dynamics and to present opinions and studies of some of the scientists engaged in the development of new ideas in the field from very different standpoints. This book will prove useful to students and researchers owing to its high content quality.

Pneumonia is an inflammatory condition of the lung that affects the alveoli. Its symptoms include chest pain, productive or dry cough, trouble breathing and fever. Pneumonia is caused by certain micro-organisms including virus and bacteria. Certain medications and autoimmune diseases also give rise to pneumonia. Some of its risk factors are cystic fibrosis, chronic obstructive pulmonary disease (COPD), asthma, diabetes, heart failure, a history of smoking, a poor ability to cough, etc. It is diagnosed on the basis of symptoms and physical examination. The diagnosis can also be done through chest X-rays, blood tests and culture of the sputum. Vaccination also prevents certain types of bacterial and viral pneumonias in children and adults. Complete treatment of pneumonia includes using oral antibiotics, analgesics, proper rest and fluids. This book contains some path-breaking studies in the field of pneumonia. The extensive content of this book provides the readers with a thorough understanding of the conditions. It will serve as a valuable source of reference for graduate and postgraduate students.

At the end, I would like to appreciate all the efforts made by the authors in completing their chapters professionally. I express my deepest gratitude to all of them for contributing to this book by sharing their valuable works. A special thanks to my family and friends for their constant support in this journey.

Editor

Cost-effectiveness of antibiotic treatment strategies for community-acquired pneumonia

Cornelis H. van Werkhoven[1†], Douwe F. Postma[1,2,3*†], Marie-Josee J. Mangen[1], Jan Jelrik Oosterheert[2], Marc J. M. Bonten[1,4] and for the CAP-START study group

Abstract

Background: To determine the cost-effectiveness of strategies of preferred antibiotic treatment with beta-lactam/macrolide combination or fluoroquinolone monotherapy compared to beta-lactam monotherapy.

Methods: Costs and effects were estimated using data from a cluster-randomized cross-over trial of antibiotic treatment strategies, primarily from the reduced third payer perspective (i.e. hospital admission costs). Cost-minimization analysis (CMA) and cost-effectiveness analysis (CEA) were performed using linear mixed models. CMA results were expressed as difference in costs per patient. CEA results were expressed as incremental cost-effectiveness ratios (ICER) showing additional costs per prevented death.

Results: A total of 2,283 patients were included. Crude average costs within 90 days from the reduced third payer perspective were €4,294, €4,392, and €4,002 per patient for the beta-lactam monotherapy, beta-lactam/macrolide combination, and fluoroquinolone monotherapy strategy, respectively. CMA results were €106 (95% CI €-697 to €754) for the beta-lactam/macrolide combination strategy and €-278 (95%CI €-991 to €396) for the fluoroquinolone monotherapy strategy, both compared to the beta-lactam monotherapy strategy. The ICER was not statistically significantly different between the strategies. Other perspectives yielded similar results.

Conclusions: There were no significant differences in cost-effectiveness of strategies of preferred antibiotic treatment of CAP on non-ICU wards with either beta-lactam monotherapy, beta-lactam/macrolide combination therapy, or fluoroquinolone monotherapy.

Keywords: Beta-lactam macrolide, Fluoroquinolone, Cost-effectiveness, Community acquired pneumonia

Background

Community-acquired pneumonia (CAP) is an important reason for hospitalization worldwide [1–3]. It has been estimated that the total costs associated with CAP amount to approximately 11 billion euros annually in Europe, with approx. 5 billion euros accounting for in-

hospital CAP costs [1]. In the Netherlands there are an estimated 25,000-36,000 hospital admissions for CAP each year, [4] with an estimated total costs of about 100 to 178 million euro annually [5, 6]. The intramural costs are mainly determined by the length of hospitalization and site of care (medical ward or intensive care unit, ICU) [5, 6].

In choosing the optimal antibiotic treatment strategy for CAP, effectiveness, cost-effectiveness and ecological effects of antibiotics should be taken into account. Optimally, this would consist of a strategy associated with the best patient outcome at the lowest price and

* Correspondence: d.f.postma@umcutrecht.nl
†Equal contributors
[1]Julius Center for Health Sciences and Primary Care, University Medical Center Utrecht, Utrecht, The Netherlands
[2]Department of Internal Medicine and Infectious Diseases, University Medical Center Utrecht, Heidelberglaan 100, 3584 CX Utrecht, The Netherlands
Full list of author information is available at the end of the article

with least selective pressure for antibiotic resistance. The three treatment strategies most widely used are beta-lactam monotherapy, beta-lactam/macrolide combination therapy, and fluoroquinolone monotherapy. From an ecological perspective beta-lactam monotherapy is preferred over beta-lactam/ macrolide combination therapy, and fluoroquinolone monotherapy, since the latter two drug classes have been associated with resistance development during treatment [7, 8].

In a cluster-randomized cross-over trial of patients hospitalized with CAP to non-ICU wards, a strategy of beta-lactam monotherapy was non-inferior to beta-lactam/macrolide combination therapy, and fluoroquinolone monotherapy in terms of all-cause day-90 mortality (CAP-START study) [9]. The quinolone monotherapy strategy was associated with a shorter length of intravenous treatment, but this was not reflected in a statistically significant shorter length of stay. In the current study, we set out to conduct a cost-minimization analysis of these different antibiotic strategies and a cost-effectiveness analysis from a third payer and a social perspective.

Methods
Intervention
The Community-Acquired Pneumonia Study on the initial Treatment with Antibiotics of Lower Respiratory Tract Infections (CAP-START, http://clinicaltrials.gov/show/NCT01660204) was a cluster-randomized cross-over trial that was performed in seven hospitals in the Netherlands between February 2011 and August 2013. Details of the study design, enrolment, and clinical outcomes have been published previously [9, 10]. In short, three strategies were compared in which one class or combination of antibiotics (beta-lactam monotherapy, beta-lactam/macrolide combination therapy or fluoroquinolone monotherapy) was the preferred empirical treatment for adult patients hospitalized to non-intensive care unit (ICU) wards with a clinical diagnosis of CAP. Hospitals were randomized to a sequence of consecutive periods of 4 months, in each of which one of the strategies were applied. Deviations from the preferred empirical treatment for medical reasons were allowed, e.g. because of contra-indications, allergy to the preferred regimen, or a suspected pathogen not covered by the preferred regimen. Physicians were encouraged to complete the preferred empirical treatment unless for a medical reason, e.g. insufficient recovery or deterioration of the patient, or detection of a pathogen for which targeted antibiotic treatment was initiated. Based on an intention-to-treat principle, inclusion of patients was independent of compliance with the strategy, which allowed us to assess the effect of the strategy as a whole.

Effects
For health outcomes we used 30- and 90-day all-cause mortality, which have been reported previously [9]. Mortality status at day 90 was recorded from the medical charts in patients that died during hospitalization, and patients that had visited the hospital after day 90 (e.g. in an out-patient clinic). The status of all other patients, except in one hospital, was checked electronically in the municipal personal records database, which is based on the citizen service number, date of birth and name. In the one hospital without electronic access to this database, research nurses contacted the general practitioner of each patient with an unknown status. In the Netherlands, every inhabitant is registered with a single general practitioner, who is routinely informed about important medical affairs.

Cost of illness
Data on healthcare resource utilization during hospitalization, e.g. hospital days, interventions, and medication (see Additional file 1: Table S2 for a complete overview), were derived from the medical records by trained research nurses using a predefined clinical record form. For other resources, patients were asked to complete a questionnaire on the 28th day after admission. This 28th day questionnaire included questions on post-discharge healthcare use such as nursing home admission, general practitioner and specialist consultations, patient costs (e.g. travel costs), and the number of days absent from paid and unpaid work for both patients and their caregivers. We defined caregivers as adult persons taking absence from paid or unpaid work in order to take care of a sick person.

Direct healthcare costs (DHC), direct non-healthcare costs (DNHC) - also referred to as patient costs -, and productivity losses (i.e. indirect non-healthcare costs-INHC) were considered in the current study. In accordance with the current Dutch guidelines for health economic evaluations, this study did not consider indirect healthcare costs [11, 12]. Indirect healthcare costs would comprise the future savings in healthcare costs in the life years lost due to premature death. DHC were composed of healthcare costs related to hospitalization, e.g. days admitted to non-ICU wards, ICU days with and without mechanical ventilation, medical interventions, antibiotic use, other medication use, and post-discharge healthcare consumption. In the DNHC category, travel costs to a general practitioner (GP), to a hospital, or over-the-counter medication were considered. Productivity losses were estimated for non-fatal CAP cases by multiplying self-reported sick leave from paid and unpaid work with the corresponding age and gender specific unit prices as reported in Additional file 1: Table S1. For fatal cases younger than 65 years, two approaches were used: the friction and the human capital approach. The friction approach, recommended in Dutch guidelines, takes into account the productivity loss from paid work due to case fatality for a period of 23 weeks from the date of admission [11, 12]. In the human capital approach, productivity losses from work due to case fatality up to the age of retirement were considered, leading to higher costs due to productivity loss for deceased patients under 65 years of age.

Costs were estimated by multiplying resources used with their corresponding unit cost prices. Additional file 1: Table S1 depicts unit cost prices for all DHC, DNHC, and INHC used in the analyses. All costs are expressed in 2012 euros and, if necessary, updated using Dutch consumer price indexes [4].

Two time horizons of 30 and 90 days were used for the economic evaluation, in accordance with the time horizons used for the effects under study, i.e. 30-day and 90-day mortality [9]. Hospital and nursing home admission costs were calculated until discharge or until the time horizon, whichever came first. For productivity losses from case-fatality, deaths falling within the defined time horizon were used, but, as explained previously, costs were extended to 23 weeks using the friction approach [11, 12], and to retirement age using the human capital approach, respectively. Discounting was only applied for productivity losses longer than 1 year (i.e. the human capital approach), using a 3% annual discount rate [13]. As in the primary analysis of clinical outcomes, the 90-day time horizon was considered for the primary analysis.

Economic evaluation
Cost-minimization analysis (CMA) and cost-effectiveness analysis (CEA) were conducted using four different perspectives. The "reduced" third payer perspective included only DHC of the CAP hospitalization. This perspective constituted the primary analysis of medical records, and as such healthcare utilization data during admission, were available for all patients. The "full" third payer perspective (referred hereafter as third payer perspective) included both DHC during admission and post-discharge. The societal perspective considered all three categories (i.e. DHC, DNHC and INHC). Two approaches were used here, the friction and the human capital approach, as explained previously.

The beta-lactam monotherapy strategy was considered the reference arm, as this is considered the first choice treatment for patients hospitalized with CAP to non-ICU wards in the Netherlands [14]. As the primary outcome of the CAP-START trial, i.e. prevented deaths per treated person, was not statistically significantly different between the strategies [9], we conducted a CMA,

assessing the incremental costs per treated case. Additionally, because small effects on clinical outcomes could not be excluded, a CEA was conducted showing the incremental costs (or savings) of the net effect (i.e. number of deaths prevented), expressed as incremental cost-effectiveness ratio (ICER) showing additional costs per prevented death.

Data analysis
Crude average costs were calculated for each antibiotic treatment strategy. For calculating incremental costs, we adjusted for the cluster-randomized design of the study, by using a mixed-effects linear regression analysis, with a random intercept for each cluster-period of 4 months, and fixed effects for hospital and treatment arm. A random intercept is used in mixed-effect models to allow for dependence of observations within one cluster [15]. For cost-minimization and cost-effectiveness analyses, differences in mortality (i.e. the incremental effect) were assessed similarly using a mixed-effects logistic regression analysis. We performed bootstrapping with 2,000 samples to obtain confidence intervals. For missing values, five imputations were performed in each bootstrapped dataset. In each of the imputed datasets, the costs and effects were compared between the treatment strategies using the aforementioned mixed-effects models. Incremental costs and effects were averaged over these 5 imputations, again resulting in 2,000 estimates of incremental costs and effects. From these, we derived incremental costs and effects which were presented as cost-effectiveness plots. 95% confidence intervals were derived from these estimates using the quantile method. Significance for cost-minimization and cost-effectiveness was defined as a 95% confidence interval not covering the null effect.

Results
Patient, data collection, and missing data
In total 656, 739, and 888 patients were included during the beta-lactam, beta-lactam/macrolide and fluoroquinolone strategies. Age, gender, and comorbidities had similar distributions in the three treatment arms (Table 1). Inclusion rates, strategy adherence, and reasons for protocol deviations and switches have been described previously [9]. Response rates for the self-reported 28th day questionnaire were comparable in all three treatment arms (42.1%, 34.2%, and 42.3% for beta-lactam monotherapy, beta-lactam/macrolide combination, and fluoroquinolone monotherapy strategy respectively).

In total, 2.1 and 6.6% of data points from the medical records and received 28th day questionnaires, respectively, were missing.

Table 1 Baseline characteristics

	Beta-lactam monotherapy (N = 656)	Beta-lactam/macrolide (N = 739)	Fluoroquinolone monotherapy (N = 888)
Median age (IQR)	70.6 (60.6–79.4)	70.7 (59.1–80.3)	71.0 (59.6–79.4)
Male gender	381 (58.1%)	431 (58.3%)	505 (56.9%)
Elderly home	32 / 644 (5.0%)	38 / 727 (5.2%)	41 / 878 (4.7%)
Hospitalization past 12 months	271 / 653 (41.5%)	298 / 722 (41.3%)	351 / 881 (39.8%)
Median number of comorbidities (IQR) [a]	1 (0–2)	1 (0–2)	1 (1–2)
Immunocompromised [b]	147 (22.4%)	173 (23.4%)	213 (24.0%)
Median CURB-65 score (IQR) [d]	1 (1–2)	1 (1–2)	1 (1–2)
Day-28 questionnaire received	276 (42.1%)	253 (34.2%)	376 (42.3%)
Reports paid work	51 / 246 (20.7%)	45 / 233 (19.3%)	78 / 342 (22.8%)
Reports volunteer work	23 / 245 (9.4%)	32 / 234 (13.7%)	35 / 340 (10.3%)

Data are reported as N (%) unless otherwise indicated. IQR: inter quartile range
[a] Reported comorbidities include chronic cardiovascular disease, heart failure, cerebrovascular disease, asthma, COPD, other chronic pulmonary disease, HIV/AIDS, diabetes mellitus, haematological malignancies[c], solid organ malignancies[c], chronic renal failure requiring dialysis, nephrotic syndrome, organ or bone marrow transplantation, alcoholism, chronic liver disease and functional or anatomic asplenia
[b] Patients were categorized as immunocompromised if any of the following conditions applied: HIV/AIDS, haematological malignancies#, solid organ malignancies[c], chronic renal failure requiring dialysis, nephrotic syndrome, organ or bone marrow transplantation, or receipt of immunosuppressive therapy (for corticosteroids this required at least 0.5 mg/kg/day prednisolone or equivalent dosage for a minimum of 14 days)
[c] Having received or been eligible for chemotherapy or radiotherapy in the past 5 years
[d] The CURB-65 score is calculated by assigning 1 point each for confusion, uraemia (blood urea nitrogen ≥20 mg per deci- liter), high respiratory rate (≥30 breaths per minute), low systolic blood pressure (<90 mm Hg) or diastolic blood pres- sure (≤60 mm Hg), and an age of 65 years or older, with a higher score indicating a higher risk of death within 30 days

Cost of illness and economic evaluation

Crude (i.e. not adjusted for the cluster-randomized cross-over design) average costs within 90 days from the reduced third payer perspective (i.e. hospitalization costs) were €4,294 (95% confidence interval, CI €3,782 to €4,952) per patient for the beta-lactam monotherapy strategy, €4,392 (95% CI €4,062 to €4,760) per patient for the beta-lactam/macrolide combination strategy, and €4,002 (95% CI €3,725 to €4,341) per patient for the fluoroquinolone mono- therapy strategy (Fig. 1). For the CMA using the reduced third payer perspective within the 90-day time horizon, estimated incremental costs, adjusted for cluster and period effects using a mixed-effects model, were €106 (95% CI -€697 to €754) per pa- tient for the beta-lactam/macrolide combination strategy and -€278 (95%CI -€991 to €396) for the fluoroquinolone monotherapy strategy, a positive number indicating higher costs as compared to the beta-lactam monotherapy strategy.

For the beta-lactam/macrolide strategy compared to the beta-lactam strategy, using the reduced third payer perspective and the 90-day time horizon, 57.8% of the bootstrap results was in the north-west quad- rant (i.e. positive incremental costs, the beta-lactam/ macrolide strategy was more costly than the beta- lactam strategy, and negative incremental effects, the beta-lactam/macrolide strategy prevented fewer deaths than the beta-lactam strategy, thus beta-lactam domi- nates the beta-lactam/macrolide strategy), 3.3% was in the north-east quadrant (i.e. "positive" incremental costs and a positive incremental effect), 35.2% was in the south-west quadrant (i.e. negative incremental costs or cost-savings and a negative incremental effect), and 3.6% was in the south-east quadrant (i.e. negative incremental costs and a positive incremental effect), with the point estimate for the ICER in the north-west quadrant (Fig. 2a). For the fluoroquinolone strategy compared to the beta-lactam strategy, using the same perspective and time window, 11.6% was in the north-west quadrant, 10.2% in the north-east quadrant, 35.3% in the south-west quadrant, and 43.0% was in the south-east quadrant, with the point estimate for ICER in the south-east quadrant (Fig. 2c). Thus, the 95% confidence interval of the ICER ranged from being dominated (positive incremental costs and negative incremental effect) to cost-saving (negative incremental costs or savings and positive incremental effects or more prevented deaths) for both comparisons.

Similar results for costs, CMA, and CEA were obtained for the third payer perspective and for the societal perspective taking the friction approach (Fig. 2, Additional file 1: Figure S1, Figure S2, and Table S3), as well as for the 30-day time horizon for these three perspectives. The societal perspective with human capital approach had large confidence intervals for costs, for both time horizons, leading to uninterpretable results for both CMA and CEA (Additional file 1: Figure S3 and Table S3).

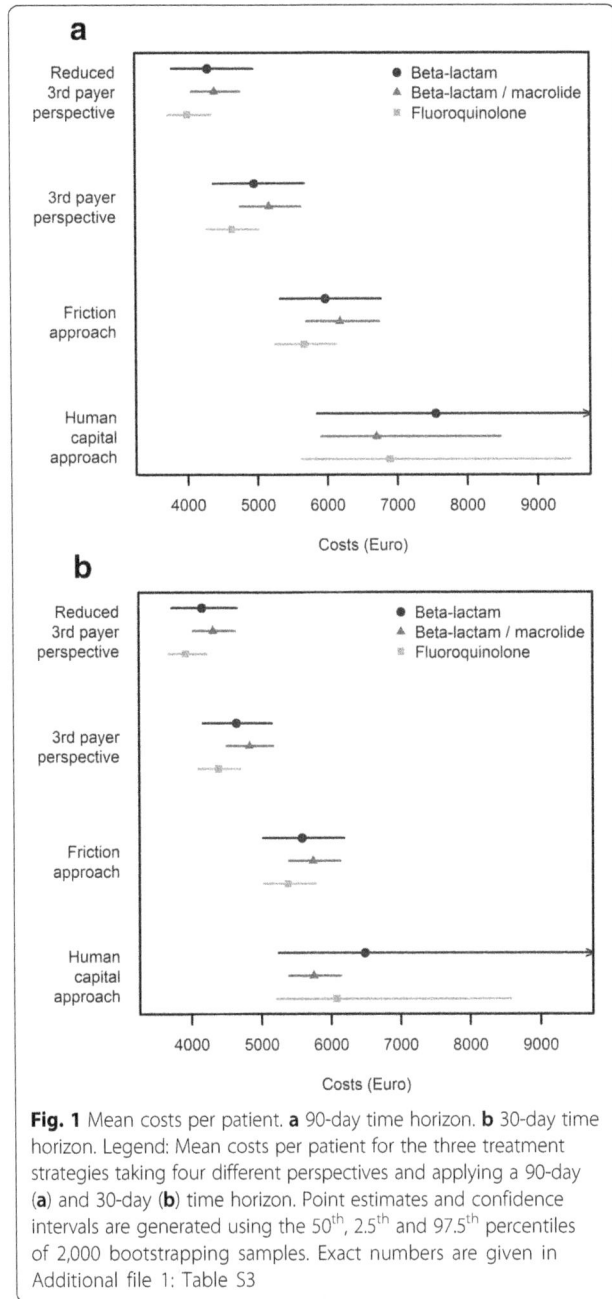

Fig. 1 Mean costs per patient. **a** 90-day time horizon. **b** 30-day time horizon. Legend: Mean costs per patient for the three treatment strategies taking four different perspectives and applying a 90-day (**a**) and 30-day (**b**) time horizon. Point estimates and confidence intervals are generated using the 50th, 2.5th and 97.5th percentiles of 2,000 bootstrapping samples. Exact numbers are given in Additional file 1: Table S3

Discussion

In these analyses, we have demonstrated that the differences in costs associated with either of three preferred empirical antibiotic treatment strategies (i.e., beta-lactam monotherapy, beta-lactam/macrolide combination therapy, or fluoroquinolone monotherapy) for patients hospitalized for community-acquired pneumonia did not reach statistical significance. Together with non-inferiority of the beta-lactam monotherapy strategy for day-90 mortality [9] and the perceived preference of beta-lactam monotherapy from an ecological perspective, the current analysis supports the use of beta-lactam

monotherapy as preferred empirical treatment for these patients.

This is the first comparison of costs and cost-effectiveness for different preferred antibiotic treatment strategies in patients hospitalized with CAP. Our study has several strengths. First, because this was a pragmatic trial, where patients were included during strategy periods regardless of the actual antibiotics used, the intention-to-treat analysis of our study is well generalizable to daily clinical practice. All patients that received antibiotic treatment for a working diagnosis of CAP and who were hospitalized to a non-ICU medical ward, were eligible. Second, the cluster-randomized design allowed the immediate start of the allocated antibiotic treatment because individual randomization was not needed. This minimizes effects of other antibiotics prescribed in the Emergency Departments before study randomization. Third, because of the cross-over design, all hospitals applied all three strategies, thus minimizing confounding bias. As a result, baseline characteristics of the three strategies were very comparable. Fourth, we have collected comprehensive data on antibiotic treatment and medical procedures that allowed us to estimate hospitalization costs per patient. Using 2,000 bootstrapping samples and five imputations per sample, we were able to provide robust estimates and confidence intervals for the different cost categories. Our estimated costs per CAP admission are in line with previously published data from the Netherlands [5, 6]. Fifth, different economic viewpoints were pursued in the current analysis. The (reduced) third payer perspective and the societal perspective taking the friction approach all gave the same direction and magnitude of effect. The large confidence intervals observed in the societal perspective with human capital approach was due to the low number of fatal cases under 65 years of age and due to working status being unknown for unreturned 28th day questionnaires. This led to unstable imputation of working status, since these variables also interact i.e. the proportion of returned questionnaires was lower for patients that had died at day 90, thus increasing confidence intervals.

Our approach had certain limitations. We had limited data on medication use other than antibiotics. Although it seems unlikely that one of the antibiotic treatment strategies would be associated with other patterns of non-antibiotic medication use, if so, we may have slightly underestimated the costs. 28th day questionnaires, used for DNHC and INHC estimation, were returned by approximately 40% of the participants. We used multiple imputation to deal with missing data because response to the 28th day questionnaire was obviously dependent on clinical outcome and was related to baseline characteristics (e.g. dependency in activities of daily living or hospitalizations in the previous year). This

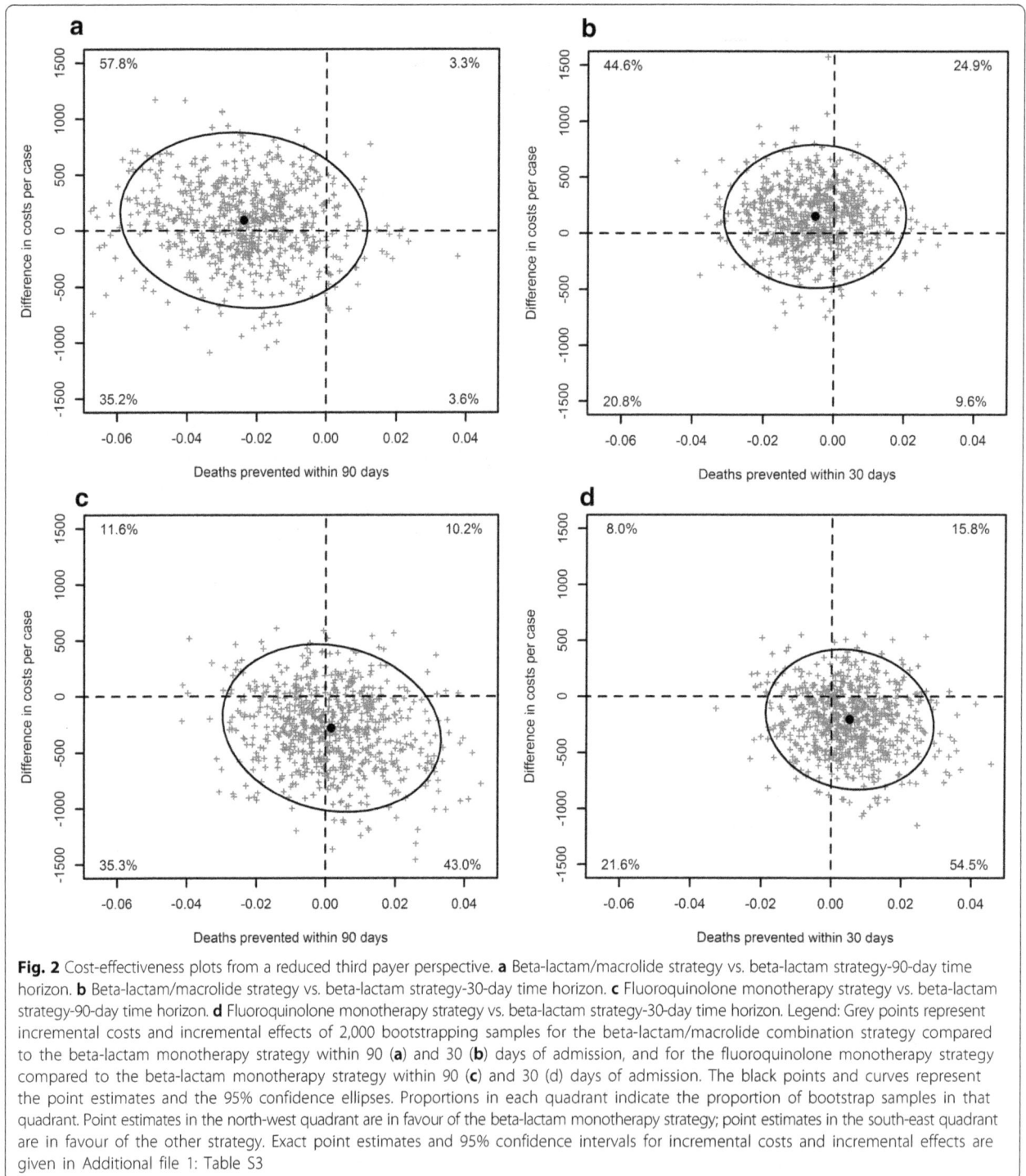

Fig. 2 Cost-effectiveness plots from a reduced third payer perspective. **a** Beta-lactam/macrolide strategy vs. beta-lactam strategy-90-day time horizon. **b** Beta-lactam/macrolide strategy vs. beta-lactam strategy-30-day time horizon. **c** Fluoroquinolone monotherapy strategy vs. beta-lactam strategy-90-day time horizon. **d** Fluoroquinolone monotherapy strategy vs. beta-lactam strategy-30-day time horizon. Legend: Grey points represent incremental costs and incremental effects of 2,000 bootstrapping samples for the beta-lactam/macrolide combination strategy compared to the beta-lactam monotherapy strategy within 90 (**a**) and 30 (**b**) days of admission, and for the fluoroquinolone monotherapy strategy compared to the beta-lactam monotherapy strategy within 90 (**c**) and 30 (d) days of admission. The black points and curves represent the point estimates and the 95% confidence ellipses. Proportions in each quadrant indicate the proportion of bootstrap samples in that quadrant. Point estimates in the north-west quadrant are in favour of the beta-lactam monotherapy strategy; point estimates in the south-east quadrant are in favour of the other strategy. Exact point estimates and 95% confidence intervals for incremental costs and incremental effects are given in Additional file 1: Table S3

may have increased uncertainty for the third payer and societal perspectives, and it certainly did for the societal perspective with human capital approach, as explained previously.

The number of days on intravenous antibiotic treatment was significantly lower during the fluoroquinolone monotherapy strategy (hazard ratio for time to switch to oral treatment 1.29, 95% CI 1.15–1.46) [9]. This was fully explained by the larger proportion of patients starting with oral treatment from the day of admission, despite the similar baseline characteristics between the different strategies, and can, therefore, not be attributed to a faster clinical response. The known high bioavailability of oral fluoroquinolones [16] may have stimulated physicians to directly start with oral antibiotics and this may have contributed to the more favourable point estimate of difference in costs seen in the fluoroquinolone monotherapy period. Whether the same proportion of patients could start with oral beta-lactam monotherapy without compromising patient outcome remains to be elucidated.

In an open-label randomized controlled trial from Switzerland, beta-lactam monotherapy was not non-inferior to beta-lactam/macrolide combination therapy in establishing clinical stability after seven days of antibiotic treatment [17]. This study was not designed to determine non-inferiority for day-30 or day-90 mortality, and there were no statistically significant or clinically relevant differences in outcome between both study arms. Time to clinical stability was not determined in our study, however, length of stay was significantly longer for the beta-lactam/macrolide combination strategy, and consequently also the costs per patient were higher, although not statistically significant. This seemingly opposite finding might in part be explained by the maximized adherence to the allocated antibiotic, i.e. the strict criteria for switching antibiotic treatment, which could only have disadvantaged the beta-lactam monotherapy arm in the Swiss study. The current analysis shows that any benefit of beta-lactam/macrolide combination treatment on time to clinical stability, if present, does not lead to cost reduction.

Generalizability of the estimated costs may depend on several factors, the most important of which are the duration of hospitalization, ICU admission, the length of intravenous and oral antibiotics, and post discharge patterns of healthcare use. Although the actual reported costs are obviously specific for the Netherlands, the relative differences in costs for medication are comparable internationally [18, 19]. As the generalizability of clinical outcome may depend on the proportion of CAP caused by pathogens not covered by beta-lactam monotherapy, as discussed previously [9], we think that the cost-efficacy will be similar in most regions with comparable etiology.

Conclusions
In conclusion, there is no significant difference in cost-effectiveness of a strategy of preferred beta-lactam monotherapy compared to beta-lactam/macrolide combination therapy or fluoroquinolone monotherapy for the empirical antibiotic treatment of CAP in non-ICU wards. Together with the preference of narrow-spectrum antibiotics from an ecological perspective, these data support the use of beta-lactam monotherapy as preferred empirical treatment for patients hospitalized with community-acquired pneumonia.

Abbreviations
CAP: Community-acquired pneumonia; CAP-START: Community-Acquired Pneumonia Study on the initial Treatment with Antibiotics of Lower Respiratory Tract Infections, http://clinicaltrials.gov/show/NCT01660204; CEA: Cost-effectiveness analysis; CER: Cost-effectiveness ratios; CMA: Cost-minimization analysis; DHC: Direct healthcare costs; DNHC: Direct non-healthcare costs; GP: General practitioner; ICU: Intensive Care Unit; INHC: Indirect non-healthcare costs

Funding
Supported financially by a grant from the Netherlands Organization for Health Research and Development (171202002).

Authors' contributions
CHvW participated in the design and conduct of the CAP-START study, performed the current analysis, and wrote the current manuscript. DFP participated in the design and conduct of the CAP-START study and wrote the current manuscript. MJM participated in the design and conduct of the CAP-START study, and revised the current manuscript. JJO participated in the design and supervision of the CAP-START study, and revised the current manuscript. MJMB participated in the design and conduct of the CAP-START study, and supervised writing of the current manuscript. All authors read and approved the final manuscript.

Competing interests
The authors declare that they have no competing interests.

Author details
[1]Julius Center for Health Sciences and Primary Care, University Medical Center Utrecht, Utrecht, The Netherlands. [2]Department of Internal Medicine and Infectious Diseases, University Medical Center Utrecht, Heidelberglaan 100, 3584 CX Utrecht, The Netherlands. [3]Department of Internal Medicine, Diakonessenhuis Utrecht, Utrecht, The Netherlands. [4]Department of Medical Microbiology, University Medical Center Utrecht, Utrecht, The Netherlands.

References
1. Welte T, Torres A, Nathwani D. Clinical and economic burden of community-acquired pneumonia among adults in Europe. Thorax. 2012;67: 71–9. Available from: http://www.ncbi.nlm.nih.gov/pubmed/20729232.
2. Jackson ML, Neuzil KM, Thompson WW, Shay DK, Yu O, Hanson CA, Jackson LA. The burden of community-acquired pneumonia in seniors: results of a population-based study. Clin Infect Dis. 2004;39:1642–50.
3. Broulette J, Yu H, Pyenson B, Iwasaki K, Sato R. The incidence rate and economic burden of community-acquired pneumonia in a working-age population. Am Heal drug benefits. 2013;6:494–503.
4. StatLine; Centraal Bureau voor de Statistiek (CBS). Statistics Netherlands. [Internet]. [cited 2015 Apr 27].Available from: http://statline.cbs.nl.
5. Spoorenberg SMC, Bos WJW, Heijligenberg R, Voorn PGP, Grutters JC, Rijkers GT, van de Garde EMW. Microbial aetiology, outcomes, and costs of hospitalisation for community-acquired pneumonia; an observational analysis. BMC Infect Dis. 2014;14:335. veilable from: https://www.ncbi.nlm.nih.gov/pmc/articles/PMC4078020/.
6. Rozenbaum MH, Mangen M-JJ, Huijts SM, van der Werf TS, Postma MJ. Incidence, direct costs and duration of hospitalization of patients hospitalized with community acquired pneumonia: A nationwide retrospective claims database analysis. Vaccine. 2015;33:3193–9. Available from: http://www.sciencedirect.com/science/article/pii/S0264410X15006131.
7. Malhotra-Kumar S, Lammens C, Coenen S, Van HK, Goossens H. Effect of azithromycin and clarithromycin therapy on pharyngeal carriage of macrolide-resistant streptococci in healthy volunteers: a randomised, double-blind, placebo-controlled study. Department of Medical Microbiology, University of Antwerp. Lancet. 2007;369:482–90.

8.   Fuller JD, Low DE. A review of Streptococcus pneumoniae infection
     treatment failures associated with fluoroquinolone resistance. ClinInfectDis.
     2005;41:118–21. Department of Microbiology, Toronto Medical Laboratories
     and Mount Sinai Hospital, Toronto, Ontario, Canada.

9.   Postma DF, van Werkhoven CH, van Elden LJR, Thijsen SFT, Hoepelman AIM,
     Kluytmans JAJW, Boersma WG, Compaijen CJ, van der Wall E, Prins JM,
     Oosterheert JJ, Bonten MJM. Antibiotic Treatment Strategies for
     Community-Acquired Pneumonia in Adults. N Engl J Med. 2015;372:
     1312–23. Available from: http://www.ncbi.nlm.nih.gov/pubmed/
     25830421.

10. Van Werkhoven CH, Postma DF, Oosterheert JJ, Bonten MJM. Antibiotic
     treatment of moderate-severe community-acquired pneumonia: design
     and rationale of a multicentre cluster-randomised cross-over trial. Neth J
     Med. 2014;72:170–8. Available from: http://www.ncbi.nlm.nih.gov/pubmed/
     24846935.

11. Hakkaart-van Roijen L, Tan S, Bouwmans C. Methoden en standaard
     kostprijzen voor economische evaluaties in de gezondheidszorg. 2010.

12. Tan SS, Bouwmans CAM, Rutten FFH, Hakkaart-van Roijen L. Update of the
     Dutch Manual for Costing in Economic Evaluations. Int J Technol Assess
     Health Care. 2012;28:152–8.

13. Tan-Torres Edejer T, Baltussen R, Adam T, Hutubessy R, Acharya A, Evans D,
     Murray C. Making choices in health: WHO guide to cost-effectiveness
     analysis. Geneva. 2003.

14. Wiersinga WJ, Bonten MJ, Boersma WG, Jonkers RE, Aleva RM, Kullberg BJ,
     Schouten JA, Degener JE, Janknegt R, Verheij TJ, Sachs AP, Prins JM. SWAB/
     NVALT (Dutch Working Party on Antibiotic Policy and Dutch Association of
     Chest Physicians) guidelines on the management of community-acquired
     pneumonia in adults. Neth J Med. 2012;70:90–101. Department of Internal
     Medicine, University of Amsterdam, Amsterdam, the Netherlands. w.j.
     wiersinga@amc.uva.nl.

15. Rietbergen C, Moerbeek M. The Design of Cluster Randomized Crossover
     Trials. J Educ Behav Stat. 2011;36:472–90.

16. Zhanel GG, Fontaine S, Adam H, Schurek K, Mayer M, Noreddin AM, Gin AS,
     Rubinstein E, Hoban DJ. A Review of New Fluoroquinolones : Focus on their
     Use in Respiratory Tract Infections. Treat Respir Med. 2006;5:437–65.

17. Garin N, Genné D, Carballo S, Chuard C, Eich G, Hugli O, Lamy O, Nendaz M,
     Petignat P-A, Perneger T, Rutschmann O, Seravalli L, Harbarth S, Perrier A.
     β-Lactam monotherapy vs β-lactam-macrolide combination treatment in
     moderately severe community-acquired pneumonia: a randomized
     noninferiority trial. JAMA Intern Med. 2014;174:1894–901. Available from:
     http://www.ncbi.nlm.nih.gov/pubmed/25286173.

18. MSH/WHO. International Drug Price Indicator Guide. Geneva: Management
     Sciences for Health/World Health Organization; 2014. Available from:
     http://erc.msh.org/dmpguide/pdf/DrugPriceGuide_2014.pdf.

19. Egger ME, Myers JA, Forest WA, Pass LA, Ramirez JA, Brock GN. Cost
     effectiveness of adherence to IDSA/ATS guidelines in elderly patients
     hospitalized for Community-Acquired Pneumonia. BMC Med Inform Decis
     Mak. 2016;16:34. doi:10.1186/s12911-016-0270-y.

2

Pneumonia caused by extensive drug-resistant *Acinetobacter baumannii* among hospitalized patients: genetic relationships, risk factors and mortality

Yu jun Li[1,2], Chu zhi Pan[3†], Chang quan Fang[4†], Zhu xiang Zhao[2†], Hui ling Chen[5†], Peng hao Guo[6†] and Zi wen Zhao[2*]

Abstract

Background: The clonal spread of multiple drug-resistant *Acinetobacter baumannii* is an emerging problem in China. We analysed the molecular epidemiology of *Acinetobacter baumanni* isolates at three teaching hospitals and investigated the risk factors, clinical features, and outcomes of hospital-acquired pneumonia caused by extensive drug-resistant *Acinetobacter baumannii* (XDRAB) infection in Guangzhou, China.

Methods: Fifty-two *A. baumannii* isolates were collected. Multilocus sequence typing (MLST) was used to assess the genetic relationships among the isolates. The $bla_{OXA-51-like}$ gene was amplified using polymerase chain reaction (PCR) and sequencing. The resistance phenotypes were determined using the disc diffusion method. A retrospective case-control study was performed to determine factors associated with XDRAB pneumonia.

Results: Most of the 52 *A. baumannii* isolates ($N = 37$, 71.2%) were collected from intensive care units (ICUs). The respiratory system was the most common bodily site from which *A. baumannii* was recovered ($N = 45$, 86.5%). Disc diffusion classified the isolates into 17 multidrug-resistant (MDR) and 35 extensively drug-resistant (XDR) strains. MLST grouped the *A. baumannii* isolates into 5 existing sequence types (STs) and 7 new STs. ST195 and ST208 accounted for 69.2% (36/52) of the isolates. The clonal relationship analysis showed that ST195 and ST208 belonged to clonal complex (CC) 92. According to the sequence-based typing (SBT) of the $bla_{OXA-51-like}$ gene, 51 *A. baumannii* isolates carried OXA-66 and the rest carried OXA-199. There were no significant differences with respect to the resistance phenotype between the CC92 and non-CC92 strains ($P = 0.767$). The multivariate analysis showed that the APACHE II score, chronic obstructive pulmonary disease (COPD) and cardiac disease were independent risk factors for XDRAB pneumonia ($P < 0.05$). The mortality rate of XDRAB pneumonia was high (up to 42.8%), but pneumonia caused by XDRAB was not associated with in-hospital mortality ($P = 0.582$).

Conclusions: ST195 may be the most common ST in Guangzhou, China, and may serve as a severe epidemic marker. SBT of $bla_{OXA-51-like}$ gene variants may not result in sufficient dissimilarities to type isolates in a small-scale, geographically restricted study of a single region. XDRAB pneumonia was strongly related to systemic illnesses and the APACHE II score but was not associated with in-hospital mortality.

Keywords: *Acinetobacter baumannii*, Extensive drug resistance, Multilocus sequence typing, $bla_{OXA-51-like}$ gene, Pneumonia

* Correspondence: zhaozw2016@163.com
†Equal contributors
2Department of Respiratory Medicine, Guangzhou First People's Hospital, Guangzhou Medical University, Panfu Road, Guangzhou, China

Background

Acinetobacter baumannii (AB) is one of the most important and common pathogens causing nosocomial outbreaks worldwide, especially in intensive care units (ICUs). The most common bodily site of *A. baumannii* infection is the respiratory tract, particularly in cases of hospital-acquired pneumonia (HAP) [1, 2]. *A. baumannii* is also notorious for its remarkable ability to acquire antibiotic resistance. Data from the CHINET surveillance system demonstrated that *A. baumannii* resistance to many important antimicrobial agents has increased, especially imipenem and meropenem, which increased from 31% in 2005 to 62.4% in 2014 and from 39% in 2005 to 66.7% in 2014, respectively [3]. Recently, the rise in the frequency of nosocomial infections caused by extremely drug resistant (XDR) *A. baumannii* strains (defined as resistance to all available antibiotics except colistin and tigecycline) has been of great concern because XDR resistance has been associated with high mortality and treatment failure [2, 4–7]. According to our previous study [5], most of the isolates (76.2%,32/42) were XDR strains, mostly recovered from the respiratory system, but at present little research concerning extensive drug-resistant *A. baumannii* (XDRAB) pneumonia has been reported.

Currently, *A. baumannii* is recognized as one of the most difficult health care-associated infections to control and treat, and the optimal treatment of infections caused by XDRAB has not been established [6]. Surveillance of *A baumannii* isolates may inform prevention and control measures for these infections. Additionally, determining the process of disease spread by routine surveillance can abrogate routes of bacterial transmission [2]. Multilocus sequence typing (MLST) is a widely used technique for bacterial typing. MLST provides a portable method that is suitable for global epidemiological studies and monitoring of the national and international spread of bacteria [8, 9]. Currently, two large national studies [10, 11] have confirmed that CC92 represents the most epidemic sequence type (ST) in China. ST92, which is the founder of CC92, is the predominant ST, whereas other STs belonging to CC92 vary by area. ST75 may be the most common epidemic ST in eastern China [12], whereas ST138 may be the most common ST in western China [13]. Our previous study discovered that ST195 and ST208 belonged to CC92 were the major clone spreading in our hospital [5]. We assumed that ST195 and ST208 may be more common in southern China Guangzhou area, but this needed to be confirmed further. These differences may be due to the different antibiotic usage habits, which possibly influenced the evolution of ST92. However, little is known about the relationship between antibiotic resistance and certain STs. Although MLST has many advantages, it is a robust

scheme that is often time-consuming, expensive, and labour-intensive [14]. Currently, several studies have reported that sequence-based typing (SBT) of $bla_{OXA-51-like}$ gene variants has potential for application to assess the epidemiological characterization of *A. baumannii* [14–16], but more data are needed.

This study investigated 52 *A. baumannii* isolates from three teaching hospitals in Guangzhou to determine the clonality of the isolates. A case-control study was conducted to evaluate the characteristics, risk factors and outcomes for hospital-acquired XDRAB pneumonia, and the relationship between antibiotic resistance and certain STs was also investigated.

Methods

Bacterial isolates and antimicrobial susceptibility testing

From April 2011 to February 2012, A total of 52 *A. baumannii* isolates were collected as part of the standard patient care regimen from three teaching hospitals (Guangzhou First People's Hospital, Guangzhou Medical University, Panfu Road, Guangzhou, China; the Third Affiliated Hospital of Sun Yat-sen University, Tian He Road, Guangzhou, China; and the First Affiliated Hospital of Sun Yat-sen University, Zhong Shan Er Road, Guangzhou, China). Among the 52 *A. baumannii* isolates, 42 isolates had been reported in our previous study [5]. All *A. baumannii* isolates derived from clinical samples (sputum,bronchoalveolar lavage fluid, blood, cerebrospinal fluid, and urine) were collected from patients hospitalized in the general wards and intensive care units (ICUs), Duplicate isolates from the same patients were excluded. The Vitek 2 (bioMerieux, Inc., Durham, NC, USA) automated microbiology system was used in identification of isolates.

According to Clinical and Laboratory Standards Institute (CLSI; M100-S22, 2012) [17], disc diffusion method were used to detect the susceptibility of 52 *A. baumannii* isolates against 15 antibiotics to determine the resistance phenotype. Isolates that showed resistance or intermediate susceptibility to imipenem, meropenem, amikacin, piperacillin/tazobactam, cefoperazone/sulbactam, ceftazidime, ceftriaxone, cefepime, aztreonam, levofloxacin, ciprofloxacin, doxycycline and tobramycin were considered XDRAB isolates. Melone Pharmaceutical Co. Ltd. (China) provided the antibiotic discs (OXOID). *Escherichia coli* ATCC 25922 and *Pseudomonas aeruginosa* ATCC 27853 were used as the control organisms.

Molecular epidemiological typing

Multilocus sequence typing (MLST) was performed on *A. baumannii*, according to Bartual et al. [18]. Seven conserved housekeeping genes (gltA, gyrB, gdhB, recA, cpn60, gpi, and rpoD) were amplified and sequencing. The allelic numbers and sequence types (STs) were identified by means of the Pubmlst database [19]. The eBURST algorithm (version 3) [20] was used to assign STs to clonal complexes (CCs) and to assess the genetic relationships among the sequences. Sequence-based typing of the $bla_{OXA\text{-}51\text{-}like}$ genes (SBT- $bla_{OXA\text{-}51\text{-}like}$ genes) was carried out as follows. The OXA-69A and OXA-69B primers [21], which were external to the $bla_{OXA\text{-}51\text{-}like}$ gene, were used to amplify the entire gene sequence, followed by sequencing. The sequences were analysed using BLAST (https://blast.ncbi.nlm.nih.gov/Blast.cgi) to determine the genetic diversity of the $bla_{OXA\text{-}51\text{-}like}$ genes [14, 15].

Case-control study

A retrospective case-control study was performed to evaluate the characteristics, risk factors and outcomes of hospital-acquired XDRAB pneumonia. The cases included patients from whom a XDRAB isolate was isolated from clinical cultures of respiratory secretions and who had been shown to have hospital-acquired pneumonia, including ventilator-associated pneumonia (VAP) defined as pneumonia that occurred more than 48 h after endotracheal intubation [22].

The inclusion criteria consisted of the following: a) diagnosis of pneumonia [23] the presence of new or progressive pulmonary infiltrates in chest radiographs, plus at least two of the following supportive clinical signs: temperature of >38 °C or <35.5 °C, leukocytosis (>12,000 WBC/mm^3) or leukopenia (<4000 WBC/mm^3), purulent bronchial secretions, or worsening oxygenation and b) at least two positive respiratory samples for A. baumannii : protected specimen brushing cultures 10^3 cfu/mL, bronchoalveolar lavage (BAL) fluid specimen 10^4 or 10^5 cfu/mL, or 10^6 cfu/mL in an endotracheal aspirate [23]. Patients <18 years of age, patients hospitalization for <48 h and patients with incomplete medical records were excluded from this study, as were patients who had other non- A. baumannii -positive cultures in addition to A. baumannii to avoid the inclusion of A. baumannii colonization.

The controls were randomly selected adult inpatients in the participating hospitals who were diagnosed with non-XDRAB hospital-acquired pneumonia during their hospital stay. The controls were matched to the cases by hospital. Two controls were recruited for each case. Computerized medical, pharmaceutical and microbiological records were reviewed. A specially designed case record form was used to collect demographic and clinical data, including age, gender, underlying diseases, severity of diseases [calculated by the Acute Physiology and Chronic Health Evaluation (APACHE) II score] while admitted to the general wards or ICU, invasive procedures (central venous and/or arterial catheter, urinary catheter, nasogastric tube and mechanical ventilation), duration of stay in the ICU, hospital stay and antibiotic exposure.

Statistical analysis

Categorical variables were compared using the Chi-square test with Yates correction or Fisher's exact test. Continuous variables were analysed using the t test. A P value <0.05 in a two-tailed test was considered statistically significant. To test the independence of the risk factors for XDRAB pneumonia, significant variables (P <0.05) in the univariate analyses were entered into a multivariate logistic regression model. SPSS (version 18.0) was used for all calculations.

Results

Characteristics of the 52 A. baumannii isolates
Most of the isolates ($N = 37$, 71.2%) were obtained from intensive care units (ICUs). The respiratory system was the most common bodily site from which A. baumannii was recovered ($N = 45$, 86.5%), followed by the blood ($N = 3$, 5.8%). Disc diffusion testing (supplementary information) classified the 52 A. baumannii isolates into 17 MDR and 35 XDR strains (Table 1).

MLST and SBT- $bla_{OXA\text{-}51\text{-}like}$ genes
According to the MLST, 52 A. baumannii isolates were grouped into 12 distinct STs, including 5 existing STs and 7 novel STs (STn1 to STn7). STn4 carried allele G1 with a T → C mutation at the 3rd nucleotide site (nt3) on the gpi111 locus. STn5 carried allele A1 with an A → C mutation at nt156 and nt159 on the gltA1 locus. ST195 and ST208 were the most common STs, accounting for 69.2% of all isolates. The clonal relationship analysis showed that ST195 and ST208 belonged to CC92. According to the sequence-based typing of the $bla_{OXA\text{-}51\text{-}like}$ genes, 51 A. baumannii isolates carried OXA-66 and the rest carried OXA-199. No significant differences with respect to the resistance phenotype were detected between the CC92 and non-CC92 strains ($P = 0.767$) (Tables 1 and 2 and Fig. 1).

Case-control study
Full medical records were available for 42 of the 52 patients from whom the A. baumannii isolates were isolated. A total of 32 patients were diagnosed with XDRAB acquisition, and 21 patients finally met the inclusion criteria and were assessed in the case-control study. Of the 21 patients with XDRAB pneumonia, 17 were men and four were women. The mean age was 77.5 years (standard deviation 11.6 years). Sixteen patients were receiving care in ICUs and 5 were in general wards during specimen collection (Tables 1 and 3).

The potential risk factors for patients with XDRAB pneumonia are shown in Table 3. The two groups were

Table 1 Characteristics of the 52 A. baumannii isolates

Number of isolates	Hospital	Specimens	Wards	gltA	gyrB	gdhB	recA	cpn60	gpi	rpoD	ST	CC	bla$_{OXA-51-like}$ genes	Phenotype	XDRAB pneumonia
1	GFPH	Sputum	ICU	1	3	3	2	2	97	3	ST208	92	OXA-66	XDR	Yes
2	GFPH	Blood	ICU	1	3	3	2	2	96	5	STn1	92	OXA-66	XDR	Yes
3	GFPH	Sputum	ICU	1	3	3	2	2	97	3	ST208	92	OXA-66	XDR	Yes
4	GFPH	Blood	ICU	1	3	3	2	2	96	3	ST195	92	OXA-66	XDR	Yes
5	GFPH	BALF	RICU	1	3	3	2	2	96	3	ST195	92	OXA-66	XDR	Yes
6	GFPH	Sputum	RICU	1	3	3	2	2	96	3	ST195	92	OXA-66	MDR	No
7	GFPH	Sputum	Respiratory	1	15	3	2	2	153	3	ST457	92	OXA-66	XDR	No
8	GFPH	Sputum	RICU	1	3	3	2	2	96	3	ST195	92	OXA-66	XDR	Yes
9	GFPH	Sputum	ICU	1	3	3	2	2	96	3	ST195	92	OXA-66	XDR	Yes
10	GFPH	Sputum	Respiratory	1	3	3	2	2	97	3	ST208	92	OXA-66	XDR	yes
11	GFPH	Sputum	Neurosurgery	1	15	3	2	2	96	3	STn2	92	OXA-199	XDR	Yes
12	GFPH	Sputum	RICU	1	3	3	2	2	96	3	ST195	92	OXA-66	MDR	No
13	GFPH	Sputum	Respiratory	1	3	3	2	2	97	3	ST208	92	OXA-66	XDR	No
14	GFPH	Sputum	ICU	1	3	3	2	2	96	3	ST195	92	OXA-66	MDR	No
15	GFPH	BALF	RICU	1	3	3	2	2	96	3	ST195	92	OXA-66	XDR	yes
16	GFPH	Sputum	ICU	1	3	3	2	2	96	3	ST195	92	OXA-66	XDR	yes
17	GFPH	Wound	Gastroenterology	1	3	3	2	2	96	3	ST195	92	OXA-66	XDR	No
18	GFPH	Sputum	Respiratory	1	3	3	2	2	97	3	ST208	92	OXA-66	XDR	No
19	GFPH	Sputum	ICU	1	3	3	2	2	97	3	ST208	92	OXA-66	XDR	yes
20	GFPH	Urine	Geriatrics ICU	21	15	3	2	35	111	4	ST254	singletons	OXA-66	XDR	No
21	GFPH	BALF	RICU	1	3	3	2	2	96	3	ST195	92	OXA-66	XDR	yes
22	GFPH	BALF	RICU	1	3	3	2	2	96	3	ST195	92	OXA-66	MDR	No
23	GFPH	Sputum	Respiratory	1	3	3	2	2	97	3	ST208	92	OXA-66	XDR	yes
24	GFPH	Sputum	ICU	1	3	3	2	2	97	3	ST208	92	OXA-66	MDR	No
25	GFPH	Sputum	RICU	1	3	3	2	2	96	3	ST195	92	OXA-66	XDR	yes
26	GFPH	Sputum	RICU	1	3	3	2	2	96	3	ST195	92	OXA-66	XDR	yes
27	GFPH	Sputum	Neurosurgery	1	81	3	2	2	96	4	STn3	singletons	OXA-66	MDR	No
28	GFPH	Sputum	Respiratory	21	15	3	2	35	111	4	ST254	singletons	OXA-66	XDR	yes
29	GFPH	Sputum	RICU	21	15	3	2	35	111	4	ST254	singletons	OXA-66	XDR	yes
30	GFPH	Sputum	RICU	1	3	3	2	2	96	3	ST195	92	OXA-66	XDR	No
31	GFPH	Sputum	Respiratory	1	3	3	2	2	97	3	ST208	92	OXA-66	XDR	yes
32	GFPH	Sputum	Neurosurgery	1	81	3	2	2	96	4	STn3	singletons	OXA-66	MDR	No
33	GFPH	Sputum	ICU	1	3	3	2	2	96	3	ST195	92	OXA-66	XDR	Yes

Table 1 Characteristics of the 52 A. baumannii isolates (Continued)

No.	Hospital	Sample	Department								ST		OXA	Type	Pneumonia
34	GFPH	BALF	RICU	1	15	3	2	2	153	3	ST457	92	OXA-66	XDR	Yes
35	GFPH	CSF	ICU	1	3	3	2	2	96	3	ST195	92	OXA-66	XDR	No
36	GFPH	Sputum	Respiratory	21	15	3	2	35	G1	3	STn4	singletons	OXA-66	MDR	No
37	GFPH	Sputum	ICU	1	3	3	2	2	96	3	ST195	92	OXA-66	XDR	No
38	GFPH	Wound	Burn	A1	15	3	2	2	153	4	STn5	92	OXA-66	XDR	No
39	GFPH	Sputum	Geriatrics ICU	21	15	3	2	35	G1	3	STn4	singletons	OXA-66	XDR	No
40	GFPH	Blood	Urinary surgery	1	3	3	2	2	96	3	ST195	92	OXA-66	XDR	No
41	GFPH	Sputum	Nephrology	1	3	3	2	2	97	3	ST208	92	OXA-66	MDR	No
42	GFPH	BALF	RICU	11	65	3	20	37	96	15	STn6	singletons	OXA-66	MDR	No
43	FAH	Sputum	ICU	1	3	3	2	2	96	3	ST195	92	OXA-66	MDR	N/A
44	FAH	Sputum	ICU	1	3	3	2	2	96	3	ST195	92	OXA-66	XDR	N/A
45	FAH	Sputum	ICU	33	31	2	28	1	96	5	STn7	singletons	OXA-66	MDR	N/A
46	FAH	Sputum	ICU	1	3	3	2	2	97	3	ST208	92	OXA-66	MDR	N/A
47	TAH	Sputum	ICU	1	3	3	2	2	96	3	ST195	92	OXA-66	MDR	N/A
48	TAH	Sputum	ICU	1	3	3	2	2	16	3	ST136	92	OXA-66	XDR	N/A
49	TAH	Sputum	ICU	1	3	3	2	2	96	3	ST195	92	OXA-66	MDR	N/A
50	TAH	Sputum	ICU	1	3	3	2	2	97	3	ST208	92	OXA-66	MDR	N/A
51	TAH	Sputum	ICU	1	3	3	2	2	96	3	ST195	92	OXA-66	MDR	N/A
52	TAH	Sputum	ICU	1	3	3	2	2	16	3	ST136	92	OXA-66	XDR	N/A

GFPH Guangzhou First People's Hospital, FAH the First Affiliated Hospital of Sun Yat-sen University, TAH the Third Affiliated Hospital of Sun Yat-sen University, BALF bronchoalveolar lavage fluid, CSF cerebrospinal fluid, ICU intensive care unit, RICU respiratory intensive care unit, G1 a new allele that has a T → C mutation at nt3 in the gpi111 locus; A1 a new allele possessing two mutations at the gltA1 locus (A → C mutations at nt156 and nt159); N/A not available

Table 2 The relationship between the clonal complex (CC) and resistance phenotype of the 52 *A. baumannii* isolates

Clonal complex	No. isolates	MDR N (%)	XDR N (%)	Statistical analysis[a]	
				χ2 -values	P values
CC92	43	14 (32.6)	29 (67.4)	0.088	0.767
ST195	24	9	15		
ST208	12	5	7		
ST457	2	0	2		
ST136	2	0	2		
STn1	1	0	1		
STn2	1	0	1		
STn5	1	0	1		
Non-CC92	9	4 (44.4)	5 (55.6)		
ST254	3	0	3		
STn3	2	2	0		
STn4	2	0	2		
STn6	1	1	0		
STn7	1	1	0		

[a] comparison of CC92 with non-CC92 strains

similar with respect to gender, days of mechanical ventilation before XDRAB pneumonia, days spent in the hospital before XDRAB pneumonia, length of stay in the ICU, and length of stay in the hospital. Additionally, no significant differences were detected with respect to malignancy, renal disease, neurological disease, urinary catheter, nasogastric tube, mechanical ventilation, or the

use of glucocorticoids, PPIs, cephalosporin, β-lactamase inhibitor, quinolone or minoglycoside. The mortality rate of XDRAB pneumonia was high (up to 42.8%), but pneumonia caused by XDRAB was not associated with in-hospital mortality ($P = 0.582$). Compared with the non-XDRAB patients, the patients with XDRAB pneumonia were significantly more likely to be older (77.5 ± 11.6 vs 68.6 ± 18.4 years, $P = 0.023$) and have a higher initial severity of illness at admission as indicated by the higher APACHE II score (21.9 ± 6.8 vs 18.0 ± 4.9, $P = 0.011$). Moreover, chronic obstructive pulmonary disease (COPD), cardiac disease and carbapenem use were risk factors for XDRAB pneumonia ($P < 0.05$).

The multivariate analysis using a logistic regression model results are presented in Table 4. The APACHE II score (OR, 1.17; 95% CI: 1.01–1.35, $P = 0.034$), COPD (OR, 7.25; 95% CI: 1.54–33.9, $P = 0.012$), and cardiac disease (OR, 6.94; 95% CI: 1.43–33.6, $P = 0.016$) were identified as independent risk factors for XDRAB acquisition.

Discussion

In this study, we examined the molecular typing and characteristics of *A. baumannii* at three teaching hospitals. In the MLST, CC92 was the most prevalent clonal complex. However, ST92, which was the predicted founder of CC92 and was reported to be one of the most epidemic STs in multiple provinces in China [1, 10, 11], was not detected in our study. ST92 was also not

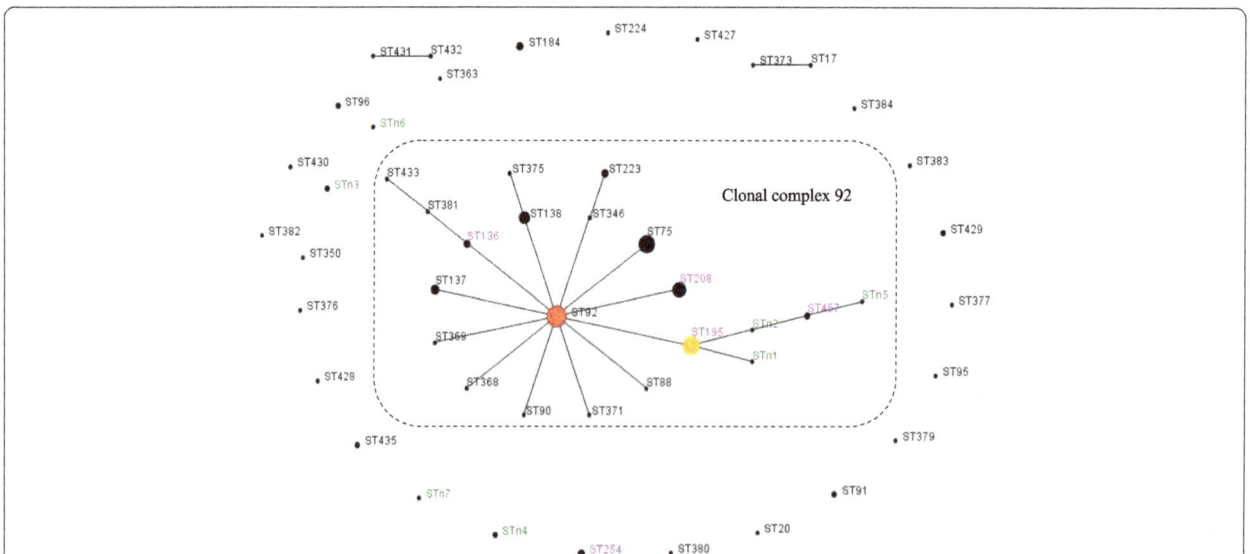

Fig. 1 Population snapshot of *A. baumannii* in this study and other existing isolates in China. Population snapshot of *A. baumannii* in this study and existing isolates in China based on the data contained in the Pubmlst database as of 27 April 2013 [5, 18] represented by an eBURST algorithm. Circles represent STs, and their sizes correspond to the numbers of isolates. The *red circle* represents the founder ST (ST92). The broken line indicates clonal complex (CC) 92. The ST labels are coloured as follows: *black*, STs found only in the Pubmlst database; *green*, STs found only in this study; and *purple*, STs found in both the Pubmlst database and this study. ST254, STn3, STn4, STn6 and STn7 were the singletons in this study

Table 3 Comparison of clinical data for pneumonia-related characteristics in HAP patients with XDRAB and non-XDRAB

	XDRAB (N = 21) N (%)	Non-XDRAB (N = 42) N (%)	P-value
Age, y[a]	77.5 ± 11.6	68.6 ± 18.4	0.023
Gender (M/F), n	17/4	23/19	0.079
APACHE II score[a]	21.9 ± 6.8	18.0 ± 4.9	0.011
Related to hospitalization[a]	18 (85.7)	30 (71.4)	0.347
Days of mechanical ventilation before XDRAB (days)	10.5 ± 11.6	5.2 ± 5.8	0.059
Hospital days before XDRAB (days)	18.3 ± 11.3	12.6 ± 11.2	0.064
Length of stay in the ICU (days)	30.1 ± 20.0	21.4 ± 21.7	0.127
Length of stay in the hospital (days)	45.5 ± 28.8	38.5 ± 24.2	0.199
Associated disease, n (%)			
COPD	13 (61.9)	9 (21.4)	0.001
Diabetes mellitus	2 (9.5)	10 (40.4)	0.307
Malignancy	2 (9.5)	9 (21.4)	0.411
Cardiac disease	13 (61.9)	6 (14.2)	0.000
Renal disease	5 (23.8)	2 (4.7)	0.065
Neurological disease	8 (38.0)	22 (52.3)	0.422
Device, n (%)			
Urinary catheter	21 (100.0)	36 (85.7)	0.172
Nasogastric tube	21 (100.0)	36 (85.7)	0.172
Mechanical ventilation	16 (76.1)	31 (73.8)	1.000
Drug usage, n (%)			
Glucocorticoids	10 (47.6)	18 (42.8)	0.720
PPIs	14 (66.7)	32 (76.1)	0.422
Antimicrobial n (%)			
Cephalosporin			
Second generation	3 (14.2)	5 (11.9)	1.000
Third generation	7 (33.3)	18 (42.8)	0.649
β-lactamase inhibitor	20 (95.2)	31 (73.8)	0.089
Quinolone	13 (61.9)	19 (45.2)	0.327
Aminoglycoside	2 (9.5)	4 (9.5)	1.000
Carbapenem	11 (52.3)	11 (26.1)	0.040
Antimicrobial Combination therapy, n (%)	11 (52.3)	19 (45.2)	0.593
Mortality, n (%)	9 (42.8)	15 (35.7)	0.582

[a]Values are presented as the mean ± standard deviation; malignancy includes haematological malignancies and solid tumours; cardiac disease includes coronary artery disease, hypertensive heart disease, valvular disease and cardiomyopathy; renal disease includes chronic renal failure; neurological disease includes cerebral haemorrhage and cerebral infarction; *PPIs* proton pump inhibitor drugs

Table 4 Multi-variate analysis of risk factors for patients with XDRAB pneumonia

Risk factor	OR (95% CI)	P-value
APACHE II score	1.17 (1.01–1.35)	0.034
COPD	7.25 (1.54–33.9)	0.012
Cardiac disease	6.94 (1.43–33.6)	0.016

detected in other studies from China [1, 5] and South Africa [24]. The lack of ST92 detection may be due to the relatively small sample size in our study, which may not accurately represent the diversity and relative abundance of *A. baumannii* STs. However, some studies [1, 5, 25] have shown that ST195, ST208, ST365, and ST191 (but not ST92) are the most common STs discovered in different hospitals across China. In this study, ST195 was the most commonly observed ST, accounting for 24/52 (46.1%) of the isolates, follow by ST208. These findings are similar to the findings of Zhou et al. [25], who found that ST195 accounted for 31/57 (54.4%) isolates. These data collectively suggest that ST195 is the most common ST and may serve as a severe epidemic marker in the Guangzhou area.

Some data are available to clarify why CC92 is predominant. Zhong et al. [12] found that ST75, which is the single locus variant (SLV) of ST92, differs in its gpi loci and belongs to CC92, has more severe imipenem resistance that might improve its chances of survival. In our study, CC92 accounted for 82.7% (43/52) of the isolates. Most of the XDR isolates (29/34, 85.3%) were from CC92. However, CC92 included 14 MDR isolates with less severe resistance, and non-CC92 had similar results. No significant differences with respect to the resistance phenotype were detected between the CC92 and non-CC92 strains ($P = 0.767$). Runnegar et al. [26] revealed that CC92 had been spread in the hospital for 9 years with variable antibiotic susceptibility. These findings may suggest that both adaptation to the hospital environment and antibiotic resistance have been important for the success of CC92.

The $bla_{OXA-51-like}$ genes are unique to *A. baumannii* and immobile and thus may be used as markers for the identification of this species [21]. Recently, sequence-based typing (SBT) of $bla_{OXA-51-like}$ gene variants was reported to have potential for use in the epidemiological characterization of *A. baumannii* isolates obtained from various locations in Europe. bla_{OXA-69}, bla_{OXA-66}, and bla_{OXA-71} are the predominant members of closely related $bla_{OXA-51-like}$ subgroups, which are associated with European clone I (EUI), EUII, and EUIII, respectively [14–16]. However, few studies have investigated the correlation between $bla_{OXA-51-like}$ variants with MLST typing.

According to a study by Hamouda et al. [14], MLST data showed that all isolates harbouring the major $bla_{OXA-51-like}$ alleles (OXA-66, OXA-69, and OXA-71) fell within the three major European clonal lineages. The SBT-$bla_{OXA-51-like}$ gene scheme produced results comparable to those produced by the Bartual MLST for the identification of the major epidemic lineages. Pournaras et al. [27] evaluated the SBT-$bla_{OXA-51-like}$ gene scheme in parallel with Pasteur's MLST. In the study, according to the SBT-$bla_{OXA-51-like}$ gene, all 585 *A. baumannii* isolates from a large international collection were typed and assigned correctly to the nine CCs and the singleton ST78. Zhou et al. [25] revealed that 52 isolates from Guangzhou city in China carrying bla_{OXA-66} were assigned to six distinct STs, which clustered into CC92; the remaining isolates belonged to four singletons that each carried a single $bla_{OXA-51-like}$ allele. The results of these studies indicate that the SBT-$bla_{OXA-51-like}$ gene scheme has the advantage of a significantly reduced

sequencing cost and assay time and may be effective for the rapid typing of *A. baumannii* strains. However, in our study, only one isolate carried OXA-199, whereas the remaining 51 *A. baumannii* isolates carried OXA-66. The SBT-$bla_{OXA-51-like}$ gene scheme failed to discriminate strains carrying the same OXA-66 allele. Similar findings reported by Wang et al. [28] showed that 18 representative isolates from different hospitals across China carried the same OXA-66 allele.

In Hamouda et al.'s study [14], the SBT-$bla_{OXA-51-like}$ method was evaluated in a large international collection of *A. baumannii* isolates including 22 countries. Similarly, Pournaras et al. [20] typed isolates obtained from various locations in Europe (Italy, Greece, Turkey, and Lebanon). Environmental differences among countries may act as natural selection forces [12] to introduce diversity among $bla_{OXA-51-like}$ genes. When confined to one city or hospital, the controlled environment and antibiotic usage habits might influence the convergent evolution of the $bla_{OXA-51-like}$ genes. As a result, single-locus sequence-based typing of the $bla_{OXA-51-like}$ genes may not be effective at distinguishing isolates in a small-scale, geographically restricted study. However, further investigation is needed to confirm this hypothesis.

Some studies have reported risk factors for antibiotic resistance in *A. baumannii* infection, which include the length of stay in an ICU, severity of the underlying disease, mechanical ventilation, invasive procedures, and prior antibiotic use [29–32]. However, the clinical characteristics of XDRAB pneumonia have rarely been reported. In our study, univariate analysis was used to identify patients at risk of acquiring XDRAB pneumonia and showed that patients with XDRAB were older and had higher APACHE II scores than patients without XDRAB, which was similar to the findings of Özgür et al. [33]. Additionally, patients who had COPD and cardiac diseases were more likely to acquire XDRAB. Multivariate analysis using a logistic regression model showed that the APACHE II score, COPD and cardiac disease were independent risk factors for XDRAB pneumonia development. Thus, XDRAB may be particularly pathogenic in patients who are immunocompromised. Our study found that carbapenem use was an important risk factor for XDRAB pneumonia ($P = 0.04$). Previous studies [29, 31, 34] have also shown that selective pressure exerted by the use of carbapenem leads to the emergence of multidrug resistant (MDR) and XDR *A. baumannii* isolates. Therefore, rational use of carbapenem is necessary to reduce the risk of generating resistant mutants.

High mortality rates have been reported for nosocomial pneumonia caused by *A. baumannii* (ranging from 28.1 to 85.3%). The independent risk factors included the severity of illness (e.g., severe sepsis, septic shock and APACHE II score) and empiric inappropriate therapy [31, 33, 35, 36]. In one study, patients with carbapenem-resistant *A. baumannii* (CRAB) pneumonia had a higher mortality rate than patients with carbapenem-susceptible *A. baumannii* (CSAB) pneumonia based on the survival analysis (29.9% vs 45.6%, respectively, $P = 0.02$) [31]. However, another study reported mortality rates for patients with MDR *A. baumannii* infections that were not significantly higher than the mortality rates in patients without MDR *A. baumannii* infections [37]. Furthermore, in a study on ventilator-associated pneumonia (VAP) due to XDRAB, the mortality rates were not significantly higher than those of non-XDRAB VAP in ICU patients [33]. Our study showed a high hospital mortality rate in patients with XDRAB pneumonia, but *A. baumannii* resistance was not associated with mortality ($P = 0.582$).

Conclusions

ST195 may be the most common ST in the Guangzhou region of China and may serve as a severe epidemic marker in this region. SBT of $bla_{OXA-51-like}$ gene variants may not be able to sufficiently distinguish isolates obtained from a small-scale, geographically restricted study. XDRAB pneumonia was strongly related to systemic illnesses and the APACHE II score but was not associated with in-hospital mortality.

Additional file

Additional file 1: 52 Isolates were tested against antibiotics by disc diffusion. All 52 of the isolates were tested against a panel of antibiotics with the disc diffusion method, as recommended by the Clinical and Laboratory Standards Institute (CLSI;M100-S22, 2012) [17], to determine the resistance phenotype. Multidrug resistance (MDR) was defined as acquired non-susceptibility to at least one agent in three or more antimicrobial categories, and extensive drug resistance (XDR) was defined as resistance to all available antibiotics except colistin and tigecycline [5]. GFPH, Guangzhou First People's Hospital; FAH, the First Affiliated Hospital of Sun Yat-sen University; TAH, the Third Affiliated Hospital of Sun Yat-sen University; R, resistance; S, sensitivity; I, intermediate; PB, polymyxin B (300 units); TGC, tigecycline (15 μg); IPM, imipenem (10 μg); AK, amikacin (30 μg); TOB, tobramycin (10 μg); MEM, meropenem (10 μg); TZP, piperacillin/tazobactam (100 / 10 μg); SCF, cefoperazone/sulbactam (70 / 35 μg); CAZ, ceftazidime (30 μg); CRO, ceftriaxone (30 μg); FEP, cefepime (30 μg); ATM, aztreonam (30 μg); LEV, levofloxacin (5 μg); CIP, ciprofloxacin (5 μg); DO, doxycycline (30 μg). (DOCX 24 kb)

Abbreviations

AB: *Acinetobacter baumannii*; APACHE II score: Acute Physiology and Chronic Health Evaluation II score; ATS/IDSA: American Thoracic Society/Infectious Diseases Society of America; BAL: Bronchoalveolar lavage; CC: Clonal complex; CLSI: Clinical and Laboratory Standards Institute; COPD: Chronic obstructive pulmonary disease; CRAB: Carbapenem-resistant *A. baumannii*; CSAB: Carbapenem-susceptible *A. baumannii*; ICUs: Intensive care units; MDR: Multidrug resistant; MLST: Multilocus sequence typing; PCR: Polymerase chain reaction; SBT: Sequence-based typing; ST: Sequence type; VAP: Ventilator-associated pneumonia; XDRAB: Extensive drug-resistant *Acinetobacter baumannii*

Acknowledgements
We thank Hui fen YE, of the Department of Clinic Laboratory, Guangzhou First People's Hospital, for technical support in culturing and reisolating strains.

Funding
This work was funded by the Guangzhou Medical and Health Science and Technology Project (no. 20151A011004).

Authors' contributions
YjL supervised the study, performed the susceptibility testing and MLST, and wrote the manuscript. CzP discussed the data and helped finalize the manuscript. CqF contributed to the case–control study and the statistical analysis. ZxZ contributed to the susceptibility testing and sequence-based typing of the $bla_{OXA-51-like}$ genes. HlC and PhG provided advice regarding the susceptibility testing technology. ZwZ planned and supervised the experiments. All authors read and approved the final manuscript.

Competing interests
The authors declare that they have no competing interests.

Consent for publication
Not applicable.

Author details
[1]The First Affiliated Hospital of Jinan University, the West of Huangpu Street, Guangzhou, China. [2]Department of Respiratory Medicine, Guangzhou First People's Hospital, Guangzhou Medical University, Panfu Road, Guangzhou, China. [3]Department of Hepatobiliary Surgery, the Third Affiliated Hospital of Sun Yat-sen University, Tian He Road, Guangzhou, China. [4]Department of Respiratory Medicine, Guangzhou Red Cross Hospital, Tong Fu Zhong Road, Guangzhou, China. [5]Department of Clinic Laboratory, Guangzhou First People's Hospital, Guangzhou Medical University, Panfu Road, Guangzhou, China. [6]Department of Clinic Laboratory, the First Affiliated Hospital of Sun Yat-sen University, Zhong Shan Er Road, Guangzhou, China.

References
1. Ying J, Lu J, Zong L, Li A, Pan R, Cheng C, et al. Molecular epidemiology and characterization of genotypes of *Acinetobacter baumannii* isolates from regions of South China. Jpn J Infect Dis. 2016;69:180–5.
2. El-Shazly S, Dashti A, Vali L, Bolaris M, Ibrahim AS. Molecular epidemiology and characterization of multiple drug-resistant (MDR) clinical isolates of *Acinetobacter baumannii*. Int J Infect Dis. 2015;41:42–9.
3. Hu FP, Guo Y, Zhu DM, Wang F, Jiang XF, Xu YC, et al. Resistance trends among clinical isolates in China reported from CHINET surveillance of bacterial resistance, 2005–2014. Clin Microbiol Infect. 2016;22 Suppl 1:S9–14.
4. Doi Y, Husain S, Potoski BA, McCurry KR, Paterson DL. Extensively drug-resistant *Acinetobacter baumannii*. Emerg Infect Dis. 2009;15:980–2.
5. Li YJ, Pan CZ, Zhao ZW, Zhao ZX, Chen HL, Lu WB. Effects of a combination of amlodipine and imipenem on 42 clinical isolates of *Acinetobacter baumannii* obtained from a teaching hospital in Guangzhou, China. BMC Infect Dis. 2013;13:548.
6. Batirel A, Balkan II, Karabay O, Agalar C, Akalin S, Alici O, et al. Comparison of colistin-carbapenem, colistin-sulbactam, and colistin plus other antibacterial agents for the treatment of extremely drug-resistant *Acinetobacter baumannii* bloodstream infections. Eur J Clin Microbiol Infect Dis. 2014;33:1311–22.

7. Apisarnthanarak A, Warren DK. Intervention to limit transmission of extremely drug-resistant *Acinetobacter baumannii* in patients who underwent surgery. Clin Infect Dis. 2013;57:1215–6.

8. Peleg AY, Seifert H, Paterson DL. *Acinetobacter baumannii*: emergence of a successful pathogen. Clin Microbiol Rev. 2008;21:538–82.

9. Karah N, Sundsfjord A, Towner K, Samuelsen Ø. Insights into the global molecular epidemiology of carbapenem non-susceptible clones of *Acinetobacter baumannii*. Drug Resist Updat. 2012;15:237–47.

10. Fu Y, Zhou J, Zhou H, Yang Q, Wei Z, Yu Y, et al. Wide dissemination of OXA-23-producing carbapenem-resistant *Acinetobacter baumannii* clonal complex 22 in multiple cities of China. J Antimicrob Chemother. 2010;65:644–50.

11. Ruan Z, Chen Y, Jiang Y, Zhou H, Zhou Z, Fu Y, et al. Wide distribution of CC92 carbapenem-resistant and OXA-23-producing *Acinetobacter baumannii* in multiple provinces of China. Int J Antimicrob Agents. 2013;42:322–8.

12. Zhong Q, Xu W, Wu Y, Xu H. Clonal spread of carbapenem non-susceptible *Acinetobacter baumannii* in an intensive care unit in a teaching hospital in China. Ann Lab Med. 2012;32:413–9.

13. He C, Xie Y, Zhang L, Kang M, Tao C, Chen Z, et al. Increasing imipenem resistance and dissemination of the ISAba1-associated blaOXA-23 gene among *Acinetobacter baumannii* isolates in an intensive care unit. J Med Microbiol. 2011;60:337–41.

14. Hamouda A, Evans BA, Towner KJ, Amyes SG. Characterization of epidemiologically unrelated *Acinetobacter baumannii* isolates from four continents by use of multilocus sequence typing, pulsed-field gel electrophoresis, and sequence- based typing of $bla_{OXA-51-like}$ genes. J Clin Microbiol. 2010;48:2476–83.

15. Evans BA, Hamouda A, Towner KJ, Amyes SG. OXA-51-like beta-lactamases and their association with particular epidemic lineages of *Acinetobacter baumannii*. Clin Microbiol Infect. 2008;14:268–75.

16. Zander E, Nemec A, Seifert H, Higgins PG. Association betweenβ-Lactamase-Encoding blaOXA-51 variants and DiversiLab rep-PCR-Based typing of *Acinetobacter baumannii* isolates. J Clin Microbiol. 2012;50:1900–4.

17. Clinical and Laboratory Standard Institute. Performance standards for antimicrobial susceptibility testing. Nineteenth informational supplement. CLSI Document M100 S22. Wayne: Clinical and Laboratory Standard Institute; 2012.

18. Bartual SG, Seifert H, Hippler C, Luzon MA, Wisplinghoff H, Rodríguez-Valera F. Development of a multilocus sequence typing scheme for characterization of clinical isolates of *Acinetobacter baumannii*. J Clin Microbiol. 2005;43:4382–90.

19. Acinetobacter baumannii MLST databases. 2016. http://pubmlst.org/abaumannii/. Accessed 3 Mar 2014.

20. eBURSTv3 algorithm. http://eburst.mlst.net/. Accessed 3 Mar 2014.

21. Héritier C, Poirel L, Fournier P-E, Claverie J-M, Raoult D, Nordmann P. Characterization of the naturally occurring Oxacillinase of *Acinetobacter baumannii*. Antimicrob Agents Chemother. 2005;49:4174–9.

22. American Thoracic Society, Infectious Diseases Society of America. Guidelines for the management of adults with hospital-acquired, ventilator-associated, and healthcare-associated pneumonia. Am J Respir Crit Care Med. 2005;171:388–416.

23. Horan TC, Andrus M, Dudeck MA. CDC/NHSN surveillance definition of health care-associated infection and criteria for specific types of infections in the acute care setting. Am J Infect Control. 2008;36:309–32.

24. Lowings M, Ehlers MM, Dreyer AW, Kock MM. High prevalence of oxacillinases in clinical multidrug-resistant *Acinetobacter baumannii* isolates from the Tshwane region, South Africa – an update. BMC Infect Dis. 2015;15:521.

25. Zhou Y, Wu X, Zhang X, Hu Y, Yang X, Yang Z, et al. Genetic characterization of ST195 and ST365 carbapenem-resistant *Acinetobacter baumannii* harboring blaOXA-23 in Guangzhou, China. Microb Drug Resist. 2015;21:386–90.

26. Runnegar N, Sidjabat H, Goh HM, Nimmo GR, Schembri MA, Paterson DL. Molecular epidemiology of multidrug-resistant *Acinetobacter baumannii* in a single institution over a 10-year period. J Clin Microbiol. 2010;48:4051–6.

27. Pournaras S, Gogou V, Giannouli M, Dimitroulia E, Dafopoulou K, Tsakris A, et al. Single-locus-sequence-based typing of blaOXA-51-like genes for rapid assignment of *Acinetobacter baumannii* clinical isolates to international clonal lineages. J Clin Microbiol. 2014;52:1653–7.

28. Wang H, Guo P, Sun H, Wang H, Yang Q, Chen M, et al. Molecular epidemiology of clinical isolates of carbapenem-resistant *Acinetobacter spp*. From Chinese hospitals. Antimicrob Agents Chemother. 2007;51:4022–8.

29. Tsai H-T, Wang J-T, Chen CJ, Chang S-C. Association between antibiotic usage and subsequent colonization or infection of extensive drug-resistant *Acinetobacter baumannii*: a matched case-control study in intensive care units. Diagn Microbiol Infect Dis. 2008;62:298–305.

30. Dent LL, Marshall DR, Pratap S, Hulette RB. Multidrug resistant *Acinetobacter baumannii*: a descriptive study in a city hospital. BMC Infect Dis. 2010;10:196.

31. Zheng YL, Wan YF, Zhou LY, Ye ML, Liu S, Xu CQ, et al. Risk factors and mortality of patients with nosocomial carbapenem-resistant *Acinetobacter baumannii* pneumonia. Am J Infect Control. 2013;41:e1–5.

32. Li Y, Guo Q, Wang P, Zhu D, Ye X, Wu S, et al. Clonal dissemination of extensively drug-resistant *Acinetobacter baumannii* producing an OXA-23 β-lactamase at a teaching hospital in Shanghai, China. J Microbiol Immunol Infect. 2015;48:101–8.

33. Özgür ES, Horasan ES, Karaca K, Ersöz G, Naycı Atış S, Kaya A. Ventilator-associated pneumonia due to extensive drug-resistant *Acinetobacter baumannii*: risk factors, clinical features, and outcomes. Am J Infect Control. 2014;42:206–8.

34. Chan MC, Chiu SK, Hsueh PR, Wang NC, Wang CC, Fang CT. Risk factors for healthcare-associated extensively drug-resistant *Acinetobacter baumannii* infections: a case-control study. PLoS One. 2014;9, e85973.

35. Yang Y-S, Lee Y-T, Huang TW, Sun J-R, Kuo S-C, Yang C-H, et al. Acinetobacter baumannii nosocomial pneumonia: is the outcome more favorable in non-ventilated than ventilated patients? BMC Infect Dis. 2013;13:142.

36. Özvatan T, Akalın H, Sınırtaş M, Ocakoğlu G, Yılmaz E, Heper Y, et al. Nosocomial *Acinetobacter* pneumonia: treatment and prognostic factors in 356 cases. Respirology. 2016;21:363–9.

37. Sunenshine RH, Wright M-O, Maragakis LL, Harris AD, Song X, Hebden J, et al. Multidrug-resistant *Acinetobacter* infection mortality rate and length of hospitalization. Emerg Infect Dis. 2007;13:97–103.

3

Incidence, temporal trend and factors associated with ventilator-associated pneumonia in mainland China

Chengyi Ding[1], Yuelun Zhang[2], Zhirong Yang[3], Jing Wang[1], Aoming Jin[1], Weiwei Wang[1], Ru Chen[1] and Siyan Zhan[1*]

Abstract

Background: Data to date is far from sufficient to describe the recent epidemiology of ventilator-associated pneumonia (VAP) in mainland China. This study aimed to estimate the overall incidence of VAP, with a special focus on its temporal trend and associated factors.

Methods: Meta-analyses of 195 studies published from 2010 to 2015 were conducted, followed by subgroup analyses by methodological quality, pre-defined setting characteristics and attributes of populations.

Results: The overall cumulative VAP incidence in mainland China was 23.8% (95% confidence interval (CI) 20.6–27.2%), with the results showing high heterogeneity. The pooled incidence densities were 24.14 (95% CI 21.19–27.51) episodes and 22.83 (95% CI 19.88–26.23) patients per 1000 ventilator-days. A decline in the cumulative incidence was observed from 2006 (49.5%, 95% CI 40.0–59.0%) to 2014 (19.6%, 95% CI 10.4–31.0%); differences in the incidence rates were also documented according to Chinese provinces and diagnostic criteria ($p < 0.001$). Older age (≥60 years), coma, re-intubation, tracheotomy and prolonged ventilation were the factors significantly associated with the occurrence of VAP.

Conclusions: The incidence of VAP remains high in mainland China but has decreased since 2006. The reported rates vary considerably across individual studies, probably due to variations in diagnosis and geographical region. More studies using standard definitions and cut-off points are needed to better clarify the epidemiology of VAP across the country.

Keywords: Ventilator-associated pneumonia, Incidence, Risk factors, Meta-analysis, China

Background

Ventilator-associated pneumonia (VAP) is the most frequent type of healthcare-associated infection (HCAI) diagnosed in developing countries and has been firmly associated with an increased mortality, a longer hospital stay and additional healthcare costs [1, 2]. However, the incidence of VAP has been defined somewhat differently from study to study; there is currently no consensus on a common numerator or denominator that represents the overall incidence of VAP on a uniform basis. Commonly reported estimates include the percentage of patients on mechanical ventilation who develop VAP (cumulative incidence) and the number of VAP episodes per 1000 ventilator-days and VAP patients per 1000 ventilator-days [3, 4].

During the past few decades, nationwide studies on the incidence of VAP have been rare in China; only three studies have calculated the incidence of VAP at a national level, including one systematic review [5–7]. Based on two multi-center studies that were both conducted from 2013 to 2014, the point estimate of the VAP

---

* Correspondence: siyan-zhan@bjmu.edu.cn
[1]Department of Epidemiology and Biostatistics, School of Public Health, Peking University, 38 Xueyuan Road, Haidian District, Beijing 100191, People's Republic of China

incidence density in intensive care units (ICUs) was 8.89 patients per 1000 ventilator-days and ranged from 4.50–32.79 patients per 1000 ventilator-days depending on the type of ICU [5, 7]. The systematic review, which included 178 studies published between 2007 and 2012, yielded a pooled VAP cumulative incidence of 33.7% in ICUs [6]. Unfortunately, data regarding the nationwide incidence of VAP outside of ICUs remain unavailable. Moreover, information on the temporal change of the VAP incidence and stratified estimates according to the characteristics of different settings (such as by Chinese province and diagnostic criteria) to date are far from sufficient to describe the epidemiology of VAP across the country.

The main risk factors for VAP, such as prolonged ventilation, pre-existing pulmonary disease, transfusion, re-intubation and enteral feeding, have been extensively described among patients receiving mechanical ventilation in mainland China [8, 9]. However, the reported risk factors were varied or discordant, and there has been no meta-analysis study on this topic until now.

Reliable and updated data on the epidemiology of VAP are needed to inform patients and clinicians, plan healthcare services and policies, ascertain the overall burden of VAP and understand its causes. Given the paucity of existing data, this systematic review aimed to estimate the incidence of VAP in mainland China as well as its temporal trend and associated factors.

Methods
Search strategy and selection criteria
This systematic review and meta-analysis followed the Preferred Reporting Items for Systematic reviews and Meta-analyses (PRISMA) statement [10]. We systematically searched five electronic databases including Medline, Embase, the Chinese BioMedical Database (CBM), the China National Knowledge Infrastructure (CNKI) and the Wanfang Database for relevant studies. Given the focus on the recent epidemiology of VAP in our review, these searches were limited to studies published between January 2010 and December 2015. MeSH and free-text terms were applied to Medline, Embase and the CBM, and free-text terms were used to search the CNKI and Wanfang databases. Detailed search strategies for each database are listed in Additional file 1: Table S1. We also hand searched reference lists of relevant studies. The reviewers were divided into two groups that worked in parallel. The titles, keywords and abstracts of each record were screened independently by reviewers according to the eligibility criteria. Potentially eligible studies were further reviewed in their entirety. Disagreements were resolved by consensus.

We placed no restrictions on patient age or diagnostic criteria of pneumonia, and included eligible studies that satisfied all following criteria:

- Involved patients with VAP defined by a joint committee of the American Thoracic Society (ATS) and the Infectious Diseases Society of America (IDSA) as "pneumonia that arises more than 48–72 hours after endotracheal intubation" [11].
- Provided sufficient data to calculate the incidence of VAP. Given the variation in the definition regarding the VAP incidence in different studies and institutions, the following incidences (one cumulative incidence and two incidence densities) were calculated for each study included in our review where applicable: the number of patients with VAP/total number of observed patients on ventilation, VAP episodes per 1000 ventilator-days and VAP patients per 1000 ventilator-days.
- Collected data in a prospective way using a surveillance study design, a cohort study or a nested case control study.
- Were conducted in mainland China. Studies dealing with the VAP incidence in Taiwan, Hong Kong and Macao in China were excluded since the socioeconomic status and healthcare policies in these regions differ from those in mainland China.
- Were published in Chinese or English.

Assessment of risk of bias
We evaluated the methodological quality of each included study using the modified Leboeuf-Yde and Lauritsen tool [12], which comprise 10 items that measure two study dimensions (external validity and internal validity) plus a summary risk of bias assessment (Additional file 2). Each item can be judged as having either a low or a high risk of bias. One point was awarded for an item if it was considered to have a low risk of bias, and the maximum possible score was 10. Scores of 8 or more, 6–7, and 5 or less were defined as having a low, moderate and high risk of bias, respectively. Graphs of the summary of risk of bias were drawn using Revman 5.3 (Cochrane's Informatics and Knowledge Management Department, London, UK).

Data extraction
An extraction form was pre-designed with EpiData 3.1 (The EpiData Association, Odense, Denmark) and then modified based on the results of a pilot test. The revised extraction form consisted of four parts: study setting, methodological quality, characteristics of the populations and data for calculating the incidences of VAP. Two groups of reviewers independently performed the data extraction, and any disagreement was resolved using

consensus as well. If possible, the corresponding authors of the included studies were contacted regarding unreported data.

Statistical analysis

All statistical analyses were carried out using R 3.2.1 (Bell Laboratories, Inc., Madison, WI, USA), and all p-values were two-tailed. Heterogeneity was assessed via Q test and I^2 statistics. $p < 0.1$ or $I^2 > 50\%$ was defined to note substantial heterogeneity [13]. The pooled estimates together with the 95% confidence intervals (CIs) of VAP incidences were obtained using a DerSimonian-Laird random-effects model to accommodate heterogeneity across all included studies [14]. To normalize the distribution of incidence, we implemented an arcsine-transformation for cumulative incidences, while a log-transformation was used to determine the incidence densities. For the log-transformation, increments of 0.5 were added to both the numerators and the denominators in studies with zero reported events. Sensitivity analyses were also conducted by omitting studies that had diagnosed VAP using unclear criteria or in those with a high risk of bias. In addition, the publication bias was examined using Egger's test [15]. The results were considered to have a probable publication bias when $p < 0.1$.

Furthermore, subgroup analyses were performed using methodological quality and pre-defined setting characteristics, including clinical department, diagnostic criteria, level of hospital, Chinese province and year of study (during which the patients are followed up and the incidence data are collected). Based on the Hospital Grade Management Regulations set by the Chinese Ministry of Health (MoH), hospitals were categorized into tertiary (>500 beds) or non-tertiary (≤500 beds) hospitals according to their size, clinical departments and healthcare personnel. When the incidence was reported for a multi-year period, the midpoint of the time interval was regarded as the year of the study [16, 17]. A line chart was created to graphically demonstrate the temporal trend of the VAP incidence. Additionally, MapInfo Professional 11.0 (Pitney Bowes Inc., Stamford, CT, US) was used to develop a map based on the subgroup analysis by province.

We also conducted subgroup analyses using the attributes of populations. Patient subgroups that were mentioned at least four times in the included studies and had been stratified using comparable cut-off points were screened to carry out the subgroup analyses regarding the attributes of populations in this review. Moreover, a Q test for heterogeneity was used to compare the incidence across subgroups, and 0.05 was defined as the threshold of the p-value for statistical significance [18].

Results

General information about the included studies

We identified a total of 8282 records and finally included 195 studies (Fig. 1), of which 93 reported the cumulative incidence of VAP, 50 had an incidence density of VAP episodes per 1000 ventilator-days and 103 reported an estimate of VAP patients per 1000 ventilator-days. The methodological quality of the included studies is illustrated in Fig. 2. Overall, most of the studies demonstrated a good or moderate methodology. A list of the included studies and a summary of their characteristics are presented in Additional file 1: Tables S2 and S3.

Overall incidence

The pooled cumulative incidence of VAP in mainland China was 23.8% (95% CI 20.6–27.2%) from 2006 to 2014 (Additional file 1: Figure S1). At the same time, the pooled incidence densities were 24.14 (95% CI 21.19–27.51) episodes and 22.83 (95% CI 19.88–26.23) patients per 1000 ventilator-days (Additional file 1: Figure S2 and S3). The Egger's test indicated that a publication bias was present when verifying the included studies that reported a cumulative incidence or an incidence density of VAP episodes per 1000 ventilator-days ($p < 0.1$ for both estimates).

Temporal trend in incidence rates

Because stratified estimates were available in most of the included studies that reported a cumulative incidence, we used the cumulative incidence to conduct all subgroup analyses. The results of the subgroup analyses by methodological quality and study settings are summarized in Table 1 and Additional file 1: Table S4. A declining trend was observed in the cumulative VAP incidence ($p < 0.001$); the pooled estimate in 2006 was 49.5% (95% CI 40.0–59.0%), which had decreased to 19.6% (95% CI 10.4–31.0%) by 2014 (Fig. 3).

Incidence rates by geographic region and diagnostic criteria

The cumulative incidence of VAP varied by geographic region (Fig. 4), with estimates that ranged from 7.5% (95% CI 5.9–9.4%) in the Fujian Province to 70.0% (95% CI 52.7–84.8%) in the Chongqing Province (Additional file 1: Table S4). Differences in incidence rates were also documented according to diagnostic algorithms ($p < 0.001$); the rate ranged from 20.0% (95% CI 15.1–25.3%) to 38.4% (95% CI 31.4–45.8%) when using the three sets of criteria published in Chinese (Table 1, Additional file 1: Table S5) [19–21].

Factors associated with the development of VAP

Table 2 displays the results of subgroup analyses based on the attributes of populations. The results indicated

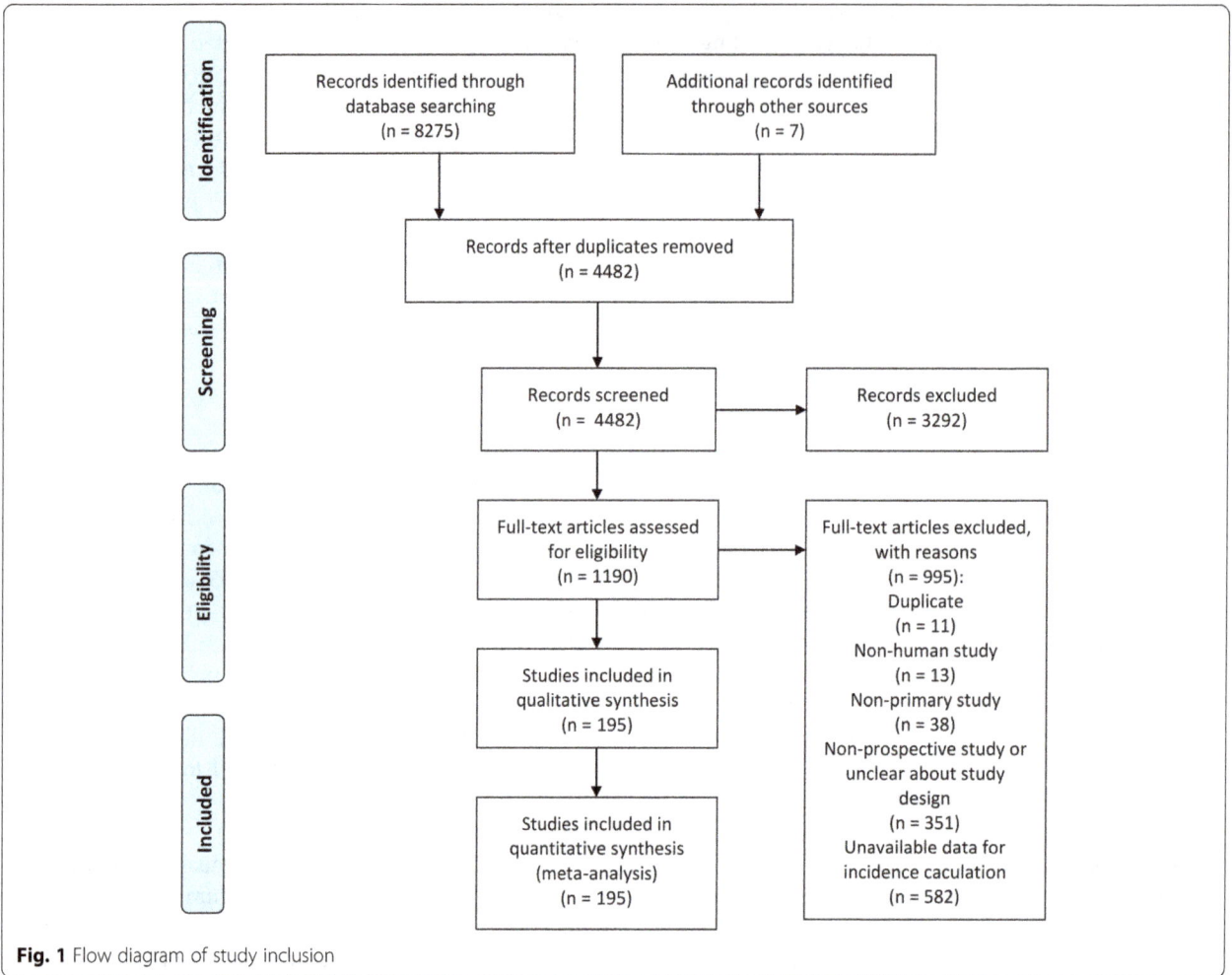

Fig. 1 Flow diagram of study inclusion

that VAP occurred more frequently in patients who received a tracheotomy, were re-intubated and were mechanically ventilated for more than two weeks. In addition, older (≥60 years of age) and comatose patients were at greater risk of developing VAP. The cumulative incidence of VAP was higher in men and in patients with diabetes, but the difference was not statistically significant.

Sensitivity analyses

In our sensitivity analyses, which excluded studies with unclear diagnostic criteria for VAP, the pooled estimates were 24.1% (95% CI 20.6–27.8%) and 23.46 (95% CI 20.53–26.81) episodes or 21.20 (95% CI 18.26–24.61) patients per 1000 ventilator-days. Sensitivity analyses were also performed by omitting studies with a high risk of bias, which resulted in pooled estimates of 23.6%

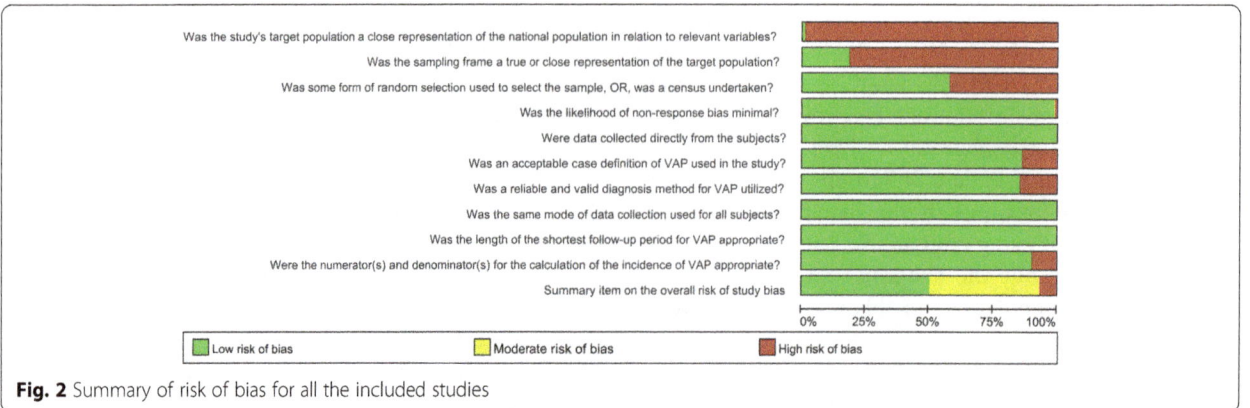

Fig. 2 Summary of risk of bias for all the included studies

Table 1 The results of subgroup analyses by methodological quality and pre-defined setting characteristics

Subgroups		Studies	Sample size	Estimate (%)[a]	95% CI (%)	I^2 (%)	p value[b]
Overall[c]		93	71,816	23.8	20.6–27.2	98.9	-
Clinical department	General ICU	11	5388	18.3	11.3–26.6	97.7	0.310
	Neonatal ward	4	136	26.1	9.4–47.6	85.5	
	Neonatal ICU	7	3938	15.7	3.2–35.0	99.4	
	Pediatric ICU	6	721	30.2	18.7–43.2	91.8	
	Respiratory ICU	5	607	27.4	23.3–31.7	15.2	
	Surgical ICU	1	85	29.4	20.3–39.5	-	
Diagnostic criteria[d]	By Chinese Critical Care Medicine Society in 2013 [26]	3	174	38.4	31.4–45.8	0.0	<0.001
	By the Chinese Ministry of Health in 2001 [25]	29	46,894	20.0	15.1–25.3	99.1	
	By Chinese Thoracic Society in 1999 [27]	35	13,979	27.2	22.2–32.5	97.6	
Hospital level	Tertiary	75	58,704	23.6	19.7–27.6	99.0	0.574
	Non-tertiary	16	2703	26.4	17.7–36.2	96.3	
Risk of bias	High	9	1286	26.3	17.1–36.6	88.2	0.687
	Moderate	43	17,973	24.6	20.8–28.5	96.8	
	Low	41	52,557	22.2	17.4–27.4	99.2	

CI confidence interval, *ICU* intensive care unit, *VAP* ventilator-associated pneumonia

[a]Pooled estimates were calculated by a random-effects model

[b]The Q test for heterogeneity was used to compare the incidence across subgroups

[c]Studies that reported the cumulative incidence of VAP

[d]A summary of diagnostic requirements for the three published sets of criteria is presented in Additional file 1: Table S5

(95% CI 20.2–27.2%) and 24.30 (95% CI 21.29–27.72) episodes or 22.61 (95% CI 19.57–26.12) patients per 1000 ventilator-days.

Discussion

In the present study, the pooled cumulative incidence of VAP in mainland China was 23.8%; the incidence density was 24.14 episodes or 22.83 patients per 1000 ventilator-days. These data appear inconsistent with previous findings obtained from two multi-center studies (7.23–8.89 patients per 1000 ventilator-days) or a systematic review (33.7%) on the nationwide VAP incidence [5–7]. The following reasons may have contributed to this

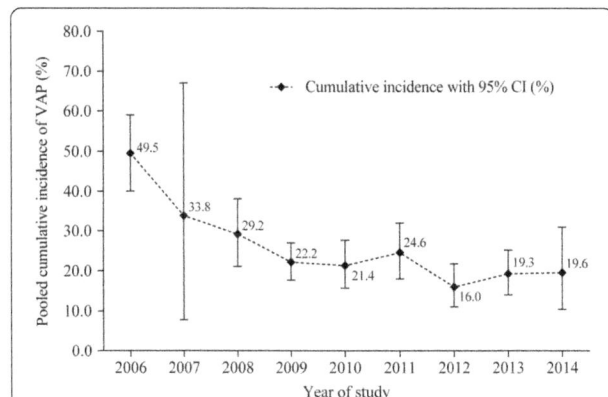

Fig. 3 Pooled cumulative incidence of VAP in mainland China at different study periods. Random-effects model was used to pool the individual cumulative incidence of each included study

inconsistency. First, the incidence of VAP varied by study setting, such as by diagnostic criteria, study period and geographic region. Therefore, variations in these settings may partly account for the differences across the estimated incidences. Second, the present meta-analysis covered approximately 71,816 patients with 1.33 million ventilator-days in mainland China. The sample sizes in our review were substantially larger than those of previous studies (35,903 patients and 101,128 total ventilator-days). A more reliable estimate could be obtained by pooling data with a larger sample size [22]. In addition, our review investigated the incidence of VAP according to characteristics of populations and thus could provide additional useful information.

Our review has shown that VAP represents a critical safety issue for hospitalized patients in mainland China. Compared with the incidence of VAP in developed countries (2.9–7.9 episodes per 1000 ventilator-days) [2, 23], the pooled incidence in mainland China was strikingly higher. The great burden of VAP in mainland China could be the result of a combination of numerous adverse factors, such as understaffing, overcrowding and a lack of knowledge and application of basic infection control measures [2]. For example, although recognized as one of the most cost-effective measures to prevent HCAI, including VAP [24], hand hygiene is very often neglected by healthcare workers in Chinese hospitals, with a suboptimal compliance of 10.6–64.6% that varies depending on clinical department [25].

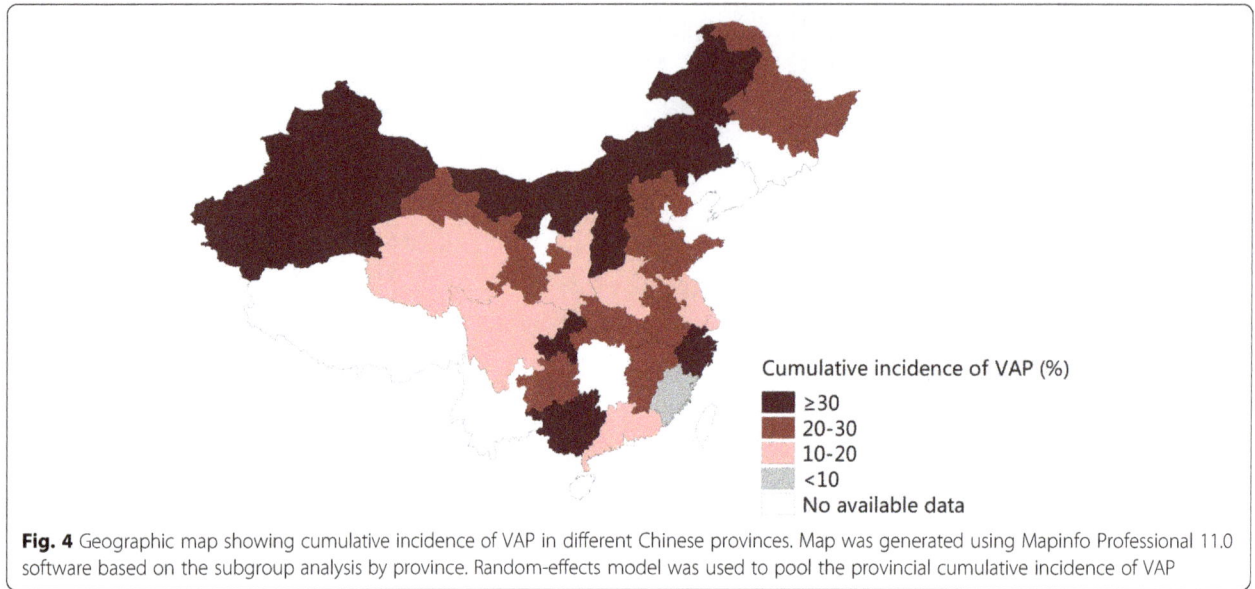

Fig. 4 Geographic map showing cumulative incidence of VAP in different Chinese provinces. Map was generated using Mapinfo Professional 11.0 software based on the subgroup analysis by province. Random-effects model was used to pool the provincial cumulative incidence of VAP

Table 2 The results of subgroup analyses by characteristics of patient populations

Subgroups	Studies	Sample size	Estimate (%)[a]	95% CI (%)	I^2 (%)	p value[b]
Overall[c]	93	71,816	23.8	20.6–27.2	98.9	-
Gender						
Male	11	2303	22.4	16.6–28.7	90.5	0.085
Female	11	1577	15.8	11.7–20.5	76.8	
Age						
<60 years	4	1219	14.0	10.5–17.9	55.6	0.039
≥60 years	6	956	30.8	15.2–49.1	96.7	
Comatose						
Yes	4	318	55.9	42.5–69.0	79.8	<0.001
No	4	2073	10.2	4.7–17.5	94.6	
Diabetes						
Yes	4	73	42.7	16.4–71.4	84.6	0.276
No	4	442	26.8	20.8–33.2	52.5	
Duration of ventilation						
< 7 days	10	3582	6.6	4.7–8.9	77.7	<0.001
7–13 days	2	208	41.3	34.8–48.1	0.0	
≥14 days	4	114	81.5	57.9–96.7	81.8	
Tracheotomy						
Yes	12	663	55.6	38.2–72.4	94.5	0.002
No	5	448	25.0	17.6–33.2	71.8	
Re-intubation						
Yes	4	209	54.6	43.9–65.2	45.9	<0.001
No	4	1233	15.7	9.9–22.5	82.4	

CI confidence interval
[a]Pooled estimates were calculated by a random-effects model
[b]The Q test for heterogeneity was used to compare the incidence across subgroups
[c]Studies that reported the cumulative incidence of ventilator-associated pneumonia

ICU beds are in short supply in resource-limited countries like China; as a result, many patients who require mechanical ventilation are hospitalized in general wards. For example, the ratio of ICU beds to general beds is 3.5% in a 1500-bed tertiary university-affiliated hospital in Beijing, whereas the figure in the United States is 5–7% [26]. Moreover, data from the same hospital showed that 24.7% of its ventilator-days during 2015–2016 occurred in general wards [27]. Despite the high percentage of patients ventilated in general wards in mainland China, studies regarding the clinical outcomes of this population remain scarce. In the present review, only four studies dealt with mechanical ventilation outside the ICU, and all focused on neonatal wards. The corresponding subgroup analysis yielded a VAP incidence of 26.1% in neonatal wards, which is much higher than the estimate in the neonatal ICU (15.7%). This finding is in line with studies from other resource-limited countries, demonstrating that ICU settings might provide better monitoring, which is associated with fewer complications and more active ventilator management [26, 28]. Given the shortage of ICU beds and the growing number of patients who need them in mainland China, future studies are needed to identify better triage criteria and alternative patient care strategies.

Our review found that the pooled cumulative incidence of VAP decreased notably from 2006 to 2014. In 2005, China committed to reduce HCAI by signing the pledge of the World Health Organization (WHO)'s First Global Patient Safety Challenge and establishing a national standard for nosocomial infection surveillance [23, 29]. According to these documents, Chinese hospitals must conduct hospital-wide surveillance of HCAI and hire at least one HCAI-control professional per 200–250 beds; a HCAI management committee is also required to supervise the implementation of these actions [29]. A meta-analysis of 11 before-after studies found that this aggressive surveillance strategy resulted in a relative risk reduction of 37% for VAP and 25% for catheter-related bloodstream infection in ICUs [30]. In addition, another meta-analysis found that the incidence of surgical site infection in mainland China has decreased significantly in recent years [31]. Therefore, we believe that these combined efforts could have contributed to the recorded decline of VAP across the country.

Although a nationwide standard for VAP monitoring has been established for many years, data on its incidence are scarce to non-existent in several Chinese provinces, including Xizang, Yunnan, Hunan and Jilin. Previous studies have suggested that the incidence of HCAI tends to be lower in eastern coastal regions relative to those of the midlands and remote western regions because the eastern coastal areas enjoy stronger economies and more abundant healthcare resources [5, 31].

However, an east-to-west gradient was not noted in our geographic mapping of the cumulative VAP incidence. The cause of these observed geographic variations therefore remains unknown but may be due to differences in diverse environmental exposures associated with lung diseases, the implementation of HCAI control measures or the availability of ventilators.

According to our review, the pooled cumulative incidence of VAP varied from 20.0–38.4% depending on which of the three diagnostic algorithms was applied for its identification. Indeed, the incidence rate calculated using the MoH criteria was much lower than the rates obtained using the other two criteria. This difference could have been because the diagnosis of a VAP episode based on the MoH criteria requires a combination of chest radiography signs, clinical symptoms and microbiological findings, while only clinical and radiological findings must be present in the other two sets of criteria; the incidence of VAP tends to decrease when more stringent criteria are applied [19–21, 32, 33]. It has been argued that microbiological findings are essential to avoid the over-diagnosis of VAP; however, the isolation of pathogens without clinical and radiological signs may simply represent colonization [34]. Thus, the diagnosis of this condition should be based on a set of criteria that includes radiological findings, clinical symptoms and microbiology. In light of the preventable nature of VAP, its incidence has served as an indicator of healthcare quality and also of the effectiveness of VAP-prevention strategies. Nevertheless, the subjectivity and discrepancies of the existing Chinese diagnostic criteria make it possible to manipulate the true incidence of this condition [35]. Therefore, relevant studies and surveillance data on this topic should be interpreted with caution.

Mechanical ventilation is a life-saving supportive intervention for critically ill patients, but it can also result in complications, such as lung injury, diaphragmatic dysfunction and VAP [36]. Since the proper identification of risk factors is essential for establishing effective strategies to prevent VAP, we performed this systematic review to resolve the uncertainties found in previous studies; the present study is the first to analyse factors predicting VAP for patients in mainland China using a meta-analysis. As expected, a considerable proportion of the included studies reported a stratified VAP incidence concerning various attributes of populations; however, the definitions or cut-off points of the grouping factors were inconsistent. As a consequence, we used the same definitions and the most common cut-off points to selectively pool stratified estimates that had been reported in at least four studies. The results of this meta-analysis indicated that advanced age (≥60 years), coma, re-intubation, tracheotomy and prolonged ventilation were the factors most frequently associated with the acquisition of VAP in mainland China.

Elderly patients have been shown to be more vulnerable to HCAI due to immunologic involution, age-associated physiological and anatomical alterations and increasingly severe chronic diseases and malnutrition [37]. Accordingly, based on our findings, VAP occurred more frequently in elderly patients than it did in younger adults. Although comatose patients represent a relatively small number of hospitalized patients, this population often comprises critically ill patients with high mortality risks [38]. Moreover, VAP is a common complication in comatose patients that may lead to a poor prognosis. Previous studies have suggested that the use of prone positioning could lower the risk of developing VAP [39, 40]. However, feasibility and safety issues may present barriers to this technique's implementation; further studies to examine the prevention of VAP in comatose patients are urgently needed.

In accordance with previous studies [41, 42], our review indicated that re-intubation could be a risk factor for VAP. The most likely mechanism underlying this risk is the aspiration of oropharyngeal or gastric secretions contaminated with potentially pathogenic organisms during the intubation procedure. Aspiration appears to play an important role in the development of VAP; therefore, medical staff members should be warned of the risk of aspiration in these patients and be trained in techniques to reduce its incidence. Several studies have proven that performing a tracheotomy earlier rather than later may decrease the incidence of VAP in patients who require prolonged intubation [43, 44]. The high overall incidence of VAP observed in tracheotomy patients in the present study indicated that the optimal timing for performing a tracheotomy in critical care settings in China must be determined; tracheotomy management should also be improved. However, a lack of sufficient data prevented a further subgroup analysis from examining the timing of the tracheotomy. In addition, the cumulative incidence of VAP in our review was highest in patients who were ventilated for more than two weeks. Those who were ventilated for 7–13 days had a lower rate of occurrence than those treated for more than two weeks, while the VAP incidence was the lowest early in the course of ventilation (<7 days). This trend could be explained by the fact that prolonged ventilation increases the risk of infection due to exposure to humidifiers and ventilator circuits that are an important source of pathogens [45]. In light of these findings, strategies to shorten the duration of ventilation may represent another key to controlling VAP, such as a daily interruption for sedative-drug infusions [46] and the application of weaning protocols [47].

There are several limitations of this study. First, about half of the included studies were of moderate or low methodological quality overall. Despite this shortcoming,

the methodological quality was not the main source of heterogeneity according to the subgroup analyses. Sensitivity analyses conducted after omitting studies with a high risk of bias showed robust results as well. Second, most of the included studies were conducted in tertiary hospitals located in big cities and therefore might not be representative of the national situation. However, in mainland China, mechanical ventilators are more readily available in tertiary hospitals [48]; our review covered hospitalized patients from more than 20 provinces at the initiation of mechanical ventilation. The risk of bias in generalizing our findings to the entire country has thus been minimized. Furthermore, although a temporal decline in the cumulative incidence of VAP was noted in our review, this result was likely biased since the mid-point of the time interval was used as the year of the study when the incidence was reported for a multi-year period [16, 17].

Conclusions

In conclusion, the incidence of VAP remains high in mainland China but has decreased since 2006. The reported rates vary widely across individual studies, which is likely due to discrepancies in diagnosis and also variations due to geographical region. Older age, coma, re-intubation, tracheotomy and prolonged ventilation were associated with an increased risk of VAP; improved management and prevention strategies that target these factors should be developed to decrease the incidence rate. In addition, more studies with standard definitions and cut-off points will be required to gain a greater understanding of the epidemiology of VAP nationwide and to provide further reliable evidence in this field.

Additional files

Additional file 1: Table S1. Search strategies and results. **Table S2.** List of all the included studies. **Table S3.** General information of all the included studies. **Table S4.** The results of subgroup analyses by Chinese provinces and years of study. **Table S5.** Summary of diagnostic requirements for the three published sets of criteria in mainland China. **Figure S1.** Forest plot of the cumulative incidence of ventilator-associated pneumonia using a random-effects model. **Figure S2.** Forest plot of the incidence density (reported as episodes per 1000 ventilator-days) of ventilator-associated pneumonia using a random-effects model. **Figure S3.** Forest plot of the incidence density (reported as patients per 1000 ventilator-days) of ventilator-associated pneumonia using a random-effects model.

Additional file 2: Risk of bias assessment tool.

Abbreviations

ATS: American Thoracic Society; CBM: Chinese BioMedical Database; CI: confidence interval; CNKI: China National Knowledge Infrastructure; HCAI: healthcare-associated infection; ICU: intensive care unit; IDSA: Infectious Diseases Society of America; MoH: Chinese Ministry of Health; PRISMA: Preferred Reporting Items for Systematic reviews and Meta-analyses; VAP: ventilator-associated pneumonia; WHO: World Health Organization

Acknowledgements
Many thanks to Xinran Liu, Yu Cao and Yuting Pan for contributing to part of work on study selection and data extraction, and to Dr. Dong Li for giving useful advice about revising the manuscript.

Funding
None.

Authors' contributions
YZ, ZY and JW performed the literature search. CD, YZ, ZY, JW, AJ, WW and RC selected the articles and collected the data. CD conducted the statistical analyses and drafted the manuscript. YZ critically revised the manuscript. YZ, ZY and SZ conceived and designed the study, and supervised the work in all phases. All authors read and approved the final manuscript.

Consent for publication
Not applicable.

Competing interests
The authors declare that they have no competing interests.

Author details
[1]Department of Epidemiology and Biostatistics, School of Public Health, Peking University, 38 Xueyuan Road, Haidian District, Beijing 100191, People's Republic of China. [2]Division of Epidemiology, The Jockey Club School of Public Health and Primary Care, The Chinese University of Hong Kong, Hong Kong, People's Republic of China. [3]Primary Care Unit, Department of Public Health and Primary Care, University of Cambridge, Cambridgeshire, UK.

References
1. Barbier F, Andremont A, Wolff M, Bouadma L. Hospital-acquired pneumonia and ventilator-associated pneumonia: recent advances in epidemiology and management. Curr Opin Pulm Med. 2013;19:216–28.
2. Allegranzi B, Bagheri Nejad S, Combescure C, Graafmans W, Attar H, Donaldson L, et al. Burden of endemic health-care-associated infection in developing countries: systematic review and meta-analysis. Lancet. 2011;377:228–41.
3. Chawla R. Epidemiology, etiology, and diagnosis of hospital-acquired pneumonia and ventilator-associated pneumonia in Asian countries. Am J Infect Control. 2008;36:S93–100.
4. Fitch ZW, Whitman GJ. Incidence, risk, and prevention of ventilator-associated pneumonia in adult cardiac surgical patients: a systematic review. J Card Surg. 2014;29:196–203.
5. Gao XD, Hu BJ, Cui YW, Sun W, Shen Y. A multicenter prospective monitoring on incidences of ventilator-associated pneumonia in 46 hospitals in China. Chinese Journal of Infection Control. 2015;14:540–3. [Chinese].
6. Zhang Y, Yao Z, Zhan S, Yang Z, Wei D, Zhang J, et al. Disease burden of intensive care unit-acquired pneumonia in China: a systematic review and meta-analysis. Int J Infect Dis. 2014;29:84–90.
7. Ren JH, Yin H, Wu AH, Hu BJ, Zhang XY, Hou TY, et al. Multicenter study on epidemiology of device-associated infection in neonatal intensive care units. Chin J Infect Control. 2015;14:530–4. [Chinese].
8. Xie DS, Xiong W, Lai RP, Liu L, Gan XM, Wang XH, et al. Ventilator-associated pneumonia in intensive care units in Hubei Province, China: a multicentre prospective cohort survey. J Hosp Infect. 2011;78:284–8.
9. Yuan TM, Chen LH, Yu HM. Risk factors and outcomes for ventilator-associated pneumonia in neonatal intensive care unit patients. J Perinat Med. 2007;35:334–8.
10. Liberati A, Altman DG, Tetzlaff J, Mulrow C, Gotzsche PC, Ioannidis JPA, et al. The PRISMA statement for reporting systematic reviews and meta-analyses of studies that evaluate health care interventions: explanation and elaboration. PLoS Med. 2009;6:e1000100.
11. American Thoracic Society, Infectious Diseases Society of America. Guidelines for the management of adults with hospital-acquired, ventilator-associated, and healthcare-associated pneumonia. Am J Respir Crit Care Med. 2005;171:388–416.
12. Hoy D, Brooks P, Woolf A, Blyth F, March L, Bain C, et al. Assessing risk of bias in prevalence studies: modification of an existing tool and evidence of interrater agreement. J Clin Epidemiol. 2012;65:934–9.
13. Higgins JP, Thompson SG, Deeks JJ, Altman DG. Measuring inconsistency in meta-analyses. BMJ. 2003;327:557–60.
14. DerSimonian R, Laird N. Meta-analysis in clinical trials. Control Clin Trials. 1986;7:177–88.
15. Egger M, Davey Smith G, Schneider M, Minder C. Bias in meta-analysis detected by a simple, graphical test. BMJ. 1997;315:629–34.
16. Tadesse G. A meta-analysis of the proportion of antimicrobial resistant human salmonella isolates in Ethiopia. BMC Pharmacol Toxicol. 2014;15:51.
17. Tong J, Zheng Q, Zhang C, Lo R, Shen J, Ran Z. Incidence, prevalence, and temporal trends of microscopic colitis: a systematic review and meta-analysis. Am J Gastroenterol. 2015;110:265–76;quiz 277.
18. Borenstein M, Hedges LV, Higgins JPT, Rothstein HR. Introduction to meta-analysis. Hoboken: John Wiley & Sons; 2009.
19. Chinese Ministry of Health. Diagnostic criteria for nosocomial infection. 2001. [Chinese]. http://www.moh.gov.cn/yzygj/s3593/200804/e19e4448378643a09913ccf2a055c79d.shtml. Accessed 13 Jun 2016.
20. Chinese Critical Care Medicine Society. Guidelines for the diagnosis, prevention and treatment of ventilator-associated pneumonia (2013). Chin J Intern Med. 2013;52:524–43. [Chinese].
21. Chinese Thoracic Society. Guidelines for the diagnosis and treatment of hospital-acquired pneumonia (Draft). Chin J Tuberc Respir Dis. 1999;22:201–3. [Chinese].
22. Yang Z, Wang J, Wang W, Zhang Y, Han L, Zhang Y, et al. Proportions of Staphylococcus aureus and methicillin-resistant Staphylococcus aureus in patients with surgical site infections in mainland China: a systematic review and meta-analysis. PLoS One. 2015;10:e0116079.
23. World Health Organization. Report on the Burden of Endemic Health Care-Associated Infection Worldwide. 2011. http://apps.who.int/iris/bitstream/10665/80135/1/9789241501507_eng.pdf. Accessed 2 Mar 2016.
24. World Health Organization. WHO Guidelines on Hand Hygiene in Health Care. 2009. http://apps.who.int/iris/bitstream/10665/44102/1/9789241597906_eng.pdf. Accessed 2 Mar 2016.
25. Li LY, Zhao YC, Jia JX, Zhao XL, Jia HX. Investigation on compliance of hand hygiene of healthcare workers. Zhongguo Yi Xue Ke Xue Yuan Xue Bao. 2008;30:546–9. [Chinese].
26. Hersch M, Sonnenblick M, Karlic A, Einav S, Sprung CL, Izbicki G. Mechanical ventilation of patients hospitalized in medical wards vs the intensive care unit–an observational, comparative study. J Crit Care. 2007;22:13–7.
27. Jia HX, Liu X, Ren JH, Jia JX, Zhao YC, Zhao XL, et al. Characteristics of device-related infections in ICUs and common wards. Chin J Nosocomiol. 2016;26:4293–5. [Chinese].
28. Wongsurakiat P, Sangsa N, Tangaroonsanti A. Mechanical ventilation of patients hospitalized on general medical Ward: outcomes and prognostic factors. J Med Assoc Thail. 2016;99:772–6.
29. Chinese Ministry of Health. Standard for nosocomial infection surveillance. 2009. [Chinese]. http://www.moh.gov.cn/zwgkzt/s9496/200904/40117/files/25b6a8b518094e00b150550fdfb0953e.pdf. Accessed 2 Mar 2016.
30. Dai FF, Zhu JQ, Lai MH, Lu SZ. Effect of infection-control practices based on targeted surveillance in intensive care units: a meta-analysis. Inter J Epidemiol Infect Dis. 2014;41:407–11. [Chinese].
31. Fan Y, Wei Z, Wang W, Tan L, Jiang H, Tian L, et al. The incidence and distribution of surgical site infection in mainland China: a meta-analysis of 84 prospective observational studies. Sci Rep. 2014;4:6783.
32. Klompas M, Magill S, Robicsek A, Strymish JM, Kleinman K, Evans RS, et al. Objective surveillance definitions for ventilator-associated pneumonia. Crit Care Med. 2012;40:3154–61.
33. Tejerina E, Esteban A, Fernandez-Segoviano P, Frutos-Vivar F, Aramburu J, Ballesteros D, et al. Accuracy of clinical definitions of ventilator-associated pneumonia: comparison with autopsy findings. J Crit Care. 2010;25:62–8.
34. Cernada M, Brugada M, Golombek S, Vento M. Ventilator-associated pneumonia in neonatal patients: an update. Neonatology. 2014;105:98–107.
35. Ego A, Preiser JC, Vincent JL. Impact of diagnostic criteria on the incidence of ventilator-associated pneumonia. Chest. 2015;147:347–55.

36. Jubran A. Critical illness and mechanical ventilation: effects on the
     diaphragm. Respir Care. 2006;51:1054–61.
37. Blot S, Koulenti D, Dimopoulos G, Martin C, Komnos A, Krueger WA, et al.
     Prevalence, risk factors, and mortality for ventilator-associated pneumonia in
     middle-aged, old, and very old critically ill patients. Crit Care Med.
     2014;42:601–9.
38. Rello J, Ausina V, Ricart M, Puzo C, Net A, Prats G. Nosocomial pneumonia in
     critically ill comatose patients: need for a differential therapeutic approach.
     Eur Respir J. 1992;5:1249–53.
39. Beuret P, Carton MJ, Nourdine K, Fowler R, Cook D, Heyland D. Prone
     position as prevention of lung injury in comatose patients: a prospective,
     randomized, controlled study. Intensive Care Med. 2002;28:564–9.
40. Muscedere J, Dodek P, Keenan S, Fowler R, Cook D, Heyland D.
     Comprehensive evidence-based clinical practice guidelines for ventilator-
     associated pneumonia: prevention. J Crit Care. 2008;23:126–37.
41. Liu B, Li SQ, Zhang SM, Xu P, Zhang X, Zhang YH, et al. Risk factors of
     ventilator-associated pneumonia in pediatric intensive care unit: a
     systematic review and meta-analysis. J Thorac Dis. 2013;5:525–31.
42. Charles MP, Kali A, Easow JM, Joseph NM, Ravishankar M, Srinivasan S, et al.
     Ventilator-associated pneumonia. Australas Med J. 2014;7:334–44.
43. Nseir S, Di Pompeo C, Jozefowicz E, Cavestri B, Brisson H, Nyunga M, et al.
     Relationship between tracheotomy and ventilator-associated pneumonia: a
     case control study. Eur Respir J. 2007;30:314–20.
44. Rumbak MJ, Newton M, Truncale T, Schwartz SW, Adams JW, Hazard PB. A
     prospective, randomized, study comparing early percutaneous dilational
     tracheotomy to prolonged translaryngeal intubation (delayed tracheotomy)
     in critically ill medical patients. Crit Care Med. 2004;32:1689–94.
45. Tan B, Zhang F, Zhang X, Huang YL, Gao YS, Liu X, et al. Risk factors for
     ventilator-associated pneumonia in the neonatal intensive care unit: a meta-
     analysis of observational studies. Eur J Pediatr. 2014;173:427–34.
46. Kress JP, Pohlman AS, O'Connor MF, Hall JB. Daily interruption of sedative
     infusions in critically ill patients undergoing mechanical ventilation.
     N Engl J Med. 2000;342:1471–7.
47. Marelich GP, Murin S, Battistella F, Inciardi J, Vierra T, Roby M. Protocol
     weaning of mechanical ventilation in medical and surgical patients by
     respiratory care practitioners and nurses: effect on weaning time and
     incidence of ventilator-associated pneumonia. Chest. 2000;118:459–67.
48. Xie JX, Zhang L. The Current Situation and Prospects of Mechanical
     Ventilator Industry. China Medical Device Information. 2014(2):10–20.
     [Chinese].

4

A comparison study between GeXP-based multiplex-PCR and serology assay for Mycoplasma pneumoniae detection in children with community acquired pneumonia

Le Wang[1], Zhishan Feng[1], Mengchuan Zhao[1], Shuo Yang[1], Xiaotong Yan[1], Weiwei Guo[1], Zhongren Shi[1*] and Guixia Li[1,2*]

Abstract

Background: Diagnosis of community-acquired pneumonia (CAP) caused by *Mycoplasma pneumoniae* (Mp) in children has been hampered by difficulty in obtaining convalescent serum and time constraints. In this study, the two diagnostic assays that targeted respectively on Mp-antibody and Mp-DNA were retrospectively investigated.

Methods: A total of 3146 children were clinically diagnosed to have CAP and were confirmed by chest X-ray during March 2015 to February 2016 in Children's hospital of Hebei Province (China). Both of the sera and sputum samples were collected in 24 h after their admission. The Mp-antibody was examined by the passive particle agglutination assay and a fourfold or greater increase of antibody titers of paired sera or $\geq$1:160 titer of single serum was set as the serology positive. Mp-DNA in the sputum samples was tested by a multiplex-PCR method named GeXP assay (multiplex PCR combined with automated capillary electrophoresis). In order to eliminate the false positive results caused by the asymptomatic carriage after infected by *M. pneumoniae,* the inconsistent samples were tested by the real-time isothermal transcription-mediated RNA amplification assay (SAT).

Results: The inter-rated agreement test was performed in 3146 CAP patients, with a highest kappa value in the school-age children as 0.783. There were 6.29% (198/3146) cases showed inconsistent results determined by GeXP and serology assay. All of the 19 GeXP(+)/Serology (−) samples and a randomly chosen 27 from 179 GeXP(−)/Serology (+) samples were tested by SAT assay, and a 97.8% diagnosis agreement was observed between SAT and GeXP assay, but not with the serology assay. In addition, patients who were detected only by serology or only by multiplex-PCR were significantly younger than those with both methods positive (3.0 and 1.5 years vs. 5.0 years, $p < 0.01$). The Viral-Mp coinfection accounted for 37.0% (97/262), which was more common in winter and spring ($p < 0.05$) and in the infantile group ($p < 0.01$), compared to the pure Mp positive ones.

Conclusion: In some children CAP cases, the Mp laboratory diagnosis was inconsistent between serology and multiplex-PCR assay. Verified by the SAT assay, the GeXP showed a more sensitive and reliable performance compared with the serology assay. Furthermore, employing the multiplex-PCR could provide more information on the associated pathogens for clinical assessment of CAP.

Keywords: *Mycoplasma pneumoniae,* Community acquired pneumonia, Multiplex-PCR, Serology

* Correspondence: lele19870204@163.com; hbetlgx@126.com
[1]Institute of Pediatric Research, Children's Hospital of Hebei Province, 133 Zhonghua South Street, Shijiazhuang, Hebei Province 050031, China

Background

Mycoplasma pneumoniae (Mp) is a leading cause (about 40%) of community-acquired pneumonia (CAP) especially in the pediatric populations [1]. The golden diagnostic criteria of *M. pneumoniae* infection has been considered as the seroconversion or rising IgG titers [2], but the antibody results are susceptible to the children's age and immunity status [3, 4], especially facing to the difficulty in obtaining convalescent serum in a pediatric hospital [5].

Due to the advantages of PCR on its sensitivity, specificity and early detection, large body of literature has been published for using PCR to detect Mp-DNA or RNA, including conventional, nested, real-time, multiplex and isothermal amplification PCR [6]. Among these, the multiplex-PCR has been accepted as a more practical diagnosis method in *M. pneumoniae* CAP, because the existence of clinical similarity resulted from Mp and other agents [7] and the common appearance of the viral co-infections [8]. Thus, in the recent study, the *M. pneumoniae* was added into our previously used pathogen panel that included 20 types/subtypes of viruses [9]. Meanwhile, several other groups have also designed the multiplex-PCR for the early detection of *M. pneumoniae* infection [10–17], but so far, the direct comparison between multiplex-PCR and serology test in larger pediatric clinical samples has rarely been reported [6]. Besides, the *M. pneumoniae* RNA detection (real-time isothermal transcription-mediated RNA amplification assay, Mp-SAT) that targeted on the specific 16SrRNA has been invented and investigated [18, 19], which could eliminate the false positive cases resulted from the previous infection or the nonpathogenic carrier state [20].

In this study, sputum samples were obtained and analyzed by a commercial multiplex-PCR kit named GeXP multiplex amplification assay for 13 types/subtypes pathogens (including *M. pneumoniae*) that were commonly detected in patients with CAP. The passive particle agglutination (PA) assay was used to examine the same patients' Mp-antibody in their serum specimens. A comparison between these two assays was conducted, and the Mp-SAT assay was used to test the inconsistent samples. The possible factors that may contribute to the disagreement results were also analyzed.

Methods

Study population

The protocols used in this retrospective study was reviewed and approved by the institutional review board of Children's Hospital of Hebei Province. The written informed consent was obtained from each patient's parent prior to enrollment. We selected specimens over a 1-year period (2015–2016) to cover all four seasons. Based on CAP Diagnosis and Management Guidelines [21], a total of 3146 otherwise healthy children aged 0.1–16.0 years (median, 2.0 years) were confirmed by the chest X-ray and finally enrolled. They respectively received the Mp-antibody and Mp-DNA testing within 24 h of admission. Patients with congenital heart or lung disease, or with immunosuppression, or had received the immunosuppressive therapy, or had been admitted to a hospital longer than 2 days within the last 90 days were excluded.

Detection of mp-antibody by the passive particle agglutination assay

The paired serum samples were taken at the presentation of pneumonia and at least 7 days after the first collection of serum. The serum was obtained from 2 mL whole blood by the separation gel tube. And the determination of Mp-specific antibody was performed using a commercially available micro-particle agglutination test Serodia-MycoII kit (Fujirebio, Tokyo, Japan) according to the manufacturer's instructions [22]. Antibody titers were measured at a range of dilutions (from 1:40 to 1:20,480). Criteria for diagnosis were defined as > or =4-found rising for paired sera of *M. pneumoniae* antibody [2] or single serum of titer > or =1:160 [23, 24].

Sputum specimen collection

Patients were asked to cough and the expectorated sputum was collected. If the child is too young to cough, a sterile negative pressure suction catheter is applied to obtain the oropharyngeal suction (OPS) into transport tube containing 1 ml DMEM medium with 2% heat-inactivated fetal calf serum, 50 IU/ml of penicillin and 100 μg/ml of streptomycin (Gibco, Beijing, China). The sample was stored at 4 °C for the same day pathogen nucleic acid extraction. Total nucleic acid (both DNA and RNA) was extracted from 200 μL sputum sample and eluted into 30 μL nuclease-free water by the EasyPure Viral DNA/RNA Kit (QSJBio, Beijing, China) in accordance with the manufacturer's instructions. Afterwards, 3 μL of extracted nucleic acid was analyzed with the GeXP-based assay. The remaining sputum samples were added into equal volume of preservative solution and stored at a – 80 °C freezer.

Detection of mp-DNA by the automated GenomeLab GeXP genetic analysis system

The GeXP assay (GenomeLab GeXP Genetic Analysis System) was performed on all specimens for the following 13 different respiratory pathogens,: Influenza A (Flu A), Influenza B (Flu B), Influenza A H1N1 pdm09 (09H1), influenza H3N2 (H3), human parainfluenza virus (HPIV), respiratory syncytial virus (RSV), rhinovirus (HRV), adenovirus (ADV), human metapneumovirus (HMPV), human bocavirus (HBoV), human coronavirus (HCoV), *Chlamydia* (*Ch*) and *Mycoplasma pneumoniae* (*Mp*), using the 13 Respiratory Pathogens Multiplex Kit (PCR-Capillary Electrophoresis Fragment Analysis) (Health Gene Tech., Ningbo, China). The reverse transcription (RT) and PCR were performed as previously described in Wang, et al. [9]. The analysis was then performed in an automated manner following the established protocol and the data were compiled by the GeXP system software provided by Beckman Coulter.

Detection of mp-rRNA by SAT

The frozen sputum specimens were thawed on the day the assays were performed. RNA extraction was performed on the MagX automated platform (Rendu Biotech., Shanghai, China), in which the targeted 16SrRNA could be enriched and purified by the magnetic particles. The final RNA was eluted into 30 μL nuclease-free water. The negative and positive controls were also introduced into the next Mp-SAT procedure. The reaction was performed as follows: incubation at 60 °C for 10 min and 42 °C for 5 min, 10 μL of SAT enzyme was added into the reaction. The Mp-SAT was completed on a real-time thermocycler (Veriti Thermal Cycler, Applied Biosystems China) in following steps: step1, 42 °C for 1 min; step2 was repeated for 40 cycles. The fluorescent light channel was set as FAM (sample channel) and HEX (internal control channel). The amplified products were then assessed using the SAT analysis system (Rendu Biotech), and a real-time PCR Ct value≦30 is defined as positive.

Statistical analysis

The Pearson and Linear-by-linear association chi-squared test was used to compare sex, admission season and age subgroups. The Kruskal-Wallis test was used to compare mean age at onset of illness. SPSS 13.0.1 statistics package (SPSS Inc., Chicago, USA) software was used for all statistical analysis. $p < 0.05$ was considered statistically significant.

Results

M. pneumoniae detection by serology versus multiplex-PCR testing

Sputum and serum specimens collected from 3146 hospitalized children were tested by GeXP assay and PA assay, respectively. A total of 243 samples (7.72%, 243/3146) were both positive and 2705 samples (85.98%, 2705/3146) were both negative based on these two methods. The inconsistent samples accounted for 6.29% (198/3146). The Kappa value was ordinary (κ = 0.677, $p< 0.01$), and the highest kappa value (κ = 0.783) was observed in the school-age children group (Table 1).

Table 1 The consistency of test results for *M. Pneumoniae* between serology and multiplex-PCR testing

MX-PRC		Serology		Kappa	P
		+	-	Value	
0-3 yr	+	52	14	0.486	<0.01
	-	78	855		
3-6 yr	+	81	3	0.723	<0.01
	-	51	910		
>6 yr	+	110	2	0.783	<0.01
	-	50	942		
Total	+	243	19	0.677	<0.01
	-	179	2705		

To better understand the discordant samples, the terms of 'false positive' and 'false negative' rates of serology were introduced. The premise to use them is to assume the results of multiplex-PCR as gold standard. If the sample is tested to be Serology (+)/Multiplex-PCR (−), it is presented as 'false positive'; to be Serology (−)/Multiplex-PCR (+), it is presented as 'false negative'. We found that both of the 'false positive' and 'false negative' rates of serology were significantly ($p< 0.001$) associated with age (Table 2). The 'false positive' samples took a proportion of 60% (78/130) in ages 0–3, 39% (51/132) in 3−6 years, and 31% (50/160) in ages >6 years. Similarly, 'false negative' samples accounted for 21% (14/66), 4% (3/84) and 2% (2/112) in ages 0–3, 3−6 and >6 years old, respectively.

Of the total 422 patients with positive serology results, paired sera were collected from 26 patients (6.2%). Interestingly, the 26 paired sera samples were in good agreement with multiplex-PCR results: 92% (24/26) cases with four fold increase titer which were corresponded to the multiplex-PCR positive.

In addition, children in whom *M. pneumoniae* was detected by serological or by multiplex-PCR alone were significantly younger than those who were detected by both methods (Z = −4.20, $p< 0.01$). But no significant differences were observed for their admission season ($p = 0.165$) or sex ($p = 0.338$) (Table 3).

Testing of specimens with mp-SAT assay

A total of 46 cases with inconsistent results were reanalyzed by the Mp-SAT assay. We randomly chose 27 samples from 179 cases that had been determined to be Serology(+)/MX-PCR (−), together with the whole 19 Serology (−)/MX-PCR(+) cases. Among the 46 sputum samples redo the Mp-SAT assay, we found 97.8% diagnosis agreement between SAT and GeXP assay. A total of 18 Serology (−)/MX-PCR (+) cases were determined to be SAT positive, and the whole 27 Serology(+)/MX-PCR

Table 2 The age-dependent false positive and false negative rates of serology assay

Age	False positive rate	Statistic value	P	False negative rate	Statistic value	P
0–3 year	60% (78/130)			21% (14/66)		
3–6 year	39% (31/132)	23.532[a]	<0.001	4% (3/84)	20.500[a]	<0.001
>6 year	31% (50/160)			2% (2/112)		

[a] Linear-by-Linear Association

(−) cases were all tested to be SAT negative (Additional file 1 Table S1).

Mp coinfection with other pathogens

Ninety-seven patients (37.0%, 97/262) had other causative pathogens besides *M. pneumoniae*. Among these patients, HRV was the most detected (20.2%, 53/262), followed with HPIV, FluB, ADV, RSV, 09H1, H3, HCoV, HBoV and HMPV (Table 4).

In the comparison of two patients groups that infected only with *M. pneumoniae* and mixed infected with other viruses, the significant discrepancies existed in different season and age subgroups, but not in the sex groups (Table 5).

The seasonal distribution analysis revealed that, patients infected only with *M. pneumoniae* were more than the mixed infection patients during summer and autumn. But in spring and winter, the mixed infection patients showed to be predominate ($\chi^2 = 5.12$, $p = 0.023$). Interestingly, the positive detection rate of school-age children was highest in the *M. pneumoniae* only group, but the lowest in the mixed infection group ($\chi^2 = 18.96$, $p< 0.01$).

Discussion

The nucleic acid amplification techniques (NAATs) targeted towards DNA or RNA have increasingly been explored for identification of pathogens including *M. pneumoniae* in infectious respiratory diseases [10–17]. So far, only a few studies have described the application of NAATs for pathogen detection in children with CAP [25–27]. Determination as well as comparison between

laboratory diagnosis methods of *M. pneumoniae* infection for childhood CAP in larger clinical database has not been reported. In the present study, we applied a multiplex-PCR, named GeXP assay, to detected 13 types of pathogens including *M. pneumoniae* in 3146 sputum samples from hospitalized CAP children. Meanwhile, their serum specimens were also collected to be tested the antibody against *M. pneumoniae*. After the comparison between serology and GeXP assays on the same patient, about 93.7% of cases were diagnosed to be either positive or negative based on these 2 methods. We randomly chose 46 samples from 198 samples that had been tested to be inconsistent by serology and GeXP assays, redo the Mp-SAT and found 97.8% diagnosis agreement between SAT and GeXP assays, but not with the serology testing. Further analysis revealed that children in whom *M. pneumoniae* was only examined to be positive by GeXP or serology were significantly younger than those of both methods positive. About 37% of patients have virus-Mp coinfection, which were most observed in infantile patients. Seasonal distribution analysis revealed that the virus-Mp coinfection were predominant in spring and winter, while Mp-only infection was more frequently identified in summer and autumn.

Only a few reports have thus far described the comparison between serology and mono-PCR assays for *M. pneumoniae* detection in pediatric CAP patients [28–31]. Using the paired sera samples, three independent research groups all observed excellent diagnosis agreement between these 2 methods [28–30], in

Table 3 Characteristics of *M. Pneumoniae* detection by serology and multiplex-PCR testing

Characteristics		Values of the Cases Tested			Statistic value	P
		Serology (+) /MX-PCR(+) (n = 243)	Serology (−) /MX-PCR(+) (n = 19)	Serology (+) /MX-PCR (−) (n = 179)		
Age (Median)		5.0	1.5	3.0	35.423[a]	<0.01
Season (n)	Spring	27	2	35	9.150[b]	0.165
	Summer	42	2	28		
	Autumn	53	7	33		
	Winter	121	8	83		
Sex (n)	Male	142	12	93	2.169[b]	0.338
	Female	101	7	86		

[a] Kruskal-Wallis test
[b] Pearson Chi-Square

Table 4 The rates of co-infection of *M. pneumoniae* CAP patients by other respiratory pathogens

	Pathogens	Positive Num.
	No other pathogens	165 (63.0%)
1	HRV	53 (20.2%)
2	HPIV	15 (5.7%)
3	FluB	12 (4.6%)
4	ADV	9 (3.4%)
5	RSV	9 (3.4%)
6	09H1	8 (3.1%)
7	H3	5 (1.9%)
8	HCoV	4 (1.5%)
9	HBoV	4 (1.5%)
10	HMPV	2 (0.8%)
11	*Ch*	0 (0.0%)

contrast to our findings and Kim's [31]. This discrepancy is mainly attributed to the proportion of paired sera. Because in our results, only 13% patients provided their second sera specimen, the good concordance could be observed between these paired sera with multiplex-PCR, On the other hand, after comparing the mono-PCR and serology assay, Kim proposed that a single titer ≥1:640 were considered to indicate the acute *M. pneumoniae* infection [31]. But in clinical, a presumptive diagnosis could be made from a single acute-phase serum titer ≥1:160 [24]. Therefore, if we interpret the Multiplex-PCR positive samples as truly indicating Mp infection, the high 'false positive rate' of serology testing (42%, 179/422) may caused by the proportion of paired sera and the criteria of diagnosis. Besides that, the serology 'false positive rate' was probably due to the other two aspects: Firstly, the serology

Table 5 Comparison of age, season and sex characteristics between children with only M. pneumoniae and those with mixed infection by at least one respiratory virus

		N	Positive rate (n)		Statistic value	P
			Mp only	Mp w/t virus		
Sex	Male	154	61.7% (95)	38.3% (59)	0.27[a]	0.606
	Female	108	64.8% (70)	35.2% (38)		
Season	Spring	32	68.8% (22)	31.2% (10)	5.12[b]	0.023
	Summer	43	72.1% (31)	27.9% (12)		
	Autumn	61	72.1% (44)	27.9% (17)		
	Winter	126	54.0% (68)	46.0% (58)		
Age	0–1 yr	16	25.0% (4)	75.0% (12)	18.96[b]	<0.01
	1–3 yr	50	46.0% (23)	54.0% (27)		
	3–6 yr	83	67.5% (56)	32.5% (27)		
	>6 yr	113	72.6% (82)	27.4% (31)		

[a] Pearson Chi-Square
[b] Linear-by-Linear Association

assay is claimed to detect both of Mp-IgM and IgG [22], the positive serology results may be caused by an earlier (not current) Mp infection, which is still detectable in the blood. Alternatively, the current infection truly exists, but the amount of organism was below the detection limit of multiplex-PCR. It has been reported that the diagnostic accuracy of PCR may decrease at ≥7 days after onset of disease in contrast to serology [32], especially patients who receive week duration of the antibiotic treatment [31].

Besides these mono-PCR studies, as reviewed by Loens et al. [6], several groups have applied the multiplex-PCR in the detection of *M. pneumoniae* infection, but the comparison assays were set as culture and/or mono-PCR, which are more suitable for accuracy validation during the methodology establishment process rather than obtaining the clinical diagnostic significance. In addition, Due to the high viral coinfection prevalence reported by Chen (25.9% [33]) and ours (37.0%), it is essential to recommend the use of multiplex-PCR assay to provide more pathogen information. More importantly, in Mp IgM-positive children, a negative PCR result was reported to be associated with coinfection by other pathogens [32]. Our results also demonstrated that the youngest children group exhibited highest Serology(+)/ Multiplex-PCR (−) rate and highest coinfection rate. In young children, since the serology positive cases may be result from other pathogen infection, the multiplex-PCR should be used to rectify these sorts of false positive cases determined by serology. Furthermore, a number of studies have demonstrated a weak or deferred antibody response to *M. pneumoniae* in young children [31–36], suggesting a possible reason leading to the highest Serology (−)/Multiplex-PCR (+) rate observed in the youngest patients group in our study. In conclusion, owing to the high coinfection rate and weak antibody response in young children, the Mp infection is needed to be monitored not only by the serology assay. A combination of serology and multiplex-PCR allows for both decreased 'false positive' and 'false negative' rates of serology assay.

In the present study, the inconsistent results were observed and took a 6.29% proportion, beside of 90% Multiplex-PCR (−)/Serology (+) samples mentioned above, the remaining 10% discordant samples were Multiplex-PCR (+)/Serology (−). Previous work has shown that the colonization of *M. pneumoniae* may cause the false positive results [37–39]. To rule out the possible false positive results of multiplex-PCR (targeting Mp-DNA) caused by colonization, the SAT assay (targeting Mp-RNA) were applied and we found that a overwhelming majority (94.7%, 18/19) of Multiplex-PCR (+)/Serology (−) sputum specimens were proved to be SAT positive. On the contrast, the randomly selected Multiplex-PCR (−)/Serology (+) sputum specimens were all observed to be SAT negative. These data suggest that the multiplex-PCR assay would be more reliable when the serology assay exhibits the opposite results. However, we felt a verification experiment with larger sample size should be used in future work. Another limitation of this work is that the highly specialized equipment is needed, namely an automated nucleic acid extraction system, which could carried out 48 samples at one time in about 1 h. Many primary hospitals or clinical laboratories do not have this equipment, and the manual work would greatly increase the turnaround time.

Abbreviations
09H1: Influenza A H1N1 pdm09; ADV: Adenovirus; CAP: Community acquired pneumonia; Ch: Chlamydia; FluA: Influenza virus A; FluB: Influenza virus B; GeXP assay: GenomeLab Genetic Analysis System; H3: Influenza H3N2; HBoV: Human bocavirus; HCoV: Human coronavirus; hMPV: Human metapneumovirus; HRV: Human rhinovirus; Mp or M: Pneumoniae, Mycoplasma pneumoniae; MX-PCR: Multiplex-PCR; NAATs: Nucleic acid amplification techniques; PA assay: Particle agglutination assay; PIV: Parainfluenza virus; RSV: Respiratory syncytial virus; RT-PCR: Reverse transcription polymerase chain reaction; SAT: Real-time isothermal transcription-mediated RNA amplification assay

Acknowledgements
We sincerely thank all the participants for their support. We also thank Dr. Hong Yan and Wenchao Zhang from the Department of Laboratory Medicine, Children's Hospital of Hebei Province, Shijiazhuang, China, for their help with recruitments of subjects.

Funding
None.

Authors' contributions
LW carried out the Ge-XP and PA assay, performed the statistical analysis and drafted the manuscript. WG participated in the validation. XY and MZ carried out the SAT assay. GL and ZS participated in the design of the study. GL conceived of the study, and participated in its design and coordination and helped to draft the manuscript. All authors read and approved the final manuscript.

Consent for publication
Not applicable.

Competing interests
All the authors declared that they have no competing interests.

Author details
[1]Institute of Pediatric Research, Children's Hospital of Hebei Province, 133 Zhonghua South Street, Shijiazhuang, Hebei Province 050031, China. [2]Department of Laboratory Medicine, Children's Hospital of Hebei Province, Shijiazhuang 050031, China.

Reference
1. Lee KY. Pediatric respiratory infections by Mycoplasma pneumoniae. Expert Rev Anti-Infect Ther. 2008;6(4):509–21.
2. She RC, Thurber A, Hymas WC, Stevenson J, Langer J, Litwin CM, Petti CA. Limited utility of culture for Mycoplasma pneumoniae and Chlamydophila pneumoniae for diagnosis of respiratory tract infections. Eur J Clin Microbiol. 2010;48(9):3380–2.
3. Han X, Li S, Lu S, Liu L, Li S, Zhang J. Amplification of 16S rDNA by nested PCR for measurement of Mycoplasma pneumoniae DNA over time: clinical application. J Med Microbiol. 2012;61(Pt 3):426–30.
4. Principi N, Esposito S. Emerging role of Mycoplasma pneumoniae and Chlamydia pneumoniae in paediatric respiratory-tract infections. Lancet Infect Dis. 2001;1(5):334–44.
5. Youn YS, Lee KY, Hwang JY, Rhim JW, Kang JH, Lee JS, Kim JC. Difference of clinical features in childhood Mycoplasma pneumoniae pneumonia. BMC Pediatr. 2010;10:48.
6. Loens K, Ieven M. Mycoplasma pneumoniae: current knowledge on nucleic acid amplification techniques and serological diagnostics. Front Microbiol. 2016;7:448.
7. Thompson KS, Yonke ML, Rapley JW, Cobb CM, Johnson V. Relationship between a self-reported health questionnaire and laboratory tests at initial office visits. J Periodontol. 1999;70(10):1153–7.
8. Bezerra PG, Britto MC, Correia JB, Duarte Mdo C, Fonceca AM, Rose K, Hopkins MJ, Cuevas LE, McNamara PS. Viral and atypical bacterial detection in acute respiratory infection in children under five years. PLoS One. 2011;6(4):e18928.
9. Wang L, Zhao M, Shi Z, Feng Z, Guo W, Yang S, Liu L, Li G. A GeXP-based assay for simultaneous detection of multiple viruses in hospitalized children with community acquired pneumonia. PLoS One. 2016;11(9):e0162411.
10. Puppe W, Weigl J, Grondahl B, Knuf M, Rockahr S, von Bismarck P, Aron G, Niesters HG, Osterhaus AD, Schmitt HJ. Validation of a multiplex reverse transcriptase PCR ELISA for the detection of 19 respiratory tract pathogens. Infection. 2013;41(1):77–91.
11. Simoes EA, Patel C, Sung WK, Lee CW, Loh KH, Lucero M, Nohynek H, Nai C, Thien PL, Koh CW, et al. Pathogen chip for respiratory tract infections. J Clin Microbiol. 2013;51(3):945–53.
12. Hirama T, Minezaki S, Yamaguchi T, Kishi E, Kodama K, Egashira H, Kobayashi K, Nagata M, Ishii T, Nemoto M, et al. HIRA-TAN: a real-time PCR-based system for the rapid identification of causative agents in pneumonia. Respir Med. 2014;108(2):395–404.
13. Weinberg GA, Schnabel KC, Erdman DD, Prill MM, Iwane MK, Shelley LM, Whitaker BL, Szilagyi PG, Hall CB. Field evaluation of TaqMan Array card (TAC) for the simultaneous detection of multiple respiratory viruses in children with acute respiratory infection. J Clin Virol. 2013;57(3):254–60.
14. Ji M, Lee NS, Oh JM, Jo JY, Choi EH, Yoo SJ, Kim HB, Hwang SH, Choi SH, Lee SO, et al. Single-nucleotide polymorphism PCR for the detection of Mycoplasma pneumoniae and determination of macrolide resistance in respiratory samples. J Microbiol Methods. 2014;102:32–6.
15. Zhao F, Liu L, Tao X, He L, Meng F, Zhang J. Culture-independent detection and genotyping of Mycoplasma pneumoniae in clinical specimens from Beijing. China PloS One. 2015;10(10):e0141702.
16. Shen H, Zhu B, Wang S, Mo H, Wang J, Li J, Zhang C, Zeng H, Guan L, Shi W, et al. Association of targeted multiplex PCR with resequencing microarray for the detection of multiple respiratory pathogens. Front Microbiol. 2015;6:532.
17. Nummi M, Mannonen L, Puolakkainen M. Development of a multiplex real-time PCR assay for detection of Mycoplasma pneumoniae, Chlamydia pneumoniae and mutations associated with macrolide resistance in Mycoplasma pneumoniae from respiratory clinical specimens. SpringerPlus. 2015;4:684.
18. Feng Xueli LQ, Xu B, Lin S, Weiwei J, Shen C, Adong S. Evaluation of RNA simultaneous amplification and testing for detection of Mycoplasma pneumoulae pneumonia in children. Chin J Appl Clin Pediatr. 2016;16(31).
19. Guo Li SL, Guo Y, Adong S. Clinical value of Mycoplasma pneumoniae RNA detection in the monitoring of Mycolasma pneumoniae pneumonia treatment in children. Chin J Evid Based Pediatr. 2016;02(11)
20. Foy HM. Infections caused by Mycoplasma pneumoniae and possible carrier state in different populations of patients. Clin Infect Dis. 1993;17(Suppl 1):S37–46.
21. He LX. Guidelines for the diagnosis and treatment of community-acquired pneumonia: learning and practicing. Zhonghua Jie He He Hu Xi Za Zhi. 2006;29(10):649–50.

22. Barker CE, Sillis M, Wreghitt TG. Evaluation of Serodia Myco II particle agglutination test for detecting Mycoplasma pneumoniae antibody: comparison with mu-capture ELISA and indirect immunofluorescence. J Clin Pathol. 1990;43(2):163–5.

23. Templeton KE, Scheltinga SA, Graffelman AW, Van Schie JM, Crielaard JW, Sillekens P, Van Den Broek PJ, Goossens H, Beersma MF, Claas EC. Comparison and evaluation of real-time PCR, real-time nucleic acid sequence-based amplification, conventional PCR, and serology for diagnosis of Mycoplasma pneumoniae. J Clin Microbiol. 2003;41(9):4366–71.

24. Matas L, Dominguez J, De Ory F, Garcia N, Gali N, Cardona PJ, Hernandez A, Rodrigo C, Ausina V. Evaluation of meridian ImmunoCard Mycoplasma test for the detection of Mycoplasma pneumoniae-specific IgM in paediatric patients. Scand J Infect Dis. 1998;30(3):289–93.

25. Juven T, Mertsola J, Waris M, Leinonen M, Meurman O, Roivainen M, Eskola J, Saikku P, Ruuskanen O. Etiology of community-acquired pneumonia in 254 hospitalized children. Pediatr Infect Dis J. 2000;19(4):293–8.

26. Cantais A, Mory O, Pillet S, Verhoeven PO, Bonneau J, Patural H, Pozzetto B. Epidemiology and microbiological investigations of community-acquired pneumonia in children admitted at the emergency department of a university hospital. J Clin Virol. 2014;60(4):402–7.

27. Rhedin S, Lindstrand A, Hjelmgren A, Ryd-Rinder M, Ohrmalm L, Tolfvenstam T, Ortqvist A, Rotzen-Ostlund M, Zweygberg-Wirgart B, Henriques-Normark B, et al. Respiratory viruses associated with community-acquired pneumonia in children: matched case-control study. Thorax. 2015; 70(9):847–53.

28. Gotoh K, Nishimura N, Ohshima Y, Arakawa Y, Hosono H, Yamamoto Y, Iwata Y, Nakane K, Funahashi K, Ozaki T. Detection of Mycoplasma pneumoniae by loop-mediated isothermal amplification (LAMP) assay and serology in pediatric community-acquired pneumonia. J Infect Chemother. 2012;18(5):662–7.

29. Chaudhry R, Sharma S, Javed S, Passi K, Dey AB, Malhotra P. Molecular detection of Mycoplasma pneumoniae by quantitative real-time PCR in patients with community acquired pneumonia. Indian J Med Res. 2013; 138:244–51.

30. Medjo B, Atanaskovic-Markovic M, Radic S, Nikolic D, Lukac M, Djukic S. Mycoplasma pneumoniae as a causative agent of community-acquired pneumonia in children: clinical features and laboratory diagnosis. Ital J Pediatr. 2014;40:104.

31. Kim NH, Lee JA, Eun BW, Shin SH, Chung EH, Park KW, Choi EH, Lee HJ. Comparison of polymerase chain reaction and the indirect particle agglutination antibody test for the diagnosis of Mycoplasma pneumoniae pneumonia in children during two outbreaks. Pediatr Infect Dis J. 2007; 26(10):897–903.

32. Chang HY, Chang LY, Shao PL, Lee PI, Chen JM, Lee CY, Lu CY, Huang LM. Comparison of real-time polymerase chain reaction and serological tests for the confirmation of Mycoplasma pneumoniae infection in children with clinical diagnosis of atypical pneumonia. *Journal of microbiology, immunology, and infection* =. Wei mian yu gan ran za zhi. 2014;47(2):137–44.

33. Chen LL, Cheng YG, Chen ZM, Li SX, Li XJ, Wang YS. Mixed infections in children with Mycoplasma pneumoniae pneumonia. Zhonghua Er Ke Za Zhi. 2012;50(3):211–5.

34. Ozaki T, Nishimura N, Ahn J, Watanabe N, Muto T, Saito A, Koyama N, Nakane K, Funahashi K. Utility of a rapid diagnosis kit for Mycoplasma pneumoniae pneumonia in children, and the antimicrobial susceptibility of the isolates. J Infect Chemother. 2007;13(4):204–7.

35. Lind K, Bentzon MW. Ten and a half years seroepidemiology of Mycoplasma pneumoniae infection in Denmark. Epidemiol Infect. 1991;107(1):189–99.

36. Bogaert D, van Belkum A, Sluijter M, Luijendijk A, de Groot R, Rumke HC, Verbrugh HA, Hermans PW. Colonisation by Streptococcus Pneumoniae and Staphylococcus Aureus in healthy children. Lancet. 2004;363(9424):1871–2.

37. Spuesens EB, Fraaij PL, Visser EG, Hoogenboezem T, Hop WC, van Adrichem LN, Weber F, Moll HA, Broekman B, Berger MY, et al. Carriage of Mycoplasma pneumoniae in the upper respiratory tract of symptomatic and asymptomatic children: an observational study. PLoS Med. 2013;10(5): e1001444.

38. Meyer Sauteur PM, van Rossum AM, Vink C. Mycoplasma pneumoniae in children: carriage, pathogenesis, and antibiotic resistance. Curr Opin Infect Dis. 2014;27(3):220–7.

39. Spuesens EB, Meyer Sauteur PM, Vink C, van Rossum AM. Mycoplasma pneumoniae infections–does treatment help? J Inf Secur. 2014;69(Suppl 1):S42–6.

5

Clinical features of community acquired adenovirus pneumonia during the 2011 community outbreak in Southern Taiwan: role of host immune response

Ching-Fen Shen[1], Shih-Min Wang[2,3], Tzong-Shiann Ho[2] and Ching-Chuan Liu[1,3,4]*

Abstract

Background: Human adenovirus 7 (HAdV-7) was responsible for a significant number of fatalities during the 2011 community outbreak in Taiwan. The mechanisms underlying the pathogenesis of severe adenovirus infections in non-immunocompromised individuals remain unclear. Adenovirus pneumonia was associated with pleural effusion in a number of patients from the 2011 outbreak suggesting that similar to bacterial pneumonia, patients diagnosed with adenovirus pneumonia who have pleural effusion are more severely and systemically infected, and may have a more protracted disease course. We hypothesized that the host immunological response determines the severity of adenoviral infection.

Methods: This retrospective case series study included patients diagnosed with severe lower respiratory tract infections at the National Cheng Kung University Hospital in southern Taiwan between December 2010 and October 2011. The main inclusion criteria were 1) presence of multifocal patchy infiltrates, lobar consolidation or reticular interstitial opacities in chest X-rays, and 2) presence of adenovirus isolated from respiratory specimens. All patients had adenovirus isolated from respiratory specimens, and were negative for other viruses. Pleural effusion was confirmed in all patients using chest echography. Clinical features and laboratory data were compared in patients with ($n = 12$) and without ($n = 15$) parapneumonic effusion.

Results: Presence of parapneumonic effusion was significantly associated with a longer febrile duration, more complicated clinical management, and a greater risk of extrapulmonary involvement, notably hepatitis. Patients without pleural effusion had significantly higher numbers of WBCs, platelets, and absolute segment cell counts (ASCs) compared to patients with pleural effusion (all $p < 0.05$). Patients without pleural effusion had significantly higher counts of CD4+, CD8+, and CD20+ T cells (all $p < 0.05$) compared to patients with pleural effusion.

Conclusion: Our data indicated that presence of parapneumonic effusion in adenoviral pneumonia was associated with longer febrile duration, more complicated clinical management, a greater risk of hepatitis, and suppression of host cellular immunity. Further prospective, large-scale studies are needed to validate our results.

Keywords: Human adenovirus, Pneumonia, Pleural effusion, Immune response, T cells

* Correspondence: liucc@mail.ncku.edu.tw
[1]Department of Pediatrics, National Cheng Kung University Hospital, College of Medicine, National Cheng Kung University, 138, Sheng Li Road, North Dist., Tainan 70403, Taiwan
[3]Center of Infectious Disease and Signaling Research, National Cheng Kung University Hospital, College of Medicine, National Cheng Kung University, Tainan, Taiwan

Background

Human adenoviruses (HAdVs) have been linked to a number of respiratory, gastrointestinal, ocular, genitourinary and neurologic diseases [1]. There are currently 60 serotypes of HAdVs identified, which are grouped into 7 species based on their morphologic, immunogenic and genomic properties [2, 3]. HAdV infections have been linked to mild upper respiratory tract infections such as pharyngitis or coryza, as well as to more severe lower respiratory tract infections (LRTIs) such as bronchiolitis, croup and pneumonia [4]. Approximately one-fifth of all HAdV infections were shown to be caused by HAdV-7, which is associated with serious LRTIs [5]. Although treatment of severe adenovirus infection is mainly supportive, antiviral agents such as acyclovir, ganciclovir, ribavirin, and cidofovir have been investigated for non-immunocompromised individuals [6, 7]. Therapeutic strategies such as extracorporeal membrane oxygenation (ECMO) with or without high frequency oscillatory ventilation (HFOV) have also been evaluated in patients with severe disease [8, 9].

Children, immunocompromised individuals, and people in crowded environments such as military recruits and hospitalized or institutionalized individuals have been shown to have a higher susceptibility to HAdV infections, especially HAdV-7 [10–13]. HAdVs 1, 2 and 5 are usually implicated in endemic or sporadic cases, while HAdVs 7 and to a lesser extent HAdV-3 have been isolated from epidemics of adenovirus LRTIs in healthy children [11, 14]. HAdV-11 and HAdV-7 were the most frequently identified pathogens in a 2011 study of community-acquired pneumonia in Beijing, China [15]. HAdV-7 was also reported as the primary pathogen in an outbreak of severe LRTI among infants in Shaanxi Province, China in 2009, and Singapore in 2012 [5, 16]. A number of adenovirus outbreaks involving HAdV-7, HAdV-3, and HAdV-4 have been reported from Taiwan between 1999 and 2005 [17, 18]. The largest reported community outbreak which occurred in Taiwan in 2011 involved co-circulating HAdV-3 and HAdV-7 [19]. Although the 2011 outbreak was associated with HAdV-3 as well as HAdV-7, patients infected with HAdV-7 had a higher fatality rate [20]. HAdV-7 isolated from the 2011 outbreak was shown to have the highest homology with HAdV-7d and HAdV-7d2, strains which had not been seen in Taiwan prior to 2011 [19].

Cellular immunity plays an important role in viral infections, and severe adenovirus infections are commonly seen in immunocompromised individuals. The mechanisms underlying the pathogenesis of severe adenovirus infections in non-immunocompromised individuals remain unclear. Production of chemokines and cytokines in response to HAdV-7 infection was shown to damage lung tissue, and result in recruitment of inflammatory cells such as neutrophils, monocytes and lymphocytes [21, 22]. Interestingly, a recent report reviewed 19 studies which evaluated immunocompetent patients with adenovirus pneumonia and showed that more than half the patients were lymphopenic [23]. A recent retrospective study also showed that non-immunocompromised patients with severe adenovirus pneumonia had lower hemoglobin levels, leucopenia, thrombocytopenia and elevated liver enzymes, suggesting a distinctive mechanism of immunopathogenesis which may contribute to the severity of the infection [7].

We hypothesized that the host immunological response determines the severity of adenoviral infection. Additionally, we observed that adenovirus pneumonia was associated with pleural effusion in a number of patients from the 2011 outbreak. We hypothesized that similar to bacterial pneumonia, patients diagnosed with adenovirus pneumonia who have pleural effusion are more severely and systemically infected, and may have a more protracted disease course. In this retrospective case series study, we evaluated the clinical manifestations of adenoviral pneumonia in a convenience sample of 27 patients from the 2011 outbreak in South Taiwan and compared clinical features and laboratory data between patients with or without parapneumonic effusion.

Methods

Materials

Blood cultures were done using the BACTEC Fx System (BD Biosciences, USA). Urine pneumococcal antigen tests were done with the BinaxNOW® *Streptococcus pneumoniae* Antigen Card (Alere Ltd, Stockport, UK), and urine Legionella antigen tests were done with the BinaxNOW *Legionella* Urinary Antigen Card (Alere Ltd, Stockport, UK). The Cryptococcus antigen test was done with the CALAS® Cryptococcal Antigen latex agglutination system (Meridian Bioscience, Inc, Cincinnati, Ohio, USA). Mycoplasma antibodies were detected using the Serodia Myco II gelatin particle agglutination kit (Fujirebio, Tokyo, Japan). The influenza rapid test was performed with the Directigen Flu A + B test (Directigen; BD Diagnostic Systems, Sparks, MD.) CDC-validated FDA-approved real time RT-PCR assays were used to detect human influenza virus (CDC influenza division, USA). The respiratory syncytial virus (RSV) antigen test was a direct fluorescent-antibody assay (DFA) by Diagnostic Hybrids Inc. (DHI; Athens, OH).

Patients

This retrospective, single-center, observational case series included a total of 27 patients who presented with severe adenovirus LRTIs at the National Cheng Kung University (NCKU) Hospital in southern Taiwan between December 2010 and October 2011. Inclusion criteria were 1) presence of multifocal patchy infiltrates, lobar consolidation or reticular interstitial opacities in chest X-rays, and 2) presence of adenovirus isolated from respiratory specimens. Pleural effusion and diagnosis of adenoviral pneumonia was confirmed in all study patients using chest echography, which is an ultrasound technique. Chest echography at the NCKU hospital is mainly performed by senior pediatric residents with at least three years of pediatric training. The results are subsequently confirmed by the attending pediatrician and another pediatric chest specialist.

All throat swabs were examined for the presence of influenza virus using PCR assays, and for the presence of RSV antigen using a direct fluorescent-antibody assay. All specimens were negative for influenza and RSV. Co-infections were excluded using blood cultures, sputum cultures, pleural effusion cultures, the urine pneumococcal antigen test, the urine Legionella antigen test, the influenza rapid test, the RSV rapid test, PCR assay for influenza and the Cryptococcus and Mycoplasma tests. Data for presence of Mycoplasma antibodies were available for 21 patients (19 patients were negative and 2 patients were positive for Mycoplasma). Data for Legionella antibodies were only available for 3 patients, all of whom were negative for Legionella. Only two cases with significantly elevated levels of mycoplasma antibody presented with simple adenovirus pneumonia. Since our results would not have changed even if we had excluded these two cases, we retained these two cases in the adenovirus pneumonia without pleural effusion group. All other viral cultures only showed the presence of adenovirus. Although the antibiotic regimen varied from patient to patient, most patients were on ampicillin/sulbactam. All patient data were recorded soon after hospitalization. It is important to note that at the NCKU Hospital, all pediatric patients except those with walking/atypical pneumonia (caused by mycoplasma) are hospitalized for evaluation and treatment, and their medical data are accessible using administrative hospital data. This decreases the likelihood of selection bias within this sample of hospitalized patients.

This study sample was a convenience sample. Patients with adenovirus pneumonia usually have prolonged fever and severe respiratory symptoms, which increases the likelihood of seeking medical care. Most patients were referred by their local practitioners if their fever did not subside on the 3rd or 4th day. Our hospital is one of the biggest and largest pediatric tertiary referral centers in southern Taiwan, and even when the study cases are sampled by convenience, they are likely to closely reflect the population of patients hospitalized with severe adenoviral infection.

This study was approved by the Institutional Review Board of the National Cheng Kung University (NCKU) Hospital.

Statistical analysis

Continuous data for the two groups of patients (patients with or without pleural effusion) were represented as either (i) mean $\pm$ SD and compared using the two-sample t-test if the data followed normal distribution or (ii) median (IQR: 1st, 3rd quartiles) and compared using the Mann-Whitney U test if the data didn't follow normal distribution. Categorical data were represented as n (%) in the two groups of patients and compared using the Fisher's exact test. All statistical assessments were two-tailed and p values <0.05 were considered significant. All statistical analyses were carried out with IBM SPSS statistical software version 22 for Windows (IBM Corp., New York, USA).

Results

This case series included a total of 27 patients who were admitted to the NCKU hospital with adenovirus pneumonia during the 2011 epidemic. Figure 1 represents the number of patients per month from whom adenoviruses were isolated at the NCKU hospital between 2007 and 2012.

In our present study, 12 study patients (44.4%) were classified into the pleural effusion group and 15 patients (55.6%) were classified into the non-pleural effusion group. The clinical characteristics of the two groups are summarized in Table 1. There were no significant differences in clinical characteristics between patients with and without pleural effusion (all $p > 0.05$). The mean age of the patients was 10 years (SD = 12.1, range: 1 to 42 years).

The study population comprised 17 males (63%). Two patients (7.4%) had underlying disease. Study patients had an average of 6 days of fever at admission (SD = 3, range: 1 to 14 days). The radiological findings showed that 12 patients (44.4%) had multifocal infiltrates, 13 patients (48.1%) had lobar pneumonia, and 2 patients (7.4%) had pneumonitis. Additionally, 6 patients (22.2%) had chest tube replacement. Genotype analysis showed that 15 patients (55.6%) had genotype 3 s, whereas 9 patients (33.3%) had genotype 7 s. Genotype data were not available for 3 patients.

Clinical findings in the two study groups are presented in Table 2. Patients without pleural effusion had a significantly lower number of febrile days (7 days vs. 10.5 days; $p = 0.022$), a significantly lower number of hospital days (5 days vs. 11 days; $p = 0.002$), a significantly lower ICU admission rate (9 out of 10 patients admitted to the ICU had pleural effusion; $p = 0.001$), and a significantly lower rate of oxygen requirement (10 out of 13 patients who required oxygen had pleural effusion; $p = 0.002$) compared to patients without pleural effusion.

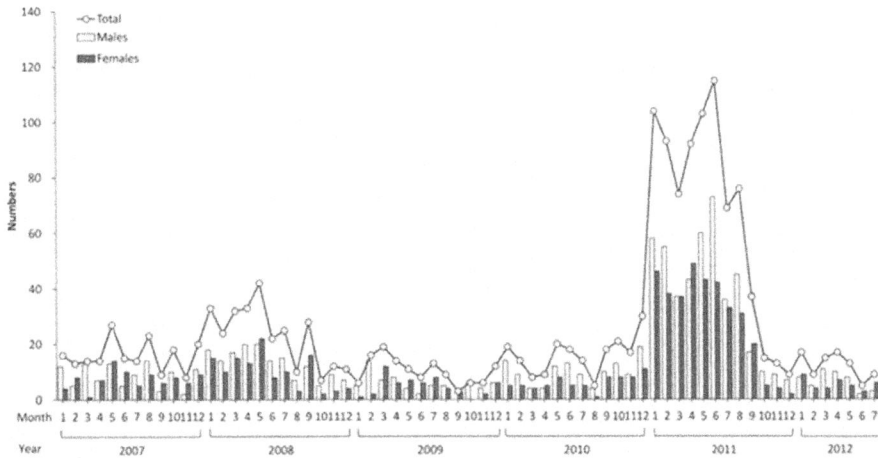

Fig. 1 Number of patients per month from whom adenoviruses were isolated at the NCKU hospital during 2007–2012/July. The number above the circle means the total number of patients for the given month

A comparison of laboratory findings in the two study groups is presented in Table 3. Our data showed that patients without pleural effusion had significantly higher WBC counts, platelet counts, and ASC compared to patients with pleural effusion (all $p < 0.05$).

White blood cell immunophenotypes were analyzed in patients with adenovirus pneumonia with and without pleural effusion. Data from 3 patients without pleural effusion and 5 patients with pleural effusion are presented in Table 4. Patients without pleural effusion had significantly higher counts of CD4+ ($p = 0.034$), CD8+ ($p = 0.031$), and CD20+ T cells ($p < 0.004$).

Discussion

In this retrospective case series study, we analyzed the data of 27 patients with adenovirus pneumonia from the 2011 outbreak in Taiwan, and compared clinical features and laboratory data between patients with or without parapneumonic effusion using pleural effusion as a marker for disease severity. Our data showed that the presence of parapneumonic effusion was significantly associated with a longer febrile duration, more complicated clinical management, and a greater risk of extrapulmonary involvement, notably hepatitis, compared to patients without parapneumonic effusion. Patients with

Table 1 Clinical characteristics of patients with adenovirus pneumonia admitted to the NCKU hospital during the 2011 epidemic ($N = 27$)

Variables	Total ($n = 27$)	Adenoviral pneumonia without pleural effusion ($n = 15$)	Adenoviral pneumonia with pleural effusion ($n = 12$)	P value
Age, years	4.1 (2.6 , 16.0)	3.7 (2.0 , 5.1)	5.6 (3.0 , 19.4)	0.213
Sex, males (%)	17 (63.0)	8 (53.3)	9 (75.0)	0.424
Underlying disease	2 (7.4)	1 (6.7)	1 (8.3)	1.000
Fever days at admission	6 (4 , 7)	5 (3 , 7)	7 (5 , 9.5)	0.092
Radiological findings				
Multifocal infiltrates	12 (44.4)	7 (46.7)	5 (41.7)	1.000
Lobar pneumonia	13 (48.1)	6 (40.0)	7 (58.3)	0.449
Pneumonitis	2 (7.4)	2 (13.3)	0 (0.0)	0.487
Chest tube replacement	6 (22.2)	0 (0.0)	6 (50.0)	NA
Genotypes				0.303
3S	15 (55.6)	10 (66.7)	5 (41.7)	
7S	9 (33.3)	3 (20)	6 (50)	
Lost	3 (11.1)	2 (13.3)	1 (8.3)	

Data were expressed as median (IQR: 1st, 3rd quartiles) for continuous variables and n (%) for categorical ones
Differences between patients with and without pleural effusion were compared using the Mann-Whitney U test for continuous variables and Fisher's exact test for categorical ones
There were no significant differences between patients with and without pleural effusion
NA not assessed

Table 2 Clinical findings in patients with adenovirus pneumonia admitted to the NCKU hospital during the 2011 epidemic based on the presence or absence of pleural effusions

Variables	Total (n = 27)	Adenoviral pneumonia without pleural effusion (n = 15)	Adenoviral pneumonia with pleural effusion (n = 12)	P value
Clinical symptoms other than respiratory tracts				
Conjunctivitis	1 (3.7)	0 (0.0)	1 (8.3)	NA
Gastroenterocolitis	11 (40.7)	7 (46.7)	4 (33.3)	0.696
Hepatitis	8 (29.6)	0 (0.0)	8 (66.7)	NA
Encephalitis	1 (3.7)	0 (0.0)	1 (8.3)	NA
Total febrile days	7 (6 , 11)	7 (5 , 9)	10.5 (7 , 12.8)	0.022[*]
Hospitalization days	7 (5 , 12)	5 (4 , 8)	11 (7.5 , 14.5)	0.002[*]
Duration for fever after admission, days	2 (0 , 4)	1 (0 , 4)	3.5 (0.3 , 4.8)	0.277
Patients with ICU admission	10 (40.7)	1 (6.7)	9 (75.0)	0.001
ICU hospitalization days[a]	6.0 (3.8 , 10.25)	9 (NA)	6 (3.5 , 11.5)	NA
Patients with ventilator	3 (11.9)	1 (6.7)	2 (16.7)	0.569
Patients with oxygen requirement	13 (48.1)	3 (20.0)	10 (83.3)	0.002[*]
Days of oxygen requirement	5 (4 , 12)	5 (4 , 14)	5 (4 , 13.3)	0.931

Data were expressed as median (IQR: 1st, 3rd quartiles) for continuous variables and n (%) for categorical ones
Difference between patients with and without pleural effusion were compared using the Mann-Whitney U test for continuous variables and Fisher's exact test for categorical ones
NA not assessed
[*]$p < 0.05$, indicates a significant difference between patients with and without pleural effusion
[a]Of 10 patients requiring ICU hospitalization, one patient had adenovirus pneumonia without pleural effusion, and nine patients had adenovirus pneumonia with pleural effusion

pleural effusion had significantly fewer leukocytes and T lymphocytes (CD4 +, CD8+, or CD20+) compared to patients without pleural effusion, suggesting that the presence of parapneumonic effusion in adenoviral pneumonia was a hallmark of depressed host cellular immunity.

It has been reported that approximately 40% of children hospitalized with pneumonia had pleural effusion [24, 25]. Pleural effusion in children is most frequently seen as a complication of bacterial pneumonia, while viral pneumonia is more frequently associated with acute respiratory distress syndrome (ARDS) than with pleural effusion. The relationship between pleural effusion and

viral pneumonia has not been fully explored. The prevalence rates of pleural effusion in influenza pneumonia and RSV pneumonia are 19.1%, and 6%, respectively [26, 27]. There are limited reports regarding the prevalence of pleural effusion in adenovirus pneumonia, with estimates ranging from 37.5 to 48%. In pneumonia associated with H1N1 influenza, patients with pleural effusion had more lymphopenia, higher C-reactive protein level and more need for oxygen therapy compared to the non-effusion group. These data suggested that there was a significant difference in immunologic response between patients in the pleural effusion group and those in the non-pleural effusion group.

Table 3 Laboratory examinations of patients with adenovirus pneumonia based on the presence or absence of pleural effusion (N = 27)

Variables	Total (n = 27)	Adenoviral pneumonia without pleural effusion (n = 15)	Adenoviral pneumonia with pleural effusion (n = 12)	P value
WBC count, cells/mm^3	9674 ± 3427	10926.7 ± 3043.6	8108.3 ± 3340.8	0.031*
Platelet, 10^3 cells/mm^3	236 ± 108	285.1 ± 108.2	175.8 ± 75.5	0.007*
ANC, cells/mm^3	7451 ± 3173	8738.4 ± 2879.7	6291.7 ± 3255.9	0.090
ASC, cells/ mm^3	6039 ± 2674	7083.4 ± 2370.8	4733.9 ± 2531.2	0.020*
ABC, cells/ mm^3	1397 ± 912	1268.1 ± 903.8	1557.8 ± 934.7	0.423
ALC, cells/ mm^3	1444 ± 1064	1677.3 ± 1204.2	1152.2 ± 814.9	0.209
CRP level, mg/L	68.9 (38.9 , 139.5)	62.9 (35.6 , 79.9)	110.8 (42.0 , 247.2)	0.082

Data were represented as mean ± SD and compared using two-sample t-test if data followed normal distribution; or median (IQR: 1st, 3rd quartiles) and compared using the Mann-Whitney U test if data didn't follow normal distribution
ANC absolute neutrophil counts, ABC absolute band form cell counts, ASC absolute segment cell counts, ALC absolute lymphocyte counts
[*]$p < 0.05$, indicates a significant difference between patients with and without pleural effusion

Table 4 Immune phenotype of white blood cells of patients with adenovirus pneumonia based on the presence or absence of pleural effusion ($n = 8$)

Variables	Adenoviral pneumonia without pleural effusion ($n = 3$)	Adenoviral pneumonia with pleural effusion ($n = 5$)	P value
WBC count, cells/mm^3	13500 (11500 , 18600)	6400 (5400 , 12800)	0.089
Lymphocyte counts, cells/mm^3	2418 (1150 , 2835)	1802 (403 , 2530)	0.451
CD4$^+$ T cells, cells/mm^3	597 (465 , 1321)	130 (102 , 319)	0.034*
CD8$^+$ T cells, cells/ mm^3	601 (284 , 621)	108 (70 , 286)	0.031*
CD20$^+$ T cells, cells/ mm^3	439 (216 , 445)	35 (14 , 112)	0.004*
NK cells, cells/ mm^3	77 (15 , 295)	23 (2 , 65)	0.393

*$p < 0.05$, indicates a significant difference between patients with and without pleural effusion

A total of 674 adenovirus isolates were identified during the 2011 outbreak, of which 215 cases were hospitalized. Our data identified 27 cases with severe adenovirus pneumonia. In contrast, 80% of hospitalized patients were diagnosed with mild to moderate upper respiratory tract infections. Our present results, showing that patients with pleural effusion had more severe disease compared to patients without pleural effusion, were consistent with previous studies analyzing the 2011 Taiwan outbreak, which showed that patients with severe infection had a longer duration of fever and higher incidence of LRTI involvement compared to patients with non-severe infection [19, 20]. Almost half the patients with severe infection from these and other studies exhibited LRTI symptoms such as pneumonic consolidation, pleural effusion, dyspnea, rales and wheezing [19]. Complications such as respiratory failure, acute respiratory distress syndrome (ARDS) and hypotension are also hallmarks of severe adenovirus infections [20, 28, 29]. Indeed, the presence of co-morbidities such as pleural effusion requiring drainage, respiratory distress, wheezing and gastroenteritis have been shown to be risk factors for severe adenovirus pneumonia [30, 31]. Our study showed that although there was no significant difference between the two groups in the number of days of oxygen requirement, a significantly higher number of patients with pleural effusion required oxygen compared to the group without pleural effusion.

The innate immune response has been shown to play an important role in the host response to HAdV infections [32, 33]. The initial inflammation in adenovirus pneumonia has been shown to begin with a neutrophilic interstitial infiltrate, followed by appearance of monocytes, then a lymphocytic infiltrate and release of IL-8 and IL-6 [21]. Other studies reported that intravenous injection of large doses of adenovirus caused leukopenia in non-human primates, humans and hamsters, with a significant decrease in the number of CD3+, CD4+ and CD8+ cells at 1 day post-challenge [34–36]. It has been suggested that adenovirus infections in immunocompetent individuals could result from inhibition of cytokine production, suppression of T cell function, and inhibition of major histocompatibility complex (MHC) expression by virulent strains like HAdV-3 and HAdV-7 [37]. Recombinant adenovirus 35 (rAd35) has been shown to inhibit DC-induced activation of CD4+ cells by specifically binding to CD46 on the surface of T cells and suppressing proliferation and cytokine production in memory cells as well as in total CD4+ cells [38]. Our study data suggested that the presence of parapneumonic effusion in adenoviral pneumonia was significantly associated with depression of host cellular immunity, and were consistent with previous findings that patients with severe infection more frequently had leukopenia and thrombocytopenia compared to patients with non-severe infection [19, 20]. It is important to note that in our study, lymphocyte counts were calculated only for cases where data for immune cell subpopulations were available ($n = 5$), whereas ALC numbers were calculated for all cases. The lymphocyte counts were therefore different from ALC counts. Since inflammation of the respiratory tract is typically associated with upregulation of ALCs, lymphocytes and T cells, we suggest that depression of host cellular immunity during parapneumonic effusion could be because of re-distribution of these immune cells. Our data indicated that patients without pleural effusion had significantly higher WBC counts compared to patients with pleural effusion. It will be interesting to validate our findings in a larger sample size to understand the association between disease severity and leukocytosis. Based on our data, it is likely that preventive measures for opportunistic infections may be effective when patients with adenovirus pneumonia present with parapneumonic effusion.

In addition to lung injury, severe adenovirus infection has been reported to also result in liver injury, with elevated levels of serum lactate dehydrogenase (LDH) and aspartate aminotransferase (AST) correlating with severity of adenovirus infection [20, 39]. In our present study, the incidence of hepatitis was significantly higher in patients with pleural effusion compared to patients without pleural effusion, suggesting the presence of a more severe systemic inflammatory process in these patients.

Conclusions

To the best of our knowledge, this study is the first to analyze T-cell profiles in relation to the presence of parapneumonic effusion in patients with adenoviral pneumonia. Our data were consistent with previous findings from the 2011 community outbreak in Taiwan, and indicated that severity of adenovirus infection correlated positively with suppression of T-cell immunity. Although the mechanism remains unclear, it is likely that T-cell depression may be due to direct inhibition by adenovirus, or non-specific inhibition associated with immunoparalysis at late sepsis. Further prospective, large-scale studies are needed to further characterize the clinical outcomes and risks for subsequent infections among these patients. An important drawback of this study was the small sample size. Therefore, although it was previously reported that patients infected with HAdV-7 had a higher mortality rate in the 2011 outbreak [20], the sample size of this study precluded our ability to stratify our study patients based on their HAdV-3 or HAdV-7 status for statistical comparison. Additionally, there were no deaths over the course of our study period. However, even with limited case numbers, we found a significant difference in immune profiles between patients with simple pneumonia and those with pleural effusion. It will be interesting to evaluate dynamic changes in immune cell profiles through the course of infection to better understand the interaction between viral and immune cells.

Abbreviations

ARDS: Acute respiratory distress syndrome; ASCs: Absolute segment cell counts; AST: Aspartate aminotransferase; DFA: Direct fluorescent-antibody assay; ECMO: Extracorporeal membrane oxygenation; HAdV: Human adenovirus; HFOV: High frequency oscillatory ventilation; LDH: Lactate dehydrogenase; LRTIs: Lower respiratory tract infections; MHC: Histocompatibility complex; NCKU: National Cheng Kung University; rAd35: Recombinant adenovirus 35; RSV: Respiratory syncytial virus

Authors' contributions

CFS is guarantor of integrity of the entire study, study concepts, carried out study design, definition of intellectual content, participate in literature research, clinical studies, experimental studies, data acquisition, data analysis, statistical analysis, manuscript preparation; SMW: participate in data acquisition, data analysis, manuscript editing, manuscript review; TSH participate in clinical studies, data acquisition; CCL participate in manuscript editing, manuscript review. All authors read and approved the study!.

Competing interests

The authors declare that they have no competing interests.

Consent for publication

We, all co-authors, agreed to publish this work once paper got formally accepted.

Author details

[1]Department of Pediatrics, National Cheng Kung University Hospital, College of Medicine, National Cheng Kung University, 138, Sheng Li Road, North Dist., Tainan 70403, Taiwan. [2]Department of Emergency Medicine, National Cheng Kung University Hospital, College of Medicine, National Cheng Kung University, Tainan, Taiwan. [3]Center of Infectious Disease and Signaling Research, National Cheng Kung University Hospital, College of Medicine, National Cheng Kung University, Tainan, Taiwan. [4]Center for Infection Control, National Cheng Kung University Hospital, College of Medicine, National Cheng Kung University, Tainan, Taiwan.

References

1. Lynch 3rd JP, Fishbein M, Echavarria M. Adenovirus. Semin Respir Crit Care Med. 2011;32:494–511.
2. Ebner K, Pinsker W, Lion T. Comparative sequence analysis of the hexon gene in the entire spectrum of human adenovirus serotypes: phylogenetic, taxonomic, and clinical implications. J Virol. 2005;79:12635–42.
3. Russell WC. Adenoviruses: update on structure and function. J Gen Virol. 2009;90:1–20.
4. Edwards KM, Thompson J, Paolini J, Wright PF. Adenovirus infections in young children. Pediatrics. 1985;76:420–4.
5. Tang L, Wang L, Tan X, Xu W. Adenovirus serotype 7 associated with a severe lower respiratory tract disease outbreak in infants in Shaanxi Province, China. Virol J. 2011;8:23.
6. Sun B, He H, Wang Z, Qu J, Li X, Ban C, et al. Emergent severe acute respiratory distress syndrome caused by adenovirus type 55 in immunocompetent adults in 2013: a prospective observational study. Crit Care. 2014;18:456.
7. Kim SJ, Kim K, Park SB, Hong DJ, Jhun BW. Outcomes of early administration of cidofovir in non-immunocompromised patients with severe adenovirus pneumonia. PLoS One. 2015;10:e0122642.
8. Low SY, Tan TT, Lee CH, Loo CM, Chew HC. Severe adenovirus pneumonia requiring extracorporeal membrane oxygenation support–Serotype 7 revisited. Respir Med. 2013;107:1810–3.
9. Hung KH, Lin LH. Adenovirus pneumonia complicated with acute respiratory distress syndrome: a case report. Medicine (Baltimore). 2015;94:e776.
10. Alcorn MJ, Booth JL, Coggeshall KM, Metcalf JP. Adenovirus type 7 induces interleukin-8 production via activation of extracellular regulated kinase 1/2. J Virol. 2001;75:6450–9.
11. Munoz FM, Piedra PA, Demmler GJ. Disseminated adenovirus disease in immunocompromised and immunocompetent children. Clin Infect Dis. 1998;27:1194–200.
12. Alpert G, Charney E, Fee M, Plotkin SA. Outbreak of fatal adenoviral type 7a respiratory disease in a children's long-term care inpatient facility. Am J Infect Control. 1986;14:188–90.
13. Klinger JR, Sanchez MP, Curtin LA, Durkin M, Matyas B. Multiple cases of life-threatening adenovirus pneumonia in a mental health care center. Am J Respir Crit Care Med. 1998;157:645–9.
14. Glezen P, Denny FW. Epidemiology of acute lower respiratory disease in children. N Engl J Med. 1973;288:498–505.
15. Gu L, Liu Z, Li X, Qu J, Guan W, Liu Y, et al. Severe community-acquired pneumonia caused by adenovirus type 11 in immunocompetent adults in Beijing. J Clin Virol. 2012;54:295–301.
16. Ng OT, Thoon KC, Chua HY, Tan NW, Chong CY, Tee NW, et al. Severe pediatric adenovirus 7 disease in Singapore linked to recent outbreaks across Asia. Emerg Infect Dis. 2015;21:1192–6.
17. Lin KH, Lin YC, Chen HL, Ke GM, Chiang CJ, Hwang KP, et al. A two decade survey of respiratory adenovirus in Taiwan: the reemergence of adenovirus types 7 and 4. J Med Virol. 2004;73:274–9.
18. Chang SY, Lee CN, Lin PH, Huang HH, Chang LY, Ko W, et al. A community-derived outbreak of adenovirus type 3 in children in Taiwan between 2004 and 2005. J Med Virol. 2008;80:102–12.
19. Tsou TP, Tan BF, Chang HY, Chen WC, Huang YP, Lai CY, et al. Community outbreak of adenovirus, Taiwan, 2011. Emerg Infect Dis. 2012;18:1825–32.
20. Lai CY, Lee CJ, Lu CY, Lee PI, Shao PL, Wu ET, et al. Adenovirus serotype 3 and 7 infection with acute respiratory failure in children in Taiwan, 2010–2011. PLoS One. 2013;8:e53614.

21. Wu W, Booth JL, Duggan ES, Patel KB, Coggeshall KM, Metcalf JP. Human lung innate immune cytokine response to adenovirus type 7. J Gen Virol. 2010;91:1155–63.
22. Ginsberg HS, Moldawer LL, Sehgal PB, Redington M, Kilian PL, Chanock RM, et al. A mouse model for investigating the molecular pathogenesis of adenovirus pneumonia. Proc Natl Acad Sci U S A. 1991;88:1651–5.
23. Clark TW, Fleet DH, Wiselka MJ. Severe community-acquired adenovirus pneumonia in an immunocompetent 44-year-old woman: a case report and review of the literature. J Med Case Rep. 2011;5:259.
24. Mocelin HT, Fischer GB. Parapneumonic pleural effusion. Pediatr Respir Rev. 2002;3:359–60.
25. Hamm H, Light RW. Parapneumonic effusion and empyema. Eur Respir J. 1997;10:1150–6.
26. Kern S, Uhl M, Berner R, Schwoerer T, Langer M. Respiratory syncytial virus infection of the lower respiratory tract: radiological findings in 108 children. Eur Radiol. 2001;11:2581–4.
27. Kim YN, Cho HJ, Cho YK, Ma JS. Clinical significance of pleural effusion in the new influenza A (H1N1) viral pneumonia in children and adolescent. Pediatr Pulmonol. 2012;47:505–9.
28. Wenman WM, Pagtakhan RD, Reed MH, Chernick V, Albritton W. Adenovirus bronchiolitis in Manitoba: epidemiologic, clinical, and radiologic features. Chest. 1982;81:605–9.
29. Hong JY, Lee HJ, Piedra PA, Choi EH, Park KH, Koh YY, et al. Lower respiratory tract infections due to adenovirus in hospitalized Korean children: epidemiology, clinical features, and prognosis. Clin Infect Dis. 2001; 32:1423–9.
30. Rajkumar V, Chiang CS, Low JM, Cui L, Lin RT, Tee NW, et al. Risk factors for severe adenovirus infection in children during an outbreak in Singapore. Ann Acad Med Singapore. 2015;44:50–9.
31. Gupta P, Goyal S, Tobias JD, Prodhan P, Purohit P, Gossett JM, et al. Risk factors associated with hospital admission among healthy children with adenovirus infection. Turk J Pediatr. 2011;53:597–603.
32. Hendrickx R, Stichling N, Koelen J, Kuryk L, Lipiec A, Greber UF. Innate immunity to adenovirus. Hum Gene Ther. 2014;25:265–84.
33. Schagen FH, Ossevoort M, Toes RE, Hoeben RC. Immune responses against adenoviral vectors and their transgene products: a review of strategies for evasion. Crit Rev Oncol Hematol. 2004;50:51–70.
34. Schnell MA, Zhang Y, Tazelaar J, Gao GP, Yu QC, Qian R, et al. Activation of innate immunity in nonhuman primates following intraportal administration of adenoviral vectors. Mol Ther. 2001;3:708–22.
35. Freytag SO, Stricker H, Movsas B, Kim JH. Prostate cancer gene therapy clinical trials. Mol Ther. 2007;15:1042–52.
36. Toth K, Lee SR, Ying B, Spencer JF, Tollefson AE, Sagartz JE, et al. STAT2 knockout Syrian hamsters support enhanced replication and pathogenicity of human adenovirus, revealing an important role of type I interferon response in viral control. PLoS Pathog. 2015;11:e1005084.
37. Hakim FA, Tleyjeh IM. Severe adenovirus pneumonia in immunocompetent adults: a case report and review of the literature. Eur J Clin Microbiol Infect Dis. 2008;27:153–8.
38. Adams WC, Gujer C, McInerney G, Gall JG, Petrovas C, Karlsson Hedestam GB, et al. Adenovirus type-35 vectors block human CD4+ T-cell activation via CD46 ligation. Proc Natl Acad Sci U S A. 2011;108:7499–504.
39. Spaeder MC, Fackler JC. Hospital-acquired viral infection increases mortality in children with severe viral respiratory infection. Pediatr Crit Care Med. 2011;12:e317–21.

6

Secondary organizing pneumonia following viral pneumonia caused by severe influenza B

Nobuhiro Asai[1], Toyoharu Yokoi[2], Naoya Nishiyama[1], Yusuke Koizumi[1], Daisuke Sakanashi[1], Hideo Kato[1], Mao Hagihara[1], Hiroyuki Suematsu[1], Yuka Yamagishi[1] and Hiroshige Mikamo[1*]

Abstract

Background: Some reported that organizing pneumonia (OP) may occur after influenza A infections including swine-origin influenza A (H1N1). However, OP associated with influenza B infection has never been reported. We report the first case of secondary OP associated with viral pneumonia caused by influenza B.

Case presentation: A 23-year old woman was diagnosed as viral pneumonia caused by type B influenza. Despite of antiviral therapy, abnormal chest shadows were not improved. Bronchoscopy and transbronchial lung biopsy showed organizing pneumonia due to viral pneumonia caused by influenza B. Corticosteroid therapy was started at 30 mg daily (0.5 mg/kg), and the dose was reduced to 25, 20, 15 or 10 mg per day every month with symptomatic and radiological resolution. Even after corticosteroid therapy was discontinued, we did not confirm disease recurrence.

Conclusions: Physicians should be aware of the possibility for SOP and severe viral pneumonia even in case of type B as well as type A influenza infections.

Keywords: Influenza pneumonia, Type B influenza virus, Organizing pneumonia

Background

Organizing pneumonia (OP) is a pulmonary inflammatory condition that occurs in certain clinical settings [1, 2]. In the appropriate clinical-radiologic context, an OP diagnosis can be confirmed with bronchoalveolar lavage fluid (BALF) and transbronchial lung biopsy (TBLB). Some reported that OP may occur after influenza A infections including swine-origin influenza A (H1N1) [3–5]. However, OP associated with influenza B infection has never been reported. We report the first case of secondary OP associated with viral pneumonia caused by influenza B.

Case presentation

A 23-year old woman without relevant medical history visited our outpatient clinic complaining fever, sorethorat and cough lasting for 3 days. She was diagnosed as influenza B infection by nasophayngeal antigen test

(Influenza B strain was not confirmed because reverse transcription-polymerase chain reaction was not performed.). She was not obese (body mass index 22.3 kg/m^2) and had not received any influenza vaccination in the past. She had no smoking history. She had an allergy history for macrolides antibiotics. Although she had received an antiviral therapy of oseltamivir 150 mg per day, flu symptoms such as fever and cough persisted and she once again came to the clinic on day 4 after starting the therapy. Also, she had an acute respiratory failure (SpO$_2$ 93% on 5 L/min O$_2$ mask) with elevation of inflammatory reactions (WBC 18,900 /μL, CRP 11.69 mg/dL). Chest radiography and chest computed tomography (CT) revealed peripheral subpleural opacities (Fig.1) and consolidations. Broad spectrum antimicrobial agent, meropenem, was empirically administered but additional antiviral therapy was not started. A rapid influenza diagnostic test showed that influenza A and B were negative and positive, respectively. Urinary streptococcal antigen and legionella antigen were both negative. No virulent pathogens were detected in the sputum. Therefore, she

* Correspondence: mikamo@aichi-med-u.ac.jp
[1]Department of Clinical Infectious Diseases, Aichi Medical University School of Medicine, 〒480-1195 1-1 Yazakokarimata, Nagakute, Aichi, Japan

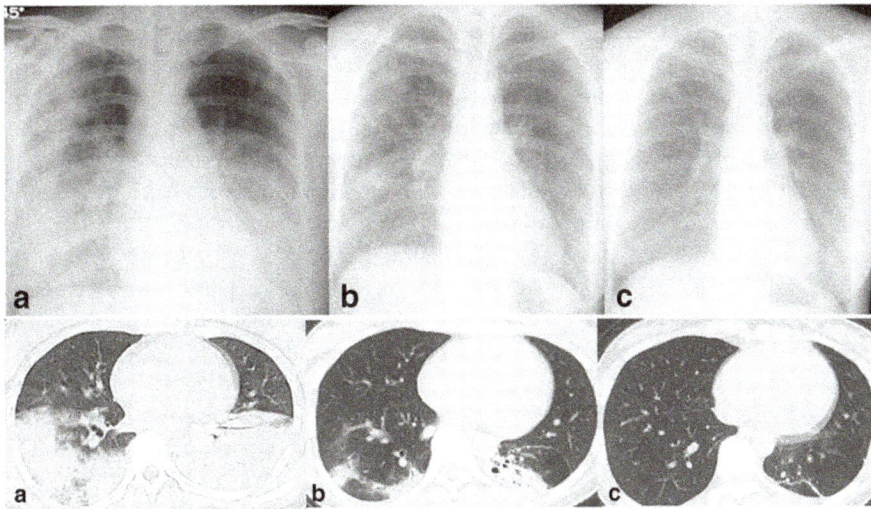

Fig. 1 Chest X-ray showed bilateral infiltrates on admission (**a** upper). After starting PSL therapy on day 25, infiltrates were improved (**b** upper). Abnormal shadows on Chest X-ray disappeared 6 months after starting corticosteroid therapy (**c** upper). Chest CT showed consolidations on both lungs on admission (**a** lower) and the shadows were improved on day 25 after starting corticosteroid therapy (**b** lower). Six months after starting corticosteroid therapy, the consolidations disappeared (**c** lower)

was diagnosed as having influenza B virus pneumonia and was referred to us. While her respiratory condition was improved, inflammatory reaction and abnormal chest radiographic shadows recurred. Transbronchial lung biopsy (TBLB) revealed lymphocytic alveolitis and organizing pneumonia (Fig 2). No pathogens were found in the BALF. She was diagnosed as secondary OP associated with influenza B pneumonia. Corticosteroid therapy was started and inflammatory reaction and chest radiography were gradually improved. The initial dose of corticosteroid was 30 mg (0.5 mg/kg) daily and tapered with improvement of inflammatory reaction and chest radiography. She was discharged on day 30. The dose was reduced to 25, 20, 15 and 10 mg per day every month with symptomatic and radiological resolution. After corticosteroid therapy was discontinued, disease recurrence was not observed.

Discussion

In general, influenza B complicating bacterial infection cause a mild disease, but severe pneumonia cases due to influenza B and *Streptococcal* co-infection have been reported [6–8].

Several mechanisms of such severe co-infection were reported in animal models. The influenza virus could damage respiratory tract epithelium and facilitate bacterial infection. The viruses also alter and/or impair ciliary function of the epithelium. It can change host immunity and inflammatory responses by impairing bacterial clearance or via the inflammatory cascade [9–11]. To the best of our knowledge, this is the first case of SOP due to influenza B virus pneumonia and the second case of severe respiratory failure due to influenza B virus infection not co-infection, following the case reported by Kato [12]. Gutierrez-Pizarraya, et al. reported that the proportion

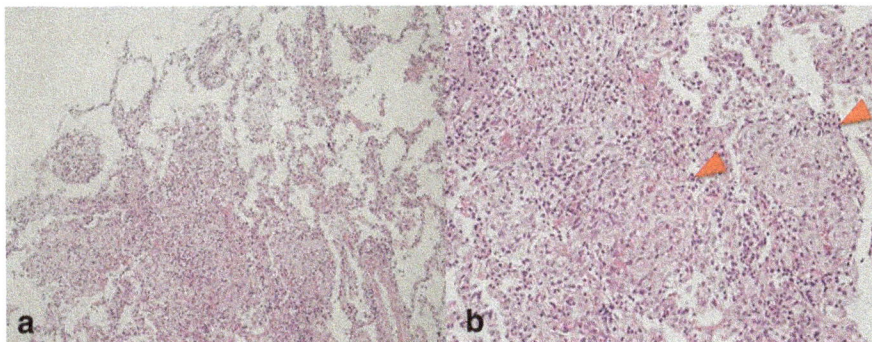

Fig. 2 TBLB specimen from the right middle lobe showed intraalveolar granulation tissue with myofibroblasts consistent with organizing pneumonia (Hematoxin-Eosin (HE) × 100) (**a**). Masson body (red arrow) was seen on the TBLB specimen (HE ×400) (**b**)

of patients with pneumonia and the rate of admission to the intensive care unit did not differ between cases of influenza A (H1N1) pdm09 and influenza B infection. Notably, the mortality rates were almost similar between patients with influenza A (16.3%) and influenza B (10%) infection [13]. Paddock, et al. documented the pathological findings of the lung autopsy cases of patients who died of influenza B virus infection and demonstrated that diffuse alveolar damage pattern were found in 17.8% of the cases [14]. These suggest that influenza B virus infection could contribute to severe respiratory failure, resulting in poor outcome that is similar to influenza A virus infection.

The standard treatment of influenza virus pneumonia is not established yet. Tanaka reported that the median survival time of post-influenza pneumococcal pneumonia in mice was longer by double dose of peramivir than by single dose of peramivir or single dose of oseltamivir group. Also, the production of inflammatory cytokines/chemokines was also significantly suppressed by double dose of peramivir compared with other two groups. These suggests that double dose of peramivir could contribute to reducing a cytokine storm by influenza virus, resulting in favorable outcomes for influenza virus pneumonia and post-influenza pneumonia patients [15]. In contrast, some demonstrated that double dose of neuraminidase inhibitors are not useful in the treatment for flu compared with the standard dose of oseltamivir [16]. In the study, they concluded that the duration of antiviral therapy was associated with the outcome. Other studies also indicate that early antiviral therapy in patients with severe influenza is associated with both clinical benefits and more rapid viral clearance from the upper respiratory tract samples [17, 18].

Some previously reported cases of SOP caused by influenza virus (Table 1) [3–5, 7, 8]. It is well known that H1N1 and avian flu could result in a cytokine storm. Thus, it is reasonable that SOP could occur in patients infected with these viruses. In terms of radiological findings of influenza A pneumonia, peripheral ground-grass opacities and consolidations has been commonly reported as in our case. Some documented a peripheral distribution of lung opacities in patients with influenza A infection mimicking OP [19–21]. SOP could be seen 2 to 3 weeks after the onset of initial influenza symptoms, whereas influenza viral pneumonia could generally occur in day 4 to 5 after the onset of illness [22, 23]. SOP should be considered if influenza patients have fever, and a dry cough after initial influenza like illness improved, and TBLB should be performed since proper OP treatment requires corticosteroid therapy. All SOP cases following severe influenza virus pneumonia were cured by corticosteroid therapy, except for the case of acute fibrosis organizing pneumonia (AFOP) associated with influenza A/H1N1 pneumonia after lung transplantation [8] as shown in Table 1. These favorable outcomes of SOP could correlate with the clinicopathological features of OP. Such features of OP might be different from that of a fatal interstitial lung disease such as diffuse alveolar damage. Ebina and colleagues reported the disappearance of subpleural and interlobular lymphatics in idiopathic pulmonary fibrosis (IPF) lungs along with a poor lymphogenesis and a significant decrease of alveolar lymphangiogenesis in comparison with cellular non-specific interstitial pneumonia and OP. These changes may exert a detrimental effect on IPF lungs by impairing alveolar clearance [24].

Table 1 Cases of secondary organizing pneumonia due to influenza virus infection

Author (Year)	Sex	Age	Type of influenza	Initial treatment	Outcome
Cornejo R [3] (2010)	Female	52	A	Steroidpulse therapy	Cure
Cornejo R [3] (2010)	Male	36	A	Steroidpulse therapy	Cure
Gómez-Gómez A [4] (2011)	Female	44	A	Corticosteoroid 0.5 mg/kg	Cure
Gómez-Gómez A [4] (2011)	Male	60	A	Corticosteoroid 0.5 mg/kg	Cure
Torrego A [5] (2010)	Female	55	A	Corticosteoroid 0.75 mg/kg	Cure
Kwok WC [7] (2016)	Female	45	B	Corticosteroid 30 mg daily	Cure[a]
Otto C [8] (2013)	Female	66	B	High dose corticosteroid	Death[b]
Asai N (2016)	Female	22	B	Corticosteroid 0.5 mg/kg	Cure

All cases were diagnosed as organizing pneumonia by transbronchial lung biopsy
[a] This is a case of secondary organizing pneumonia associated with influenza B and *Streptococcal* co-infection
[b] This is a case of acute fibrinous and organizing pneumonia associated with influenza A/H1N1 pneumonia after lung transplantation

AFOP is a distinct reaction pattern in acute respiratory failure with high mortality rate of up to 90%. Current literature reported that cause of AFOP are idiopathic, or collagen vascular diseases, or bacterial infection, drug exposure (e.g. amiodarone, abacavir or statins) [8, 25]. Physicians should know that influenza infection could induce AFOP, resulting in a poor outcome.

Conclusions

Physicians should be aware of the possibility of severe respiratory failure due to influenza B virus infection and secondary OP following influenza B infection, even though once influenza infection was cured.

Abbreviations
BALF: Bronchoalveolar lavage fluid; CT: Computed tomography; IPF: Idiopathic pulmonary fibrosis; OP: Organizing pneumonia; TBLB: Transbronchial lung biopsy

Acknowledgments
We are grateful for the diligent and thorough critical reading of our manuscript by Dr. Yoshihiro Ohkuni, Chief Physician, Taiyo and Mr. John Wocher, Executive Vice President and Director, International Affairs/ International Patient Services, Kameda Medical Center (Japan).

Funding
None declared.

Authors' contributions
NA, NN, YK, YY, HM carried out the clinical follow up. NA draft the manuscript. DS and HS performed microbial testing and NA, NN, YK, YY, HM performed laboratory analysis. HK and MH supervised the antibiotic and antiviral therapy. All authors read and approved the final manuscript.

Consent for publication
Written informed consent was obtained from the patient for publication of this report.

Competing interests
The authors declare that they have no competing interests.

Author details
[1]Department of Clinical Infectious Diseases, Aichi Medical University School of Medicine, 〒480-1195 1-1 Yazakokarimata, Nagakute, Aichi, Japan. [2]Department of Pathology, Nagoya Ekisaikai Hospital, Nagoya, Aichi, Japan.

References
1. Cordier JF. Organizing pneumonia. Thorax. 2000;55:318–28.
2. Vasu TS, Cavallazzi R, Hirani A, Sharma D, Weibel SB, Kane GC. Clinical and radiologic distinctions between secondary bronchiolitis obliterans organizing pneumonia and cryptogenic organizing pneumonia. Respir Care. 2009;54:1028–32.
3. Cornejo R, Llanos O, Fernández C, Carlos Díaz J, Cardemil G, Salguero J, et al. Organizing pneumonia in patients with severe respiratory failure due to novel a (H1N1) influenza. BMJ Case Rep. 2010;21:2010. pii: bcr0220102708
4. Gómez-Gómez A, Martínez-Martínez R, Gotway MB. Organizing pneumonia associated with swine-origin influenza a H1N1 2009 viral infection. AJR Am J Roentgenol. 2011;196:W103–4.
5. Torrego A, Pajares V, Mola A, Lerma E, Franquet T. Influenza A (H1N1) organising pneumonia. BMJ Case Rep. 2010;27:2010. pii: bcr1220092531
6. Lam KW, Sin KC, Au SY, Yung SK. Uncommon cause of severe pneumonia: co-infection of influenza B and streptococcus. Hong Kong Med J. 2013;19:545–8.
7. Kwok WC, Lam SH, Wong MP, Ip MS, Lam DC. Influenza B/streptococcal co-infection complicated by organizing pneumonia. Respirol Case Rep. 2016; 4(5):e00170.
8. Otto C, Huzly D, Kemna L, Hüttel A, Benk C, Rieg S, et al. Acute fibrinous and organizing pneumonia associated with influenza a/H1N1 pneumonia after lung transplantation. BMC Pulm Med. 2013;13:30.
9. Park K, Bakaletz LO, Coticchia JM, Lim DJ. Effect of influenza a virus on ciliary activity and dye transport function in the chinchilla eustachian tube. Ann Otol Rhinol Laryngol. 1993;102:551–8.
10. Echchannaoui H, Frei K, Schnell C, Leib SL, Zimmerli W, Landmann R. Toll-like receptor 2-deficient mice are highly susceptible to Streptococcus Pneumoniae meningitis because of reduced bacterial clearing and enhanced inflammation. J Infect Dis. 2002;186:798–806.
11. Dallaire F, Ouellet N, Bergeron Y, Turmel V, Gauthier MC, Simard M, et al. Microbiological and inflammatory factors associated with the development of pneumococcal pneumonia. J Infect Dis. 2001;184:292–300.
12. Kato S, Fujisawa T, Enomoto N, Inui N, Nakamura Y, Suda T. Severe respiratory failure associated with influenza B virus infection. Respirology case report. 2015;3:61–3.
13. Gutiérrez-Pizarraya A, Pérez-Romero P, Alvarez R, Aydillo TA, Osorio-Gómez G, Milara-Ibáñez C, et al. Unexpected severity of cases of influenza B infection in patients that required hospitalization during the first postpandemic wave. J Inf Secur. 2012;65:423–30.
14. Paddock CD, Liu L, Denison AM, Bartlett JH, Holman RC, Deleon-Carnes M, et al. Myocardial injury and bacterial pneumonia contribute to the pathogenesis of fatal influenza B virus infection. J Infect Dis. 2012;205:895–905.
15. Tanaka A, Nakamura S, Seki M, Iwanaga N, Kajihara T, Kitano M, et al. The effect of intravenous peramivir, compared with oral oseltamivir, on the outcome of post-influenza pneumococcal pneumonia in mice. Antivir Ther. 2015;20:11–9.
16. South East Asia Infectious Disease Clinical Research Network. Effect of double dose oseltamivir on clinical and virological outcomes in children and adults admitted to hospital with severe influenza: double blind randomised controlled trial. BMJ. 2013;30:346.
17. Neuraminidase Inhibitor Flu Treatment Investigator Group. Efficacy and safety of oseltamivir in treatment of acute influenza: a randomised controlled trial. Lancet. 2000;355:1845–50.
18. McGeer A, Green KA, Plevneshi A, Siddiqi N, Raboud J, Low DE, et al. Antiviral therapy and outcomes of influenza requiring hospitalization in Ontario, Canada. Clin Infect Dis. 2007;45:1568–75.
19. Valente T, Lassandro F, Marino M, Squillante F, Aliperta M, Muto R. H1N1 pneumonia: our experience in 50 patients with a severe clinical course of novel swine-origin influenza a (H1N1) virus (S-OIV). Radiol Med. 2012;117:165–84.
20. Ajlan AM, Quiney B, Nicolaou S, Müller NL. Swine-origin influenza a (H1N1) viral infection: radiographic and CT findings. AJR Am J Roentgenol. 2009; 193:1494–9.
21. Marchiori E, Zanetti G, Hochhegger B, Rodrigues RS, Fontes CA, Nobre LF, et al. High-resolution computed tomography findings from adult patients with influenza a (H1N1) virus-associated pneumonia. Eur J Radiol. 2010;74:93–8.
22. Influenza Investigators ANZIC, Webb SA, Pettilä V, Seppelt I, Bellomo R, Bailey M, et al. Critical care services and 2009 H1N1 influenza in Australia and New Zealand. N Engl J Med. 2009;361:1925–34.
23. Kumar A, Zarychanski R, Pinto R, Cook DJ, Marshall J, Lacroix J, et al. Critically ill patients with 2009 influenza a(H1N1) infection in Canada. JAMA. 2009;302:1872–9.
24. Ebina M, Shibata N, Ohta H, Hisata S, Tamada T, Ono M, et al. The disappearance of subpleural and interlobular lymphatics in idiopathic pulmonary fibrosis. Lymphat Res Biol. 2010;8:199–207.
25. Beasley MB, Franks TJ, Galvin JR, Gochuico B, Travis WD. Acute fibrinous and organizing pneumonia: a histological pattern of lung injury and possible variant of diffuse alveolar damage. Arch Pathol Lab Med. 2002;126:1064–70.

7

First report of cavitary pneumonia due to community-acquired *Acinetobacter pittii*, study of virulence and overview of pathogenesis and treatment

Romaric Larcher[1*] (iD), Alix Pantel[2], Erik Arnaud[1], Albert Sotto[3] and Jean-Philippe Lavigne[2]

Abstract

Background: *Acinetobacter pittii* is a nosocomial pathogen rarely involved in community-acquired infections. We report for the first time that *A. pittii* can be responsible for cavitary community-acquired pneumonia and study its virulence, and discuss its pathogenesis and treatment options.

Case presentation: A 45-year-old woman with a history of smoking and systemic lupus was admitted to Nimes University Hospital (France) with coughing and sputum lasting for three weeks. Thoracic CT scanner showed cavitary pneumonia. Broncho-alveolar lavage cultures found community-acquired *Acinetobacter calcoaceticus-baumannii* complex. The clinical outcome was favourable after twenty-one days of antimicrobial treatment by piperacillin/tazobactam and amikacin then cefepime. Multilocus sequence typing (MLST) analyses identified an *A. pittii* ST249. Despite the atypical clinical presentation with an unexpected partial destruction of lung parenchyma, we found very low virulence potential of the *A. pittii* strain with nematode killing assays and biofilm formation test. The median time required to kill 50% of the nematodes was 7 ± 0.3 days for *A. pittii* ST249, 7 ± 0.2 days for *A. baumanii* NAB ST2 and 8 ± 0.2 days for *E. coli* OP50, ($p > 0,05$). *A. pittii* ST249 showed significantly slower biofilm formation than *A. baumanii* NAB ST2: BFI = 8.83 ± 0.59 vs 3.93 ± 0.27 at 2 h ($p < 0.0001$), BFI = 6.3 ± 0.17 vs 1. 87 ± 0.12 at 3 h ($p < 0.0001$) and BFI = 3.67 ± 0.41 vs 1.7 ± 0.06 after 4 h of incubation ($p < 0.01$).

Conclusions: Community-acquired *A. pittii* should be considered as possible cause of sub-acute cavitary pneumonia particularly in a smoking and/or immunocompromised patient despite its low virulence potential.

Keywords: Community-acquired pneumonia, Cavitary pneumonia, Cavitation, *Acinetobacter pittii*, *Acinetobacter calcoaceticus-baumannii* complex, Virulence, Biofilm

Background

The classic underlying causes of lung abscess or cavitary lung lesions are anaerobes, *Streptococcus pneumonia*, *Streptococcus milleri* group, *Staphylococcus aureus* and *Klebsiella pneumoniae*. More rarely *Pseudomonas aeruginosa* and other aerobic Gram-negative bacilli, *Nocardia* spp., *Aspergillus* spp. and *Cryptococcus* spp. could be identified [1]. To our knowledge, *Acinetobacter pittii*, formerly known as *Acinetobacter* genomospecies 3, has not been described as a cause of cavitary pneumonia before and it appears to be an unusual cause of community-acquired infections [1–3]. However, it is increasingly described as a cause of hospital-acquired infection particularly in intensive care unit setting [4]. Here, we report the first case of cavitary community-acquired pneumonia due to *A. pittii* in a patient with a systemic lupus and study the virulence profile of *A. pittii*.

Case presentation

A 45-year-old woman, was admitted to Nimes University Hospital (France) for a cough and sputum lasting for three weeks with an unfavourable outcome despite

---
* Correspondence: romaric.larcher@gmail.com
[1]Department of Internal Medicine, Caremeau University Hospital, 29 place du Professeur Debre, Nimes, France
Full list of author information is available at the end of the article

prescription of antibiotics (cefixime then pristinamycin). She had a medical history of smoking and systemic lupus diagnosed in 1991 with moderately reduced glomerular filtration rate (57 ml/min/1.73m^2), stroke and right nephrectomy in 2011. Her usual treatment included hydroxychloroquine, clopidogrel and atorvastatine.

At admission, she presented dyspnoea, crackles of the right lung field and normal temperature. The white blood cell count was 19×10^3 cells/µL and C reactive protein was high at 144 mg/L. Chest X-ray showed a large pulmonary cavity of the right lower lobe (Fig. 1) and computed tomography (CT-scan) showed four large cavities and nodules of the right lower lobe (Figs. 2 and 3). Blood cultures remained negative. A fibroscopy with broncho-alveolar lavage (BAL) showed local inflammation with sputum. Piperacillin/tazobactam plus amikacin was administered as empirical treatment. The BAL culture was positive with more than 10^4 CFU/mL of Gram negative bacilli.

MALDI-TOF (Matrix Assisted Laser Desorption Ionisation/Time Of Flight) analysis (Vitek MS, bioMérieux) identified *A. calcoaceticus-baumannii* complex (99%). Antimicrobial susceptibility was tested by disc diffusion in accordance with EUCAST (European Committee on Antimicrobial Susceptibility Testing) recommendations (version 5.0, 2015; http://www.eucast.org). The isolate was susceptible to ticarcillin, piperacillin, third and fourth generation cephalosporins, imipenem, ciprofloxacin and amikacin. Cultures for mycobacteria, *Nocardia* spp., *Aspergillus* spp. and *Cryptococcus* spp. were negative. Bronchial biopsy was normal.

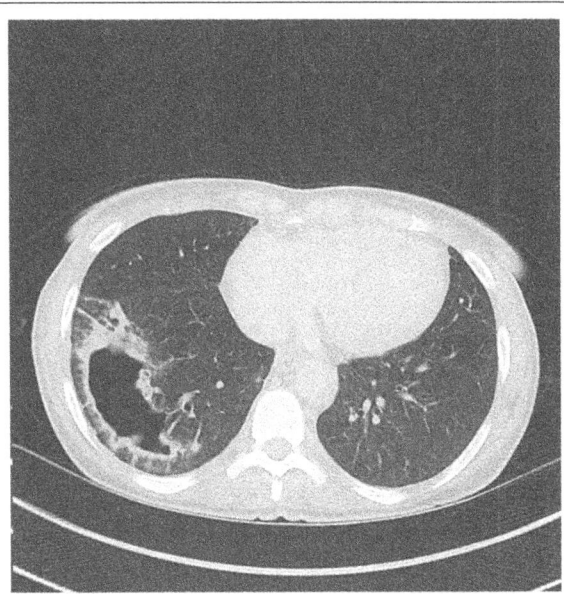

Fig. 2 Thoracic CT scan showing a cavitary community-acquired pneumonia due to *A. pittii* with the largest cavitation of the right lower lobe, three days after admission

Cavitary community-acquired pneumonia due to *A. calcoaceticus-baumannii* complex was considered. The antimicrobial treatment was changed to cefepime after seven days of piperacillin/tazobactam and two days amikacin. After twelve days of antimicrobial treatment (including five days cefepime) the CT-scan showed persistent excavated lung lesions. Size of the largest cavity was slightly reduced and the walls were thinner.

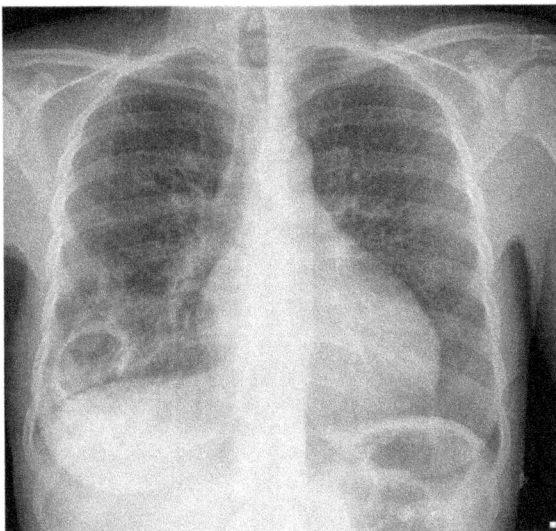

Fig. 1 Chest X-ray showing a community-acquired pneumonia due to *A. pittii* with a large pulmonary cavity of the right lower lobe, at hospital admission

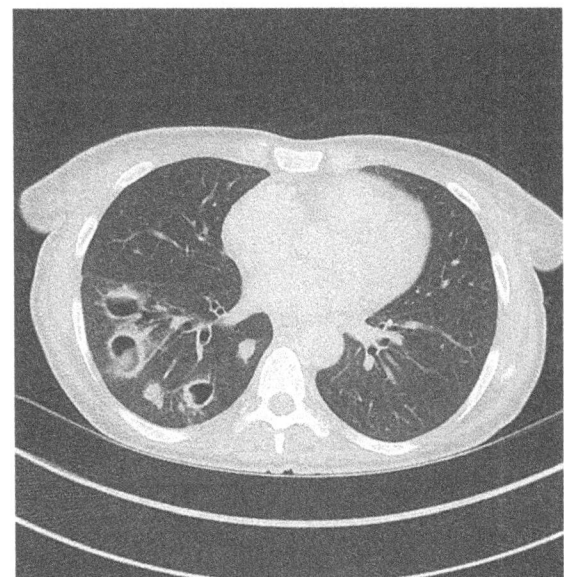

Fig. 3 Thoracic CT scan showing a cavitary community-acquired pneumonia due to *A. pittii* with the three others cavitations and nodules of the right lower lobe, three days after admission

The clinical outcome was favourable after twenty-one days of antimicrobial treatment (including fourteen days cefepime). The Positon Emission Tomography - Computed Tomography performed at the end of the antimicrobial therapy did not find hypermetabolic fixation. Six months later, CT-scan showed residual excavated lung lesions of the right lower lobe. The bronchoscopy with biopsies was normal and the BAL cultures were negative.

Species identification

As species included in *A. calcoaceticus-baumannii* complex are closely related, rpoB sequencing and multilocus sequence typing (MLST) (bigsdb.web.pasteur.fr) [5] were performed to characterize the taxonomic status of the strain and the clone involved in this case. The isolate was identified as *A. pittii* belonging to ST249.

Virulence study

To evaluate the virulence of the *A. pittii* strain, we conducted a *Caenorhabditis elegans* nematode killing assay, a virulence model well described to study *Acinetobacter* spp. virulence [6]. The median time required to kill 50% of the Fer-15 *C. elegans* population (LT50) was compared between *A. pittii* isolate and an *A. baumannii* strain belonging to international clone II/ST2 isolated in our laboratory (NAB ST2). In vivo kinetics of killing of *C. elegans* infected by *A. pittii* and NAB ST2 were compared with the survival curve for worms fed on non-pathogenic *E. coli* (OP50) using a log-rank (Mantel-cox) test.

There was no significant difference between kinetics of killing of *C. elegans* infected by *A. pittii* ST249 and NAB ST2 compared with those fed on non-pathogenic *E. coli*

OP50, showing a very low virulence potential for the two strains equivalent to the standard feeding strain *E. coli* OP50 for nematodes (Fig. 4). The LT50 were 7 ± 0.3 days, 7 ± 0.2 days and 8 ± 0.2 days respectively for *A. pittii* ST249, NAB ST2 and *E. coli* OP50, ($p > 0,05$).

Given that biofilm formation is reported to favour bacterial colonization and persistence, biofilm-forming ability was investigated and kinetics of *A. pittii* ST249 and NAB ST2 were compared. The kinetics of the early phase of biofilm formation for *A. pittii* and NAB ST2 were studied using the BioFilm Ring Test® (BioFilm Control, Saint Beauzire, France) [7]. A high BioFilm Index (BFI) value (>8) corresponds to high mobility of free beads under magnetic attraction (no biofilm), while a low value (≤ 2) corresponds to complete immobilisation of beads (strong biofilm) [8]. BFI values between 2 and 8 indicate that biofilm formation is in progress. Three experiments with two repeats were performed per strain and per incubation time. Mean BFI were compared between each strain after 1, 2, 3, 4 and 5 h, using two-way Anova test followed by Bonferroni's multiple comparisons test. Statistics and graphs were prepared using the software package GraphPad Prism 6.0®.

There were no significant differences between the two strains at the very beginning of kinetics (BFI = 9.27 ± 0.27 for *A. pittii* and 8.63 ± 0.37 for NAB ST2 at 1 h of incubation, $p > 0,05$) (Fig. 5). However, at the next time points, *A. pittii* ST249 showed a significantly slower biofilm formation than NAB ST2: BFI = 8.83 ± 0.59 vs 3.93 ± 0.27 respectively at 2 h ($p < 0.0001$), BFI = 6.3 ± 0.17 vs 1.87 ± 0.12 at 3 h ($p < 0.0001$) and BFI = 3.67 ± 0.41 vs 1.7 ± 0.06 after 4 h incubation

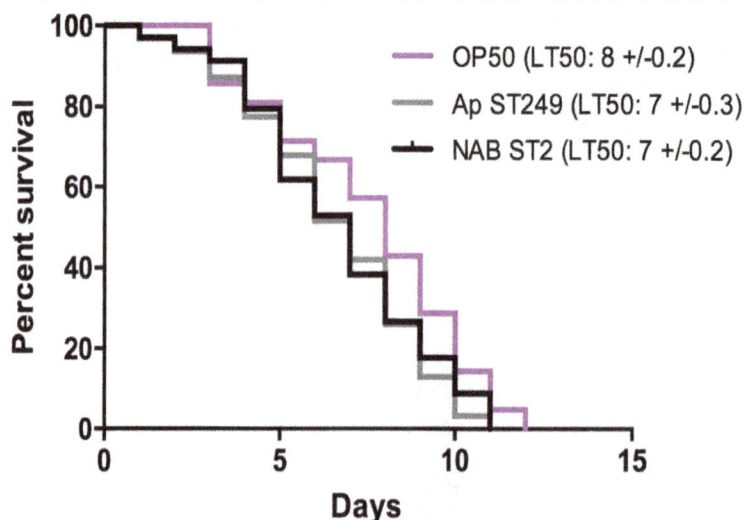

Fig. 4 In vivo kinetics of killing of *C. elegans* infected by *A. pittii* ST249 (Ap ST249) and *A. baumannii* ST2 (NAB ST2) compared with the survival curve for worms fed on non-pathogenic *E. coli* (OP50) using a log-rank (Mantel-cox) test to evaluate differences in survival rates between the different strains (*p* non-significant)

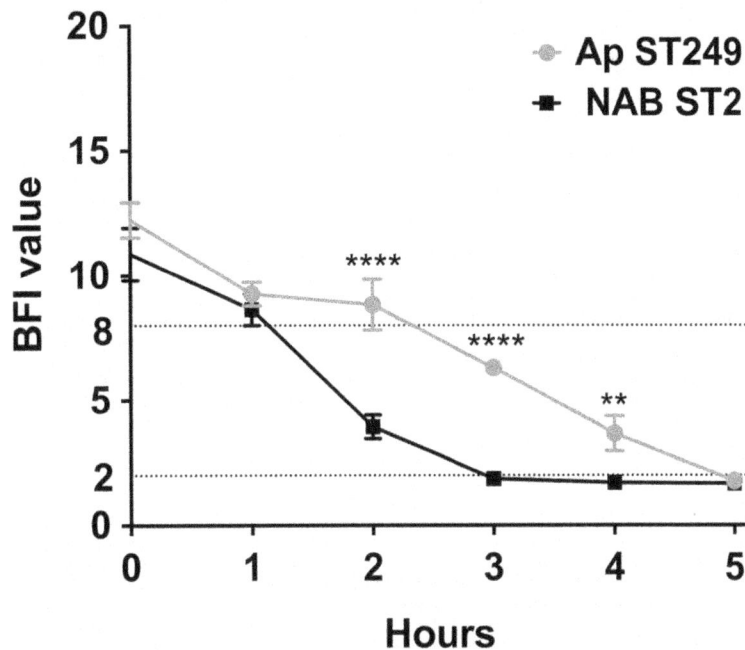

Fig. 5. Comparison between the kinetics of the early phase of biofilm formation for *A. pittii* ST249 (Ap ST249) and *A. baumannii* ST2 (NAB ST2). Means ± standard deviations of BioFilm Indice (BFI) for at least three independent replicates are presented and significant differences between each strain at each time using two-way Anova test, followed by Bonferroni's multiple comparisons test are indicated by ** ($p < 0.01$) and **** ($p < 0.0001$)

($p < 0.01$). *A. pittii* biofilm was constituted after 5 h of incubation (BFI = 1.77 ± 0.09).

Discussion and conclusions

We report the first case of cavitary community-acquired pneumonia due to an *A. pittii* strain with low virulence potential, in a smoking patient with systemic lupus.

A. pittii is a member of the *A. calcoaceticus-baumannii* complex which also includes *A. baumannii*, *A. calcoaceticus* and *A. nosocomialis*. As a result of advances in molecular biology, *A. pittii* is increasingly recognized as a significant cause of nosocomial infection, particularly in intensive care unit setting, but nevertheless remains uncommon [3]. This bacterium is rarely observed to cause community-acquired infections notably cavitary pulmonary disease [1]. *A. pittii* ST249 has been described only twice, in two patients with hospital-acquired infection in Germany, a country where the prevalence of *A. pittii* seems high among species of *A. calcoaceticus-baumannii* complex [9]. The proportion of *A. pittii* community-acquired infections is not defined because of technological limitations in species identification across laboratories worldwide [5, 10]. Prevalence may also be under-evaluated in healthy individuals because the low virulence profile does not result in clinical disease.

The large destruction of lung parenchyma with both cavitary lung lesions and pulmonary nodules in this case suggests that *A. pittii* is highly virulent. However, the *C.*

elegans killing assays and the BioFilm Ring Test® showed very low virulence potential and a poor ability to form biofilm as recently observed [11, 12]. The significant variability of virulence described among *A. baumannii* complex species probably explains the sub-acute clinical course unlike the fulminant evolution usually associated with *Acinetobacter* community-acquired pneumonia in tropical areas [12–14]. Moreover, the mortality rate for patients infected with *A. pittii* seems to be lower than for *A. baumannii* (15% versus 40%) [4, 10]. Finally, the hosts' immune status and tobacco consumption seem to play a crucial role to facilitate infection. *A. pittii* and *A. baumannii* appear genetically and metabolically similar [15] and probably share the same risk factors for causing community-acquired infections: smoking, excessive alcohol consumption, diabetes mellitus and chronic lung disease [13, 14]. In this case, the patient is diabetic, smokes and also has lupus, a condition known to increase the risk of infection with or without immunosuppressive drugs [16]. *A. pittii* is widely distributed in the environment and may contaminate food and animals, thus humans could acquire skin and/or oral carriage which subsequently favours infection [13, 17]. A study with more patients would allow us to better characterize the virulence of *A. pittii* and the host-pathogenic interaction but seems difficult due to the low prevalence of this type of infection.

With regard to drug choice, on the one hand, initial empiric antimicrobial therapy may be inappropriate if following standard practice guidelines for community acquired pneumonia, except if a fluoroquinolone is chosen [18]. On the other hand, second line treatment is ultimately most often appropriate because *A. pittii* is relatively susceptible to antibiotics used in this case [4, 6]. The most effective drugs are carbapenems [5, 10]. Piperacillin/tazobactam, ticarcillin/clavulanate, ceftazidime or fluoroquinolone are alternative choices [10, 19]. However, carbapenem resistance does occur frequently in the *A. calcoaceticus-baumannii* complex [5] and *A. pittii* ST249 has been described in association with the production of a carbapenemase GIM-1 [9]. In these cases, amikacin or colistin often remain the only therapeutic option.

In conclusion, one case of *A. pittii* community-acquired pneumonia revealed by cavitary lung lesions with a sub-acute clinical course lead to describing its low virulence profile. In the setting of immunocompromised patients and tobacco consumption, evaluation of *A. pittii* as a possible cause of community-acquired pneumonia should be considered, particularly in case of unsatisfactory response to first line antimicrobial therapy. The clinical course seems to be less severe than when caused by *A. baumannii*. As we can now more easily identify *A. pittii* in the *A. calcoaceticus-baumannii* complex, studying more patients could be interesting to asses the clinical features of this type of pneumonia.

Abbreviations
BAL: Broncho-alveolar lavage; BFI: BioFilm Indice; CFU: Colony Forming Unit; CT-scan: Computed tomography; EUCAST: European Committee on Antimicrobial Susceptibility Testing; LT50: Median time required to kill 50% of the Fer-15 *C. elegans* population; MALDI-TOF: Matrix Assisted Laser Desorption Ionisation/Time Of Flight; MLST: MultiLocus Sequence Typing; NAB ST2: *A. baumannii* strain belonging to international clone II/ST2; OP50: Non-pathogenic *E. coli*

Acknowledgements
Dr. Julie Carr, for reviewing this manuscript.

Funding
This research did not receive any specific grant from funding agencies in the public, commercial, or not-for-profit sectors.

Authors' contributions
RL contributed to study design, literature search, data collection, analysis and interpretation, and writing. AP contributed to literature search, analysis and interpretation, and writing. EA contributed data collection and critical revision. JPL contributed to study design, literature search, data analysis and interpretation, writing and critical revision. AS contributed to study design, writing and critical revision. All authors read and approved the final manuscript.

Consent for publication
Written consent for potentially identifying information being published as a case report was obtained from patient during admission. Consent was also reconfirmed verbally prior to submission of written article for publication.

Competing interests
None of the authors has any conflict of interest to declare that could influence this work.

Author details
[1]Department of Internal Medicine, Caremeau University Hospital, 29 place du Professeur Debre, Nimes, France. [2]Department of Microbiology, Caremeau University Hospital, 29 place du Professeur Debre, Nimes, France. [3]Department of Infectious Diseases, Caremeau University Hospital, 29 place du Professeur Debre, Nimes, France.

References
1. Gadkowski LB, Stout JE. Cavitary pulmonary disease. Clin Microbiol Rev. 2008;21:305–33.
2. Lee Y-C, Huang Y-T, Tan C-K, Kuo Y-W, Liao C-H, Lee P-I, et al. Acinetobacter Baumannii and Acinetobacter genospecies 13TU and 3 bacteraemia: comparison of clinical features, prognostic factors and outcomes. J Antimicrob Chemother. 2011;66:1839–46.
3. Nemec A, Krizova L, Maixnerova M, van der Reijden TJK, Deschaght P, Passet V, et al. Genotypic and phenotypic characterization of the Acinetobacter calcoaceticus–Acinetobacter Baumannii Complex with the proposal of Acinetobacter pittii sp. nov. (formerly Acinetobacter genomic species 3) and Acinetobacter nosocomialis sp. nov. (formerly Acinetobacter genomic species 13TU). Res. Microbiol. 2011;162:393–404.
4. Chusri S, Chongsuvivatwong V, Rivera JI, Silpapojakul K, Singkhamanan K, McNeil E, et al. Clinical outcomes of hospital-acquired infection with Acinetobacter nosocomialis and Acinetobacter pittii. Antimicrob Agents Chemother. 2014;58:4172–9.
5. De Vos D, Pirnay J-P, Bilocq F, Jennes S, Verbeken G, Rose T, et al. Molecular epidemiology and clinical impact of Acinetobacter calcoaceticus-baumannii complex in a Belgian burn wound center. PLoS One. 2016;11:e0156237.
6. Vila-Farrés X, Ferrer-Navarro M, Callarisa AE, Martí S, Espinal P, Gupta S, et al. Loss of LPS is involved in the virulence and resistance to colistin of colistin-resistant Acinetobacter nosocomialis mutants selected in vitro. J Antimicrob Chemother. 2015;70:2981–6.
7. Chavant P, Gaillard-Martinie B, Talon R, Hébraud M, Bernardi T. A new device for rapid evaluation of biofilm formation potential by bacteria. J Microbiol Methods. 2007;68:605–12.
8. Olivares E, Badel-Berchoux S, Provot C, Jaulhac B, Prévost G, Bernardi T, et al. The BioFilm ring test: a rapid method for routine analysis of Pseudomonas Aeruginosa biofilm formation kinetics. J Clin Microbiol. 2016;54:657–61.
9. Kaase M, Szabados F, Pfennigwerth N, Anders A, Geis G, Pranada AB, et al. Description of the metallo-β-lactamase GIM-1 in Acinetobacter pittii. J Antimicrob Chemother. 2014;69:81–4.
10. Wisplinghoff H, Paulus T, Lugenheim M, Stefanik D, Higgins PG, Edmond MB, et al. Nosocomial bloodstream infections due to Acinetobacter Baumannii, Acinetobacter pittii and Acinetobacter nosocomialis in the United States. J Inf Secur. 2012;64:282–90.
11. Lázaro-Díez M, Navascués-Lejarza T, Remuzgo-Martínez S, Navas J, Icardo JM, Acosta F, et al. Acinetobacter Baumannii and A. Pittii clinical isolates lack adherence and cytotoxicity to lung epithelial cells in vitro. Microbes Infect. 2016;18:559–64.
12. Na IY, Chung ES, Jung C-Y, Kim DH, Shin J, Kang K, et al. Comparison of the virulence-associated phenotypes of five species of Acinetobacter Baumannii Complex. J Microbiol Biotechnol. 2016;26:171–9.
13. Anstey NM, Currie BJ, Hassell M, Palmer D, Dwyer B, Seifert H. Community-acquired Bacteremic Acinetobacter pneumonia in tropical Australia is caused by diverse strains of Acinetobacter Baumannii, with carriage in the throat in at-risk groups. J Clin Microbiol. 2002;40:685–6.
14. Antunes LCS, Visca P, Towner KJ. Acinetobacter Baumannii: evolution of a global pathogen. Pathog Dis. 2014;71:292–301.
15. Peleg AY, Seifert H, Paterson DL. Acinetobacter Baumannii: emergence of a successful pathogen. Clin Microbiol Rev. 2008;21:538–82.
16. Luijten RK Cuppen BV, Bijlsma JW, Derksen RH Serious infections in systemic lupus erythematosus with a focus on pneumococcal infections. Lupus 2014; 23:1512–1516.

17. Al Atrouni A, Joly-Guillou M-L, Hamze M, Kempf M. Reservoirs of non-baumannii Acinetobacter species. Front Microbiol. 2016;7:49.

18. Mandell LA, Wunderink RG, Anzueto A, Bartlett JG, Campbell GD, Dean NC, et al. Infectious Diseases Society of America/American Thoracic Society consensus guidelines on the Management of Community-Acquired Pneumonia in adults. Clin Infect Dis. 2007;44:S27–72.

19. Burgess DS, Frei CR. Comparison of beta-lactam regimens for the treatment of gram-negative pulmonary infections in the intensive care unit based on pharmacokinetics/pharmacodynamics. J Antimicrob Chemother. 2005;56:893–8.

Distribution of *Streptococcus pneumoniae* serotypes in the northeast macro-region of São Paulo state/Brazil after the introduction of conjugate vaccine

Marta Inês Cazentini Medeiros[1], Samanta Cristine Grassi Almeida[2], Maria Luiza Leopoldo Silva Guerra[2], Paulo da Silva[3], Ana Maria Machado Carneiro[3] and Denise de Andrade[4,5*] (ID)

Abstract

Background: Infections caused by *Streptococcus pneumoniae* (Spn) still challenge health systems around the world, even with advances in vaccination programs. The present study evaluated the frequency of various Spn serotypes isolated in Regional Health Care Network 13 (RRAS 13), which includes the regional health departments (RHDs) of Araraquara, Barretos, Franca and Ribeirão Preto, especially after the introduction of 10-valent pneumococcal conjugate vaccine (PCV10) in 2010.

Methods: The analyzed Spn strains were isolated from patients with invasive pneumococcal diseases (IPDs) and then sent to Adolfo Lutz Institute (ALI) for further confirmative identification tests during the period from 1998 to 2013. The samples were from the cities in RRAS13, which is located in the Northeast region of São Paulo State, and totals 90 municipalities.

Results: We analyzed strains isolated from 796 patients. They were predominantly: men (58.9%); 20 to 60 years old (32.2%); evaluated from 2003 to 2010 (60.2%); and diagnosed with meningitis (45.7%) and pneumonia (45.0%), the most common invasive pneumococcal diseases. In 2010, serotypes 3, 19F, 1, 23F, 6A and 6B were among the most frequent, while serotypes 3, 12F, 14, 6A, 18C, 8 and 6B were more common after the introduction of PCV10. Serotypes 14, 19F and 3 were more frequent in meningitis, while serotypes 14, 3 and 1 prevailed in pneumonia. After 2010, there was a decrease in serotypes 14, 1, 23F and 5 and an increase in serotypes 3, 12F, 11A and 8, which were not present in the vaccine.

Conclusions: The present study noted the increase in serotypes 3, 12F, 11A and 8 after vaccination. None of those serotypes are included in the available conjugate vaccines, which highlights the importance of continued monitoring of IPDs in order to measure the disease burden in the population in the long term and provide new epidemiological information to determine the impact of PCV10 in Brazil.

Keywords: *Streptococcus pneumoniae*, pneumococcus, serotype, conjugate vaccine

* Correspondence: dandrade@eerp.usp.br
[4]Ribeirão Preto College of Nursing at University of São Paulo - Ribeirão Preto, São Paulo, Brazil
[5]Ribeirão Preto College of Nursing, University of São Paulo, Ribeirão Preto, São Paulo, Brazil

Background[1]

Streptococcus pneumoniae, or pneumoccocus, represents a big threat to human health. Invasive pneumococcal diseases (IPDs) are the most serious form of pneumococcal disease, and involve pneumonia accompanied by bacteremia, meningitis, peritonitis, bacteremia, sepsis, and arthritis, among others [1]. Around 30 to 50% of pneumococcal pneumonia cases are associated with bacteremia. In the Latin American region, pneumonia is among the leading causes of hospitalization and death in children under 5 years old and the elderly over 60 years old. Bacterial meningitis is less common than pneumonia, but has a higher risk of sequelae and death [2].

Ninety-four pneumococcal serotypes have been identified, after the inclusion of serotypes 6C, 6D, 11E and 20A/20B [3–6]. They are part of the normal ecological environment of the nasopharynx, with pathogenic potential for humans when they reach normally sterile parts of the body. The serotypes are variably distributed according to region, age, and clinical syndrome over time, and they vary in virulence, invasiveness and ability to acquire drug resistance [7].

Due the increasing spread of pneumococcal resistance to antibiotics, there is heightened interest in preventing infections by using vaccination. The use of conjugate vaccines, in addition to decreasing the incidence of pneumococcal infection, reduces the consumption of antibiotics and consequently the circulation of resistant strains [8]. There are different types of pneumococcal vaccines, classified by the amount of serotypes in their composition [9]. Vaccination is unquestionably the best tool to prevent pneumococcal disease, but immunity develops specifically according to serotype [10].

Limited vaccine coverage represents a big obstacle to controlling the diseases associated with pneumococcus, as does the difficulty of including a greater number of antigens in conjugated vaccines. This means that vaccinated individuals remain susceptible to non-vaccine serotypes, which may be capable of causing diseases [10]. Therefore, there is a need to know the epidemiological profile of different communities in order to provide data to support the development of vaccines [11].

The present study aimed to describe the distribution of cases of IPDs in the Northeast region of São Paulo State according to demographic characteristics and pneumococcal serotype strains isolated from 1998 to 2013, in order to relate it to the National Vaccination Program that was implemented in 2010.

Methods

This was a retrospective follow-up study, based on microbiological information for pneumococci isolated from individuals with IPDs during the 16-year period from 1998 to 2013. Analysis was performed on strains of

S. pneumoniae isolated from sterile sites. The patients included in this study lived in the northeast region of São Paulo State - Brazil, in cities belonging to Regional Health Network 13 (RRAS 13), with approximately 90 municipalities, covering the Regional Health Departments (RHDs) of Araraquara, Barretos, Franca and Ribeirão Preto [12].

Microbiological information on the serotypes was collected (Serotype and antimicrobial susceptibility profile) from the database of the Regional Laboratory Center/ALI of Ribeirão Preto and the Central ALI/São Paulo.

Statistical analysis used the chi-square test between two or more independent samples to verify the dependence or independence of the variables. Thus, possible associations between the presence of specific serotypes and age, distribution of cases according to period and age, and clinical diagnosis and serotype were investigated; a p value of <0.05 was adopted. The Statistical Package for Social Sciences (SPSS) version 19.0 was used.

The study was approved by a Research Ethics Committee, linked to Ribeirão Preto College of Nursing, University of São Paulo and obtained permission from regional health departments for their achievement.

Results

For the 796 strains of *S. pneumoniae* analyzed, the age range of the patients was from less than 1 month up to 93 years old (mean = 25.1, SD = 25.9, median = 13.0). A total of 58.9% of the isolates were from male patients. There was a higher number of cases in the age group of 20 to 60 years old (32.2%) and in the period from 2003 to 2010 (60.2%).

The most frequent IPDs were meningitis (45.7%) and pneumonia (45.0%), while others represented 9.3% of the cases. The RHD of Ribeirão Preto had higher occurrence of pneumonia (56.3%), differing from the other municipalities, where meningitis was more frequent (92.6% - Araraquara, 88.6% - Franca, 93.6% - Barretos). Blood was the biological material most often used for diagnosis (45.6%).

The distribution of IPDs by age changed over time, with a progressive decrease in the percentage of IPDs in individuals under 20 years old and an increase in those over 20 years old. From 1998 to 2002, the highest frequency of IPDs was observed in children under 5 years old, with a predominance in those less than 1 year old. From 2010 on, besides a decrease in the proportion of IPDs in the age groups covered by the vaccine, there was a reduction of cases in individuals under 20 years old (Table 1).

We found 59.4% of IPDs in individuals 5 years and older. Of these, 16.0% had meningitis. Among children under 5 years old, meningitis affected more of those under 1 year of age (8.2%) (Table 2). There was no significant change in the serotypes included in the 7-valent

Table 1 Age and major invasive pneumococcal diseases (IPDs) in patients treated in Regional Health Care Network 13, according to the isolation period, 1998–2013

Age group (years)	Period						Total	
	1998–2002		2003–2010		2011–2013			
	n°	%*	n°	%*	n°	%*	n°	%
<1	51	23.5	54	11.8	7	7.4	112	14.5
1–2	36	16.6	49	10.7	3	3.1	88	11.4
2–5	37	17.1	52	11.3	9	9.5	98	12.7
Subtotal (<5)	124	57.1	155	33.8	19	20.0	298	38.7
5–20	36	16.6	68	14.8	6	6.3	110	14.3
20–60	45	20.7	164	35.7	47	49.5	256	32.2
≥60	12	5.5	72	15.7	23	24.2	107	13.9
Subtotal (≥5)	93	42.9	304	66.2	76	80.0	473	61.3
Ignored[a]	5	0.6	20	2.5	0	0.0	25	31
IPD								
Meningitis	124	55.8	195	40.7	45	47.4	364	45.7
Pneumonia	79	35.6	240	50.1	39	41.0	358	45.0
Bacteremia/sepsis	7	3.2	34	7.1	8	8.4	49	6.2
Other[b]	12	5.4	10	2.1	3	3.2	25	3.1
Total	222	100.0	479	100.0	95	100.0	796	100.0

%* refers to the total IPD cases in each period
[a]Patients without information on their age
[b]Abscess, arthritis, peritonitis, pancreatitis, cirrhosis, surgical site infection and appendicitis

Table 2 Age groups of patients who received care in Regional Health Care Network 13, according to main IPDs, from 1998 to 2013

Age group (years)	Diagnosis								Total	
	Meningitis		Pneumonia		Bact/sepsis		Other[b]			
	n°	%*	n°	%*	n°	%*	n°	%*	n°	%
<1	65	8.2	42	5.3	5	0.6	0	0.0	112	14.1
1–2	29	3.6	54	6.8	4	0.5	1	0.1	88	11.0
2–5	33	4.1	59	7.4	4	0.5	2	0.3	98	12.3
Subtotal < 5	127	16.0	155	19.5	13	1.6	3	0.4	298	37.4
5–20	57	7.2	44	5.5	4	0.5	5	0.6	110	13.8
20–60	127	16.0	101	12.7	19	2.4	9	1.1	256	32.2
≥60	42	5.3	50	6.3	9	1.1	6	0.8	107	2.1
Subtotal ≥ 5	226	28.4	195	24.5	32	4.0	20	2.5	473	59.4
Ignored[a]	11	1.4	8	1.0	4	0.5	2	0.3	25	3.1
Total	364	45.7	358	45.0	49	6.2	25	3.1	796	100.0

%* refers to the total cases
[a]Patients without information on their age
[b]Abscess, arthritis, peritonitis, pancreatitis, cirrhosis, surgical site infection and appendicitis

pneumococcal conjugated vaccine (PCV7) between 1998 and 2002 (45.9%) and 2003–2010 (48.2%) (Table 3).

After the introduction of PCV10, considering the periods 2003–2010 and 2011–2013, the total number of IPDs decreased from 479 to 95, associated mainly with the reduction of vaccine serotypes. The proportion of serotypes included in 13-valent pneumococcal conjugate vaccine (PCV13) increased from 2003 to 2010 to 2011–2013, as well as non-vaccine serotypes 12F, 11A, 8, 9 N, 15C and 6C. From 1998 to 2010, serotype 14 was the most prevalent, but after 2010 this serotype decreased from 19.6 to 6.3% (Table 3).

Fifty-four pneumococcus serotypes were identified. Serotypes 14, 3, 19F, 1, 6A, 6B, 23F, 9 V, 18C, 19A, 12F, 4, 7F, 5, 11A, 22F, 8 and 9 N represented 83.3% of the cases. Serotype 14 was the most common serotype in the four RHDs studied. In descending order, serotypes 3, 1, 19F, 6A, 6B, 19A, 23F and 9 V were the most isolated in the RHD of Ribeirão Preto; 3, 18C, 19F, 9 V, 11A, 6A, 17F and 23F in the RHD of Araraquara; 23F, 3, 19F, 22F, 6A, 6B and 7F in the RHD of Franca; and 6B, 3, 19F, 1, 18C, 19A and 23F in the RHD of Barretos. Note that serotypes 14, 3, 19F and 23F were the most frequent in the four RHDs.

In the period preceding the introduction of PCV10, there was predominance, in descending order, of serotypes 14, 3, 19F, 1, 23F, 6B and 6A. After the introduction of vaccination, there was a predominance of serotypes 3, 12F, 14, 6A, 18C, 8 and 6B. Up to 2010, serotype 14 was the most frequent, with a significant decrease in the last studied period; it was surpassed by serotype 3 after 2011. Evaluating all age groups and serotypes with 10 or more isolates, there was a statistically significant decrease in serotypes 14, 1, 23F and 5 and increase in serotypes 3, 12F, 11A and 8 (Table 4).

Serotypes 14 and 3 were the most often associated with meningitis and pneumonia. Serotype 1 was not detected among the main causes of meningitis (Table 5). Serotype 1 greatly affected patients from 2 to 20 years old (Table 6).

Serotype 3 occurred mostly in adults. However, its importance was also noted in children under 2 years old. In children under 5 years old, 83% of the isolates were of serotypes 14, 6A, 6B, 3, 1, 18C, 19A, 23F, 19F and 9 V. In children over 5 years of age, 71% of pneumococci were related to serotypes 3, 19F, 14, 1, 23F, 9 V, 12F, 4, 6A, 6B, 19A, 18C, 7F and 11A (Table 6).

During the study, prevalence of serotype 19A did not change, being more isolated in children under 5 years of age, especially in those less than 1 year old. Serotypes 14, 6B, 6A, 19A and 3 were among the main causes of IPDs in children under 2 years old. In the age group of 60 years old or older, serotypes 3, 9 V, 19F and 23F were the most common (Table 6).

Table 3 Vaccine and non-vaccine serotypes of *S. pneumoniae* identified in patients with invasive pneumococcal disease cared for in Regional Health Care Network 13, according to the isolation period, 1998 to 2013

Serotypes	Periods						Total	
	1998–2002		2003–2010		2011–2013			
	n°	%*	n°	%*	n°	%*	n°	%
PCV7								
14	45	20.3	94	19.6	6	6.3	145	18.2
19F	15	6.8	28	5.8	3	3.2	46	5.8
6B	7	3.2	27	5.6	4	4.2	38	4.8
23F	8	3.6	29	6.1	0	0.0	37	4.6
9V	6	2.7	25	5.2	3	3.2	34	4.3
18C	13	5.9	15	3.1	5	5.3	33	4.1
4	8	3.6	13	2.7	3	3.2	24	3.0
Total PCV7	102	45.9	231	48.2	24	25.3	357	44.8
Included PCV10								
1	12	5.4	31	6.5	0	0.0	43	5.4
7 F	7	3.2	12	2.5	2	2.1	21	2.6
5	14	6.3	1	0.2	2	2.1	17	2.1
Total PCV10	33	14.9	44	9.2	4	4.2	81	10.2
Included PCV13								
3	14	6.3	42	8.8	17	17.9	73	9.2
6A	13	5.9	20	4.2	6	6.3	39	4.9
19A	13	5.9	18	3.8	2	2.1	33	4.1
Total PCV13	40	18.0	80	16.7	25	26.3	145	18.2
Non-vaccine								
12F	1	0.5	18	3.8	9	9.5	28	3.5
11A	0	0.0	12	2.5	3	3.2	15	1.9
22F	3	1.4	12	2.5	0	0.0	15	1.9
8	2	0.9	5	1.0	5	5.3	12	1.5
9N	1	0.5	6	1.3	3	3.2	10	1.3
10A	3	1.4	5	1.0	1	1.1	9	1.1
15C	2	0.9	3	0.6	4	4.2	9	1.1
17F	3	1.4	5	1.0	0	0.0	8	1.0
6C	1	0.5	3	0.6	4	4.2	8	1.0
18A	4	1.8	3	0.6	0	0.0	7	0.9
18B	2	0.9	5	1.0	0	0.0	7	0.9
23B	1	0.5	5	1.0	0	0.0	6	0.8
NT	3	1.4	3	0.6	0	0.0	6	0.8
NR	0	0.0	2	0.4	0	0.0	2	0.3
Other[a]	21	9.5	37	7.7	13	13.7	71	8.9
Total non- vaccine	47	21.2	124	25.9	42	44.2	215	27.0
Total	222	100.0	479	100.0	95	100.0	796	100.0

%* refers to the total casos of IPDs in each period, Other [a]serotypes with less than 6 isolates
NT Non-typable, *NR* Not carried out (unviable strain)
PCV7 – valent pneumococcal conjugate vaccine
PCV10–10-valent pneumococcal conjugate vaccine
PCV13–13-valent pneumococcal conjugate vaccine

Considering the most common serotypes and cross-immunity between 6A and 6B, the estimated vaccine serotypes isolated from children under 5 years old reached 69.2% for PCV10 and 87.0% for PCV13. However, for those over 5 years old, the percentage of serotypes present in PCV10 and PCV13 was 46.0% and 65.2%, respectively. In the analyzed period, serotypes 6A, 3 and 19A represented 17.8%, 15.9 and 19.2%, respectively, in patients younger than 5 years old and older than 5 years old (Table 6).

Discussion

In the present study, blood was the biological material most often used for diagnosis. The isolation of pneumococcus in culture is considered the gold standard for the definition of pneumococcal disease, although the positivity of blood culture is low, especially in children [13]. It is worth highlighting the importance of routine blood culture for patients suspected of having bacteremia, particularly in relation to the meningitis diagnosis, in which blood culture is often neglected when just the culture of cerebrospinal fluid is targeted [14].

Besides the low positivity of blood culture, another aggravating factor for proper diagnosis, especially for pneumonia, is cases that are cared for in clinics and treated empirically, without collection of biological samples for identification of microorganisms. Diagnosis is also hampered by previous use of antibiotics before the collection of biological material [15]. It is estimated that around 50% of cases of pneumonia remain undiagnosed [16]. Therefore, the extent of pneumococcal disease is underestimated and difficult to assess.

In the present study, one possible reason for the higher frequency of meningitis is its compulsory notification and a more active surveillance system when compared to pneumonia.

After the introduction of PCV7 in the United States, beyond the direct effect on the reduction of cases of pneumococcal disease in the vaccinated population, the herd effect was also observed, which acted indirectly to prevent disease in non-vaccinated individuals as a consequence of reduced circulation of vaccine serotypes [10]. The data presented in the current study were through 2013, so a further observation period in the unvaccinated population would be necessary to detect the full effect of herd immunity.

In Brazil, PCV7 was introduced in 2002, and was provided free of charge only to people at high risk of acquiring IPD and in private clinics, reaching a small portion of the population, verifying the absence of response to this intervention.

In 2010, Brazil introduced PCV10 into its routine National Immunization Program, aiming to minimize the impact of pneumococcal disease. Research on the

Table 4 Main serotypes of *S. pneumoniae* isolated from patients with invasive pneumococcal disease cared for in Regional Health Care Network 13, according to the isolation period,1998 to 2013

Serotypes	1998–2002 n = 222		Period				2011–2013 n = 95		Total n = 796		p value
			2003–2010 n = 479		Subtotal n = 701						
	n°	%*	n°	%*	n°	%	n°	%*	n°	%	
14	45	20.3	94	19.6	139	19.8	6	6.3	145	18.2	**0.006**
3	14	6.3	42	8.8	56	8.0	17	17.9	73	9.2	**0.004**
19F	15	6.8	28	5.8	43	6.1	3	3.2	46	5.8	0.451
1	12	5.4	31	6.5	43	6.1	0	0.0	43	5.4	**0.039**
6A	13	5.9	20	4.2	33	4.7	6	6.3	39	4.9	0.501
6B	7	3.2	27	5.6	34	4.9	4	4.2	38	4.8	0.344
23F	8	3.6	29	6.1	37	5.3	0	0.0	37	4.6	**0.026**
9V	6	2.7	25	5.2	31	4.4	3	3.2	34	4.3	0.262
18C	13	5.9	15	3.1	28	4.0	5	5.3	33	4.1	0.205
19A	13	5.9	18	3.8	31	4.4	2	2.1	33	4.1	0.245
12F	1	0.5	18	3.8	19	2.7	9	9.5	28	3.5	**<0.001**
4	8	3.6	13	2.7	21	3.0	3	3.2	24	3.0	0.811
7F	7	3.2	12	2.5	19	2.7	2	2.1	21	2.6	0.832
5	14	6.3	1	0.2	15	2.1	2	2.1	17	2.1	**<0.001**
11A	0	0.0	12	2.5	12	1.7	3	3.2	15	1.9	**0.047**
22F	3	1.4	12	2.5	15	2.1	0	0.0	15	1.9	0.206
8	2	0.9	5	1.0	7	1.0	5	5.3	12	1.5	**0.006**
9N	1	0.5	6	1.3	7	1.0	3	3.2	10	1.3	0.140

%* refers to the total IPD cases in each period
p values in bold are significant

effectiveness of PCV10 implementation for public health services in Brazil has indicated a reduction in children's hospitalizations for pneumonia [17]; protection of nasopharyngeal pneumococcal carriers against vaccine serotypes [18]; and reduction of IPDs cases in all age groups, especially in children under 2 years old [19].

In 2011 and 2012, vaccination coverage of PCV10 in Brazil was 82.1% and 88.4%, respectively [20]. In the cities of Ribeirão Preto, Araraquara, Franca and Barretos, the coverage of PCV10 in children under 5 years old was around 86% [21], not reaching the ideal rate of 95% recommended by the Ministry of Health for efficient vaccination coverage for PCV10. In addition, completion of 3 doses of the vaccine was necessary in order to ensure the reduction of IPD cases [22], which explains the persistence after 2010 of some serotypes contained in the vaccine.

Classically, pneumococcal diseases mainly affect children and the elderly [1]. However, an understanding of pneumococcal epidemiology should involve all age groups. In mid-2012 in Argentina and Bolivia, most cases of IPDs occurred in patients between 2 and 5 years old. In Brazil, there was a higher incidence in people between 30 and 49 years old [23], coinciding with our data.

Meningitis is commonly associated with children under 2 years old, and mostly under 1 year old [14]. Contradicting our data, in Uberlândia, the Federal District [24] and Rio Grande do Norte [25], pneumococcal meningitis prevailed in children under 5 years old. In the region studied, meningitis occurred mainly in adults.

From 2001 to 2011 in Brazil, 282,593 cases of meningitis were identified; 100,559 of those were bacterial meningitis, of which 13,469 were related to *S. pneumoniae* [14]. From 1999 to 2010, it was observed that 32.5% of bacterial meningitis in Rio Grande do Sul was caused by pneumococcus [26]. In the present study, the percentage of patients with meningitis was higher than that.

Considering that in Brazil, PCV10 is given free only to children under 2 years old, the occurrence of IPDs in patients over 5 years old is relevant information, especially taking into account that in recent decades, increases in the elderly Brazilian population have accelerated [27]. This highlights the importance of constant surveillance, aiming to detect changes in the circulation of serotypes in this age group.

With the use of conjugate vaccines, a decrease in vaccine serotypes, and an increase in those not included in the vaccines, a phenomenon known as serotype

Table 5 *S. pneumoniae* serotypes isolated from patients with invasive pneumococcal disease cared for in Regional Health Care Network 13 according to the main IPDs diagnosed, 1998 to 2013

Serotype	Meningitis		Pneumonia		Bact/sepsis		Other		Total	
	n°	%*	n°	%*	n°	%*	n°	%*	n°	%*
14	45	5.7	95	11.9	3	0.4	2	0.3	145	18.2
3	34	4.3	35	4.4	4	0.5	0	0.0	73	9.2
19F	30	3.8	12	1.5	3	0.4	1	0.1	46	5.8
1	7	0.9	33	4.1	1	0.1	2	0.3	43	5.4
6A	22	2.8	12	1.5	0	0.0	5	0.6	39	4.9
6B	15	1.9	19	2.4	3	0.4	1	0.1	38	4.8
23F	16	2.0	16	2.0	3	0.4	2	0.3	37	4.6
9V	19	2.4	12	1.5	3	0.4	0	0.0	34	4.3
18C	22	2.8	8	1.0	2	0.3	1	0.1	33	4.1
19A	15	1.9	14	1.8	3	0.4	1	0.1	33	4.1
12F	21	2.6	4	0.5	2	0.3	1	0.1	28	3.5
4	7	0.9	14	1.8	2	0.3	1	0.1	24	3.0
7F	8	1.0	9	1.1	2	0.3	2	0.3	21	2.6
5	4	0.5	12	1.5	0	0.0	1	0.1	17	2.1
11A	10	1.3	5	0.6	0	0.0	0	0.0	15	1.9
22F	8	1.0	7	0.9	0	0.0	0	0.0	15	1.9
8	4	0.5	6	0.8	2	0.3	0	0.0	12	1.5
9N	2	0.3	5	0.6	3	0.4	0	0.0	10	1.3
Other	75	9.4	40	5.0	13	1.6	5	0.6	133	16.7
Total	364	45.7	358	45.0	49	6.2	25	3.1	796	100.0

%* refers to the total cases

replacement has been observed in several countries [28–33]. Therefore, when evaluating the effect of pneumococcal vaccines, the overall rate of disease occurrence may not decrease significantly, because of an increase in other non-vaccine serotypes [29].

The increase in non-vaccine serotypes detected in the present study suggests serotype replacement. This conflicts with a study done in São Paulo that showed no significant increase in non-vaccine serotypes in IPDs after the introduction of PCV10 [19]. Fluctuations in the occurrence of serotypes can happen naturally or by selective pressure caused by vaccines, so increases in non vaccine serotypes should be carefully evaluated. Complexes and varied factors are involved in the replacement phenomenon, making it difficult to analyze [34].

Currently, the most advanced technology for pneumococcal vaccine is polysaccharides containing capsular conjugate vaccines linked to a carrier protein. However, there have been studies of the implementation of a new generation of vaccines based on common protein components of *S. pneumoniae* that provide serotype independent immunity [35]. According to the World Health Organization, adoption of this new technology will need to provide equivalent or greater benefit than that obtained with conjugate vaccines to prevent pneumococcal disease [36].

Thus, changes in the incidence of pneumococcal serotypes associated with the disease after the use of conjugate vaccines must be distinguished from normal serotype temporal changes [1].

In this scenario, serotype replacement after vaccination may raise questions regarding the effect of this intervention. However, some non-vaccine serotypes seem to be less invasive than those present in the vaccine, so that reduction of IPDs becomes a more positive effect than eventual serotype replacement [37].

The target for prevention of pneumococcal diseases with vaccines is the bacterial capsule. The effect of vaccination can be reduced by the classical phenomenon of capsular exchange, in which a vaccine serotype changes its capsular locus and begins to express other non-vaccine serotypes [38].

Noteworthy is an increase in serotypes 3, 12F, 11A and 8, reinforcing the need for continued vigilance. With the exception of Serotype 3 included in PCV13, no other serotypes are included in the available vaccine formulations (PCV10 and PCV13).

An example of serotype replacement is what happened with 19A, which is cited as one of the emerging serotypes in the United States since the introduction of PCV7 [30]. However, it stabilized after an increase in the use of PCV13, in which it is included [39]. During the present study, prevalence of serotype 19A did not change, which is similar to what was reported in São Paulo [19]. There was a predominance of 19A in children under 5 years old. This is similar to results found in the United States, where the frequency of this serotype in children under 6 years old was substantial [40].

In Brazil, as in the Caribbean and some other Latin American countries, there is low frequency of serotype 19A [2]. Although a case-control study on the impact of PCV10 in Brazil showed cross-protection between serotypes 19F and 19A [41], an increase in the circulation of Serotype 19A was reported in 2012 [23].

In the Central Laboratory of Paraná, in 2001–2002, pneumococcus was the most common etiologic agent in acute bacterial meningitis, with higher incidence of serotypes 14, 23F and 3 [42]. In our study, serotypes 14, 3 and 19F were more involved in meningitis. The potential for invasion expressed by Serotype 1 has been linked to outbreaks and fatal cases of meningitis in Africa [43] and in some countries in Europe [44], but in the present study, Serotype 1 was not detected among the main causes of meningitis. In Latin America, this serotype has been considered a major cause of IPDs in all ages [45].

Serotype 3 has a specific virulence factor for pneumonia associated with severe disease cases [46], especially

Table 6 Main *S. pneumoniae* serotypes isolated from patients with invasive pneumococcal disease cared for in Regional Health Care Network 13, according to age, from 1998 to 2013

Serotype	Age group (years)																Total		p value
	<1 n = 112		1 2 n = 88		2 5 n = 98		Subtotal < 5 n = 298		5 20 n = 110		20 60 n = 256		≥60 n = 107		Subtotal ≥ 5 n = 473		n = 771		
	n°	%*	n°	%*	n°	%	n°	%*	n°	%*	n°	%*	n°	%*	n°	%	n°	%	
14	37	33.0	36	40.9	38	38.8	**111**	**37.2**	8	7.3	15	5.9	7	6.5	**30**	**6.3**	141	18.3	**<0.001**
3	8	7.1	5	5.7	3	3.1	**16**	**5.4**	5	4.5	34	13.3	17	15.9	**56**	**11.8**	72	9.3	**0.001**
19F	3	2.7	1	1.1	5	5.1	**9**	**3.0**	11	10.0	13	5.1	9	8.4	**33**	**7.0**	42	5.4	**0.005**
1	3	2.7	2	2.3	11	11.2	**16**	**5.4**	16	14.5	7	2.7	3	2.8	**26**	**5.5**	42	5.4	**<0.001**
6A	10	8.9	3	3.4	8	8.2	**21**	**7.0**	7	6.4	9	3.5	2	1.9	**18**	**3.8**	39	5.1	**0.079**
6B	6	5.4	10	11.4	3	3.1	**19**	**6.4**	0	0.0	13	5.1	5	4.7	**18**	**3.8**	37	4.8	**0.012**
23F	4	3.6	5	5.7	2	2.0	**11**	**3.7**	6	5.5	12	4.7	7	6.5	**25**	**5.3**	36	4.7	0.696
9V	4	3.6	4	4.5	3	3.1	**11**	**3.7**	5	4.5	8	3.1	10	9.3	**23**	**4.9**	34	4.4	0.167
18C	6	5.4	4	4.5	6	6.1	**16**	**5.4**	8	7.3	5	2.0	3	2.8	**16**	**3.4**	32	4.2	0.174
19A	10	8.9	3	3.4	3	3.1	**16**	**5.4**	2	1.8	9	3.5	6	5.6	**17**	**3.6**	33	4.3	0.123
12F	1	0.9	1	1.1	1	1.0	**3**	**1.0**	4	3.6	15	5.9	4	3.7	**23**	**4.9**	26	3.4	**0.074**
4	0	0.0	0	0.0	2	2.0	**2**	**0.7**	2	1.8	16	6.2	4	3.7	**22**	**4.7**	24	3.1	**0.007**
7F	2	1.8	2	2.3	1	1.0	**5**	**1.7**	3	2.7	9	3.5	3	2.8	**15**	**3.2**	20	2.6	0.825
5	2	1.8	3	3.4	1	1.0	**6**	**2.0**	3	2.7	6	2.3	0	0.0	**9**	**1.9**	15	1.9	0.531
11A	0	0.0	0	0.0	0	0.0	**0**	**0.0**	2	1.8	10	3.9	2	1.9	**14**	**3.0**	14	1.8	**0.036**
22F	1	0.9	0	0.0	1	1.0	**2**	**0.7**	1	0.9	7	2.7	3	2.8	**11**	**2.3**	13	1.7	0.404
8	1	0.9	0	0.0	0	0.0	**1**	**0.3**	0	0.0	9	3.5	1	0.9	**10**	**2.1**	11	1.4	**0.027**
9N	0	0.0	1	1.1	0	0.0	**1**	**0.3**	3	2.7	5	2.0	1	0.9	**9**	**1.9**	10	1.3	0.357

%* refers to the total number of cases in each age group - 25 patients were excluded for lack of information regarding the age range
p values in bold are significant

in the elderly [47]. This corroborates the present study, in which this serotype was important in pneumonia.

In RRAS 13, serotypes 14, 6B, 6A, 19A and 3 were among the leading causes of IPDs in children younger than 2 years old. Serotypes 14 and 6B are included in PCV10; the remaining serotypes are included only in PCV13. In 2010, countries like Italy [48] and the U.S. [49] replaced PCV7, in use since 2000, with PCV13 because of its higher serotype coverage.

In the age group of 60 years old or older, serotypes 3, 9 V, 19F and 23F were the most common. One study found that in Argentina, most IPDs were caused by serotypes 14, 1 and 5, and in Bolivia the most frequent serotypes were 14, 6B and 18F [23].

Among the specific serotypes of PCV13, serotypes 6A and 19A did not present a significant increase during the course of the present study. Serotype 3 presented a progressive increase (Tables 3 and 4), especially in cases of meningitis and pneumonia (Table 5), with emphasis on patients over 20 years old (Table 6). This increase should be monitored to evaluate the circulation of this serotype in the community.

This research has limitations. Because it is a retrospective study, results and conclusions are based on social and microbiological pre-existing information, thus are subject to information bias. In addtion, there is to consider the use of sampling related to convenience criterion adopted for the study.

Conclusions

After the introduction of PCV10, there was a decrease in the overall percentage of vaccine serotypes and an increase in some non-PCV10 serotypes. Of note is the increase in serotypes 3, 12F, 11A and 8 after vaccination. Considering that 12F, 11A, and 8 are not included in the available conjugate vaccines, and the possibility of serotype replacement after the use of conjugated vaccines, it is necessary to implement studies of new vaccine generation based on the common protein component of *S. pneumoniae*, which is capable of providing serotype-independent immunity. The finding of a high percentage of IPDs patients in the 20 to 60 age group highlights the importance of continuous monitoring of IPDs to assess the long-term disease burden in the population, especially in adult patients, who are not routinely covered by vaccination. Such monitoring would provide new epidemiological information to determine the impact of PCV10 in Brazil. Due to the significant increase in

Serotype 3 found in the present study, the use of PCV13 as an alternative to PCV10 in public health services in Brazil could reduce the percentage of IPDs in the studied region.

Abbreviations

ALI: Adolfo Lutz Institute; IPD: Invasive pneumococcal disease; OPAS: Pan American Health Organization; PCV: Valent pneumococcal conjugate vaccine; RHD: Regional health department; RRAS: Regional Health Care Network; SD: standard deviation; Spn: *S. pneumoniae*; SPSS: Statistical Package for Social Sciences; WHO: World Health Organization

Acknowledgements

We thank PROEX-CAPES for financial support.

Funding

Financial support - PROEX-CAPES.

Authors' contributions

MICM, DA and SCGA carried out conception, design, acquisition, analysis and interpretation of study data. MLLSG and PS contributed with the study by participating in its design analysis and helped to draft the manuscript. AMMC contributed to the organization of the ideas that originated the research project, in the analysis and interpretation of the results obtained, as well as in the successive revisions of the manuscript. All authors read and approved the final version of the manuscript.

Consent for publication

Not applicable.

Competing interest

The authors declare that they have no competing interest.

Author details

[1]Regional Laboratory Center of Instituto Adolfo Lutz - Ribeirão Preto and student at College of Nursing at University of São Paulo - Ribeirão Preto, São Paulo, Brazil. [2]Bacteriologic Center of Instituto Adolfo Lutz Central–São Paulo, São Paulo, Brazil. [3]Regional Laboratory Center of Instituto Adolfo Lutz - Ribeirão Preto, São Paulo, Brazil. [4]Ribeirão Preto College of Nursing at University of São Paulo - Ribeirão Preto, São Paulo, Brazil. [5]Ribeirão Preto College of Nursing, University of São Paulo, Ribeirão Preto, São Paulo, Brazil.

References

1. World Health Organization (WHO). Measuring impact of *Streptococcus pneumoniae* and *Haemophilus influenza* type b conjugate vaccination; 2012. http://www.who.int/iris/bitstream/10665/75835/1/WHO_IVB_12.08_eng.pdf Accessed 05.01.14.
2. Organização Panamericana da Saúde (OPAS). Informe regional de SIREVA II, 2009. Tecnologia de Salud para la Calidad de la Atención (THR/HT), OPS/OMS. Washington - D.C, 2010. http://antimicrobianos.com.ar/ATB/wp-content/uploads/2013/01/Informe-Regional-SIREVAII-2009.pdf. Accessed 20.06.4.

3. Calix JJ, et al. Differential occurrence of *Streptococcus pneumoniae* serotype 11E between asymptomatic carriage and invasive pneumococcal disease isolates reflects a unique model of pathogen microevolution. Clin Infect Dis. 2012a;54:794–9.
4. Calix JJ, et al. Biochemical, genetic and serological characterization of two capsule subtypes among *Streptococcus pneumoniae* serotype 20 strains: discovery of a new pneumococcal serotype. J Biol Chem. 2012b;287:27885–94.
5. Jin P, et al. First report of putative *Streptococcus pneumoniae* serotype 6D among nasopharyngeal isolates from Fijian children. J Infect Dis. 2009;200:1375–80.
6. Park IH, et al. Discovery of a new capsular serotype (6C) within serogroup 6 of *Streptococcus pneumoniae*. J Clin Microbiol. 2007;45:1225–33.
7. Valenzuela MT et al. The burden of pneumococcal disease among Latin American and Caribbean children: review of the evidence. Rev Panam Salud Publica 2009;25(3):270–279.
8. Ferigolo LP, Perez VP. Fatores bacterianos de virulência associados a pneumonias e doenças invasivas pelo *Streptococcus pneumoniae*: uma revisão. Rev Fasem Ciências. 2013:4(2).
9. Song JY, Nahm MH, Moseley MA. Clinical implications of pneumococcal serotypes: invasive disease potential, clinical presentations, and antibiotic resistance. J Korean Med Sci. 2013;28:4–15.
10. Centers for Disease Control and Prevention (CDC). Direct and indirect effects of routine vaccination of children with 7-valent pneumococcal conjugate vaccine on incidence of invasive pneumococcal disease – United States, 1998–2003. Morbidity and Mortality Weekly Report (MMWR) 2005; 54(36):893-7 http://www.cdc.gov/mmwr/preview/mmwrhtml/mm5436a1.htm. Accessed 02.01.14.
11. Verani, J.R. et al. Indirect cohort analysis of 10-valent pneumococcal conjugate vaccine effectiveness against vaccine-type and vaccine-related invasive pneumoccal disease. Vaccine, v. 33, p. 6145–6148, 2015.
12. Secretaria de Estado da Saúde (SES). Mapa regional de Saúde. RRAS 13 - Araraquara - Barretos - Franca - Ribeirão Preto. São Paulo 2012. Available from: http://www.fosp.saude.sp.gov.br:443/boletinsRaas/Boletim-RRAS13.pdf. Accessed 06.12.13.
13. Werno AM, Murdoch DR. Medical microbiology: laboratory diagnosis of invasive pneumococcal disease. Clin Infect Dis. 2008;46(6):926–32.
14. Ministério da Saúde - DATASUS. Meningite. Brasília 2011. Available from: http://tabnet.datasus.gov.br/cgi/deftohtm.exe?sinannet/meningite/bases/meninbrnet.def.
15. Sousa AFL, et al. Social representations of community-acquired infection by primary care professionals. Acta paul enferm. 2015;28(5):454–9.
16. Filet Junior TM, MarrieTJ. Burden of community-acquired pneumonia in north American adults. Postgraduate Med J. 2010;122:130–41.
17. Afonso ET, et al. Effect of 10-valent pneumococcal vaccine on pneumonia among children. Brazil Emerg Infect Dis. 2013;19(4):589–97.
18. Andrade AL, et al. Direct effect of 10-valent conjugate pneumococcal vaccination on pneumococcal carriage in children Brazil. PLoS One. 2014;9 http://www.ncbi.nlm.nih.gov/pmc/articles/PMC4043727/pdf/pone.0098128.pdf. Accessed 20.04.15.
19. Santos SR, et al. Serotype distribution of *Streptococcus pneumoniae* isolated in Brazil before and after tem-pneumococcal conjugate vaccine implementation. Vaccine. 2013;31(51):6150–4.
20. Kfouri RA. Construindo um País mais Saudável 40 anos do Programa Nacional de Imunizações 2014. http://www.acaoresponsavel.org.br/40anospni/images/Renato_Kfouri.pdf. Accessed 15.04.15.
21. Ministério da Saúde - DATASUS - PNI -Sistema de Informação do Programa Nacional de Imunizações. Brasília 2014. http://pni.datasus.gov.br/consulta_mrc_13_selecao.php?sel=C02&uf=SP&municipio. Accessed 16.04.15.
22. Scotta MC, et al. Impact of 10-valent pneumococcal non-typeable Haemophilus influenzae protein D conjugate vaccine (PHiD-CV) on childhood pneumonia hospitalizations in Brazil two years after introduction. Vaccine. 2014;32:4495–9.
23. Organização Panamericana da Saúde (OPAS). Informe regional de SIREVA II, 2011. Tecnologia de Salud para la Calidad de la Atención (THR/HT), OPS/OMS. Washington - D.C, 2012. Available from: http://www.paho.org/hq/index.php?option=com_content&view=article&id=5536%3A2011-sirevaii&catid=1591%3Aabout&Itemid=3966&lang=pt.
24. Vieira AC, et al. *Streptococcus pneumoniae*: a study of strains isolated from cerebrospinal fluid. J Ped. 2007;83(1):71–8.
25. Silva WA, et al. Epidemiological profile of acute bacterial meningitis in the state of Rio Grande do Norte. Brazil Rev Soc Bras Med Trop. 2010;43(4):455–7.

26. Schossler JGS, et al. Perfil etiológico das meningites bacterianas, notificadas entre 1999 e 2010 no Rio Grande do Sul. Rev Saúde 2012;38(2):65-76.

27. Instituto Brasileiro de Geografia e Estatística (IBGE). Pesquisa Nacional por Amostra de Domicílios- Censo. Brasil 2010. http://censo2010.ibge.gov.br/resultados.html. [Accessed 13.12.13].

28. Guevara M, et al. Changing epidemiology of invasive pneumococcal disease following increased coverage with the heptavalent conjugate vaccine in Navarre, Spain. Clin Microbiol Infect Dis. 2009;15:1013–9.

29. Aguiar SI, et al. Serotypes 1, 7F and 19A became the leading causes of pediatric invasive pneumococcal infections in Portugal after 7 years of heptavalent conjugate vaccine use. Vaccine. 2010;28(32):5167–73.

30. Hicks LA, et al. Incidence of pneumococcal disease due to non-pneumococcal conjugate vaccine (PCV7) serotypes in the United States during the era of widespread PCV7 vaccination, 1998-2004. J Infect Dis. 2007;196(9):1346–54.

31. Olivier CW. Ten years of experience with the pneumococcal conjugate 7-valent vaccine in children. Méd Malad Infect. 2013;43:309–21.

32. Parra EI, et al. Changes in *Streptococcus pneumoniae* serotype distribution invasive disease and nasopharyngeal carriage after the heptavalent pneumococcal conjugate vaccine introduction in Bogotá, Colombia. Vaccine. 2013;31:4033–8.

33. Wenger JD et al. Invasive pneumococcal disease in Alaskan children: impact of the seven-valent pneumococcal conjugate vaccine and the role of water supply. Pediatr Infect Dis J. 2010;.29:251–6.

34. Iisaacman DJ, McIntosh ED, Reinert RR. Burden of invasive pneumococcal disease and serotype distribution among *Streptococcus pneumoniae* isolates in young children in Europe: impact of the 7-valent pneumococcal conjugate vaccine and considerations for future conjugate vaccines. Intern J Infect Dis. 2010;14(3):197–209.

35. Miyaji EN, et al. Serotype-independent pneumococcal vacines. Cell Mol Life Sci. 2013;70(18):3303–26.

36. World Health Organization (WHO). Relevé épidémiologique hebdomadaire. Pneumococcal conjugate vaccine for childhood immunization – Wkly Epidemiol. Rec Geneva. 2007;12(82):93–104. Available from: http://www.who.int/wer/2012/wer8714.pdf.

37. Scott JR, et al. Impact of more than a decade of pneumococcal conjugate vaccine use on carriage and invasive potential in native American communities. J Infect Dis. 2012;205:280–8.

38. Brueggemann AB, et al. Vaccine escape recombinants emerge after pneumococcal vaccination in the united states. PLoS Patho. 2007;3(11):e 168.

39. Richter SS, et al. Pneumococcal serotypes before and after introduction of conjugate vaccines. Emerg Infect Dis. 2013;19(7):1074–83.

40. Pai R, et al. Postvaccine genetic struture of *Streptococcus pneumoniae* serotype 19A from children in the United States. J Infect Dis. 2005;192(11):1988–95.

41. Domingues CMAS, et al. Effectiveness of ten-valent pneumococcal conjugate vaccine against invasive pneumococcal disease in Brazil: a matched case-control study. Lancet. 2014;2(6):464–71.

42. Rossoni AMO et al. Acute bacterial meningitis caused by *Streptococcus pneumoniae* resistant to the antimicrobian agentes and thir serotypes. Arq Neuro-Psiq. 2008;66(3a):509–15.

43. Gessner BD, Mueller JE, Yaro S. African meningitis belt pneumococcal disease epidemiology indicates a need for an effective serotype 1 containing vaccine, including for older children and adults. J Infect Dis. 2010;10(22):1–10.

44. Motlová J. Distribution of *Streptococcus pneumoniae* serotypes and serogroups among patients with invasive pneumococcal diseases in the Czech Republic in 1996-2003: background data for vaccination strategy. J Epidemiol, Microbiol Immunology. 2005;54(1):3–10.

45. Castañeda E, et al. Laboratory-based surveillance of *Streptococcus pneumoniae* invasive disease in children in 10 Latin American countries: SIREVA II project group, 2000-2005. Pediatr Infect Dis J. 2009;28:265–70.

46. Bender JM, et al. Pneumococcal necrotizing pneumonia in Utah: does serotype matter? Clin Infect Dis. 2008;46(9):1346–52.

47. Miranda JMD. Infecções pneumocócicas invasivas no idoso em Portugal em 2008 e 2009. 2012. Dissertação (Mestrado em Microbiologia Aplicada - Faculdade de Ciências da Universidade de Lisboa), 2012.

48. Martinelli D, et al. Towards the 13-valent pneumococcal conjugate universal vaccination: effectiveness in the transition era between PCV7 and PCV13 in Italy, 2010-2013. Hum Vaccin and Immunotherapy. 2014;10(1):33–9.

49. American Academy of Pediatrics. Policy statement—recommendations for the prevention of *Streptococcus pneumoniae* infections in infants and children: use of 13-valent pneumococcal conjugate vaccine (PCV13) and pneumococcal polysaccharide vaccine (PPSV23). J Pediatr. 2010;126(1):186–90.

Clinical failure with and without empiric atypical bacteria coverage in hospitalized adults with community-acquired pneumonia

Khalid Eljaaly[1,2]* (iD), Samah Alshehri[1,2], Ahmed Aljabri[1,2], Ivo Abraham[2], Mayar Al Mohajer[3], Andre C. Kalil[4] and David E. Nix[2,3]

Abstract

Background: Both typical and atypical bacteria can cause community-acquired pneumonia (CAP); however, the need for empiric atypical coverage remains controversial. Our objective was to evaluate the impact of antibiotic regimens with atypical coverage (a fluoroquinolone or combination of a macrolide/doxycycline with a β-lactam) to a regimen without atypical antibiotic coverage (β-lactam monotherapy) on rates of clinical failure (primary endpoint), mortality, bacteriologic failure, and adverse events, (secondary endpoints).

Methods: We searched the PubMed, EMBASE and Cochrane Library databases for relevant RCTs of hospitalized CAP adults. We estimated risk ratios (RRs) with 95% confidence intervals (CIs) using a fixed-effect model, but used a random-effects model if significant heterogeneity (I^2) was observed.

Results: Five RCTs with a total of 2011 patients were retained. A statistically significant lower clinical failure rate was observed with empiric atypical coverage (RR, 0.851 [95% CI, 0.732–0.99; $P = 0.037$]; $I^2 = 0\%$). The secondary outcomes did not differ between the two study groups: mortality (RR = 0.549 [95% CI, 0.259–1.165, $P = 0.118$], $I^2 = 61.434\%$) bacteriologic failure (RR = 0.816 [95% CI, 0.523–1.272, $P = 0.369$], $I^2 = 0\%$), diarrhea (RR = 0.746 [95% CI, 0.311–1.790, $P = 0.512$], $I^2 = 65.048\%$), and adverse events requiring antibiotic discontinuation (RR = 0.83 [95% CI, 0.542–1.270, $P = 0.39$], $I^2 = 0\%$).

Conclusions: Empiric atypical coverage was associated with a significant reduction in clinical failure in hospitalized adults with CAP. Reduction in mortality, bacterial failure, diarrhea, and discontinuation due to adverse effects were not significantly different between groups, but all estimates favored atypical coverage. Our findings provide support for the current guidelines recommendations to include empiric atypical coverage.

Keywords: Community-acquired pneumonia, Antibiotics, Atypical, Macrolides, Fluoroquinolones

* Correspondence: keljaaly@kau.edu.sa; eljaaly@pharmacy.arizona.edu
[1]Department of Clinical Pharmacy, King Abdulaziz University, P.O. Box 80200, Jeddah Postal code 21589, Saudi Arabia
[2]College of Pharmacy, University of Arizona, Drachman Hall – B306, 1295 N Martin Ave, P.O.Box 210202, Tucson, AZ, USA

Background

Community-acquired pneumonia (CAP) is one of the leading causes of mortality [1–4]. This disease can be caused by a variety of pathogens, including typical and atypical bacteria. The most common typical bacteria causing CAP are *Streptococcus pneumoniae* and *Haemophilus influenzae*. The need to include empiric coverage for atypical bacteria, such as *Mycoplasma pneumoniae*, *Chlamydophila pneumoniae* and *Legionella spp.*, for all hospitalized adult patients is controversial. Adding antibiotics to cover atypical bacteria might increase the likelihood of adverse effects, bacterial resistance, and cost; However, routine empiric atypical coverage is recommended by the current major guidelines for CAP [1–4].

Prior meta-analyses of randomized clinical trials (RCTs) of atypical coverage for CAP have not demonstrated the benefit of empiric atypical coverage in the treatment of hospitalized adults with CAP. It should be noted, however, that these meta-analyses had major limitations despite including a large number of trials [5–7]. The two meta-analyses that found mortality benefit of empiric atypical coverage were based mainly on observational studies [8, 9].

The primary objective of this meta-analysis was to evaluate the impact of atypical coverage on rates of clinical failure with guideline-recommended antibiotic regimens. Rates of mortality, bacteriologic failure, and adverse events were evaluated as secondary outcomes. The meta-analysis was limited to RCTs comparing treatments with atypical coverage (a fluoroquinolone or combination of a macrolide/doxycycline with a β-lactam) to a regimen without atypical antibiotic coverage (β-lactam monotherapy).

Methods

The meta-analysis was conducted according to the Preferred Reporting Items for Systematic Reviews and Meta-Analyses (PRISMA) guidelines (Additional file 1: Table S1).

Search strategy and data extraction

An independent librarian helped to formulate the appropriate search strategy (provided in the Additional file 1). Two authors (S.A. and A.A.) independently searched the PubMed, Embase, and Cochrane Library biomedical databases without date restrictions through December 11, 2016 using a standard form for data extraction. Languages were limited to English, Spanish, Arabic, French, German, Italian, and Dutch. The references of included studies were checked to identify additional clinical trials. In addition, the ClinicalTrials.gov website was searched for unpublished trials through December 11, 2016. We only considered the results from the intention-

to-treat analysis reported in each study. Any disagreement between the authors was resolved through discussion.

Study selection

RCTs of hospitalized adult patients with CAP that compared empiric antibiotic regimens with atypical coverage (a respiratory fluoroquinolone or combination of a macrolide/doxycycline with a β-lactam) to a regimen without atypical antibiotic coverage (β-lactam monotherapy) were identified and included. The respiratory fluoroquinolones included levofloxacin, moxifloxacin, and gemifloxacin. The macrolides included azithromycin, clarithromycin, or erythromycin. β-lactam agents with >85% coverage against *S. pneumoniae* were allowed and this included amoxicillin, amoxicillin/clavulanate, ampicillin, ampicillin/sulbactam, piperacillin, piperacillin/tazobactam, cefuroxime, cefpodoxime, cefdinir, cefditorin, cefotaxime, ceftriaxone, cefepime, ceftaroline, imipenem, meropenem, and ertapenem. We excluded studies published as abstracts only; studies that deviated from the assigned empiric β-lactam monotherapy (permitted adding empiric atypical bacterial coverage); studies including >25% outpatients and/or >10% of patients with nosocomial pneumonia; and if the target population had conditions other than CAP but did not report separate outcomes for the CAP group.

Data synthesis and analysis

The primary outcome was the rate of clinical failure of CAP. Secondary outcomes included rates of mortality, bacteriologic failure, and adverse events. Outcome rates assessed early during treatment or end of treatment were preferred over assessments at follow up post therapy. Heterogeneity (I^2) was assessed by using a Cochran's chi-squared test. The risk ratios (RRs) with 95% confidence intervals (CIs) were estimated using fixed-effect models, but the random-effects models were used when significant heterogeneity between the studies was observed (*P*-value less than 0.1 in the chi-squared test for heterogeneity). We assessed the quality of studies by using the Cochrane risk of bias tool for RCTs (low, unclear or high) [10]. Funnel plot was used to evaluate publication bias, and this plot was provided as Additional file 1. All analyses were conducted using Comprehensive Meta-Analysis Version 3 software (Biostat, Englewood, NJ, USA).

Results

Search results

The search process identified 1105 articles (PubMed 785; Embase 119; Cochrane Library 201) of duplicates for a total of 910 articles after removal [Fig. 1]. Fifteen full-text articles were assessed for eligibility after screening by title and/or abstract. After searching ClinicalTrials.gov

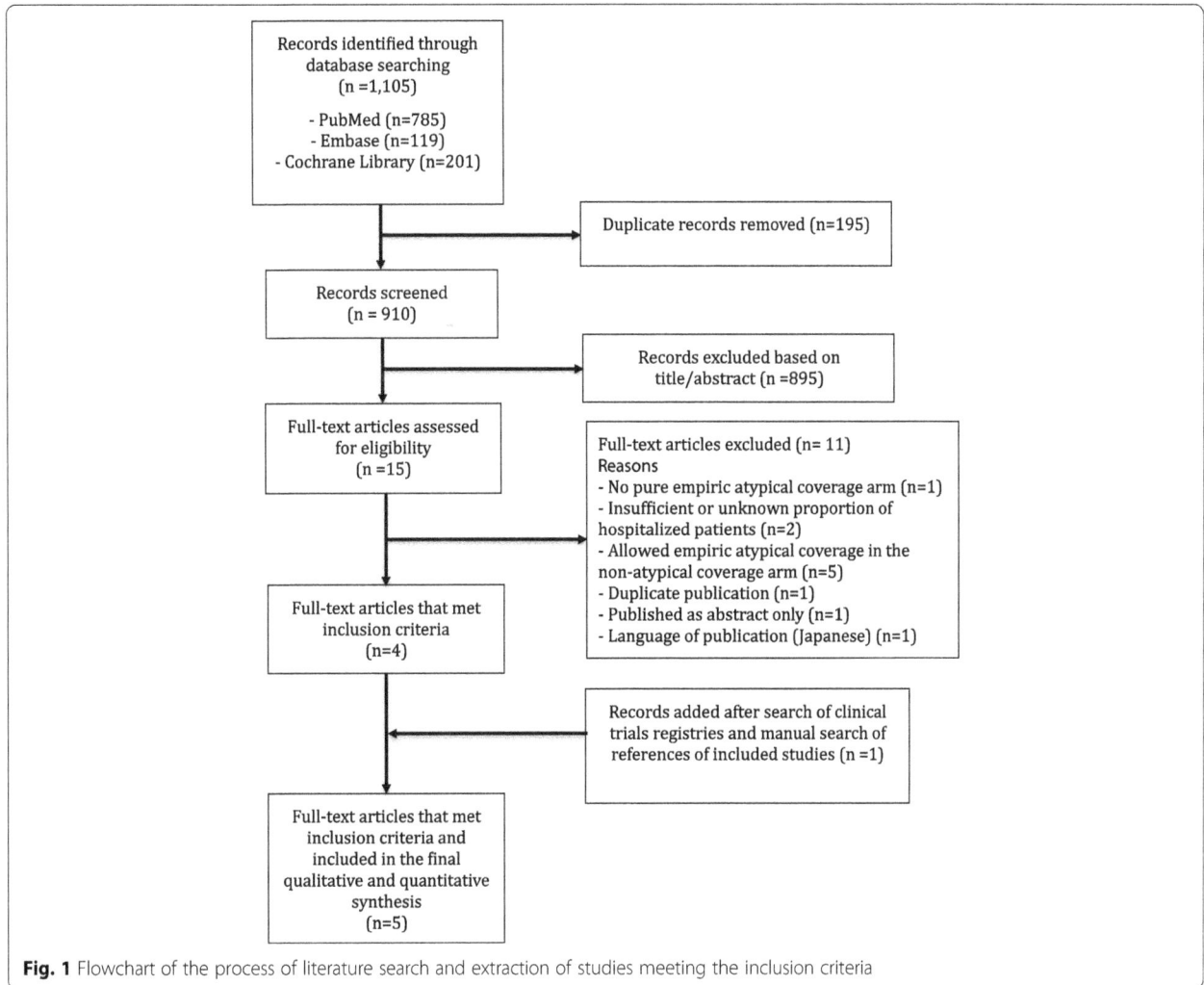

Fig. 1 Flowchart of the process of literature search and extraction of studies meeting the inclusion criteria

and a manual search of references of included studies, five RCTs (with 2011 patients) were retained. A total of 998 patients treated with empiric atypical bacterial coverage were compared to 1013 patients treated without empiric atypical bacterial coverage.

Study characteristics
The characteristics of the five included studies are summarized in Table 1. They were conducted between 1998 and 2014. Two studies were double-blinded [11, 12]; four were multicenter [11–14]; three were multinational and multicontinental [11–13]; one was funded by industry [13]; and four were in English [11–14] and one was in Spanish [15]. One study was excluded because of language (Japanese) [16]. The mean subject age in three studies was under 65 years [11, 12, 15]. Only one study included outpatients, who represented <25% of patients [12]. Two studies excluded patients with severe CAP [11, 15]. The regimen of β-lactams combined with a macrolide was used only in one study [14]. This study is the most recent one and included 580 patients). The

other four studies included fluoroquinolones as the atypical bacterial coverage arm [11–13, 15]. The assessments of bias risk are summarized in the Additional file 1. All five studies were RCTs; the risks of selection bias (random sequence generation and allocation concealment) and detection bias (blinding of outcome assessment) were low in three studies; the risk of performance (blinding of participants and personnel) bias was low in two studies; and the risk of reporting bias was low in all studies.

Primary outcome: clinical failure
Clinical failure rates were reported in all 5 RCTs [Fig. 2]. Two of the studies reported early clinical outcomes at 72 h and 7 days. The remaining three trials assessed outcomes within a few days after end of treatment. A statistically significant lower clinical failure rate was observed with empiric atypical coverage (RR, 0.851 [95% CI, 0.732–0.99; $P = 0.037$]; $I^2 = 0\%$; Q = 1.564 [$P = 0.815$]) in fixed-effect and random-effects model.

Table 1 Characteristics of Included Studies

Study	Study Period; Publication Year	Design	Location	Funding Source	Enrolled Patients[a]; ITT	Age (years)	PNA Characteristics	Antibiotic Regimen[a]	Duration of Therapy (days)	Outcomes Definitions
Grain et al.	2009–2013; 2014	Non-inferiority open-label, RCT	6 sites in 1 country (Switzerland)	Non-industry	602; 580 (289 vs. 291)	76 (median)	Moderately severe PNA	BL (IV cefuroxime 1.5 G X 3/d or IV amoxicillin/ clavulanate 1.2 G X 4/d) vs BL + ML (IV/PO clarithromycin 500 mg X 2/d)	10	Mortality = 30-day. Failure = no clinical stability at day 7
Petitpretz et al.	1997–1998; 2001	Superiority, double-blind, RCT	82 sites in 20 countries (Europe, South America, Australia, Africa)	Non-industry	411; 408 (200 vs. 208)	51 (mean)	Mild-moderate PNA; suspected pneumococcal PNA; 79% hospitalized/21% outpatients	BL (PO amoxicillin 1 G X 3/d) vs FQ (PO moxifloxacin 400 mg X 1/d)	10	Mortality = during the study (38-day). Failure = no clinical/bacteriological response 3–5 days after end of therapy
Norby et al.	Not reported; 1998	Superiority, open-label, RCT	64 sites in 13 countries (Europe, North and South America, Africa, Asia)	Industry	625; 619 (314 vs. 305)	65 (median)	Moderately severe PNA; excluded strongly suspected mycoplasma, chlamydia or legionella PNA; 94% CAP and 6% nosocomial PNA	BL (IV ceftriaxone 4 G X 1/d) vs FQ (IV levofloxacin 500 mg X 2/d, followed by PO levofloxacin 500 mg X 2/d)	8	Mortality = during the study (29-day). Failure = no clinical/bacteriological response 2–5 days after end of therapy
Leophonte et al.	1998–1999; 2004	Superiority, double-blind, RCT	102 sites in 3 countries (Europe, Africa)	Non-industry	324; 320 (167 vs. 153)	54 (mean)	Mild-moderate PNA; suspected pneumococcal PNA; 94% hospitalized	BL (PO amoxicillin/ clavulanate 1.2 G X 3/d) vs FQ (PO gemifloxacin 320 mg X 1/d)	7 for FQ; 10 for B-lactam	Mortality = during the study (30-day). Failure = no clinical/ bacteriological response at end of therapy
Kalbermatter et al.	1998; 2000	Superiority, open-label, RCT	1 site in 1 country (Argentina)	Non-industry	84; 84 (28 vs. 56)	60 (mean)	Mild-moderate PNA	BL (IV ceftriaxone 1 G X 2/d or IV amoxicillin/ clavulanate 1.2 G X 3/d) vs FQ (PO levofloxacin 500 mg X 2/d)	7–10 if favorable response	Failure = no clinical response at 72 h

[a] atypical bacterial coverage arm vs non-atypical bacterial coverage arm. *Abbreviations: PNA* pneumonia, *RCT* randomized clinical trial, *BL* β-lactam, *ML* Macrolide, *PO* orally, *IV* intravenously, *CAP* community-acquired pneumonia

Clinical failure with and without empiric atypical bacteria coverage in hospitalized adults...

67

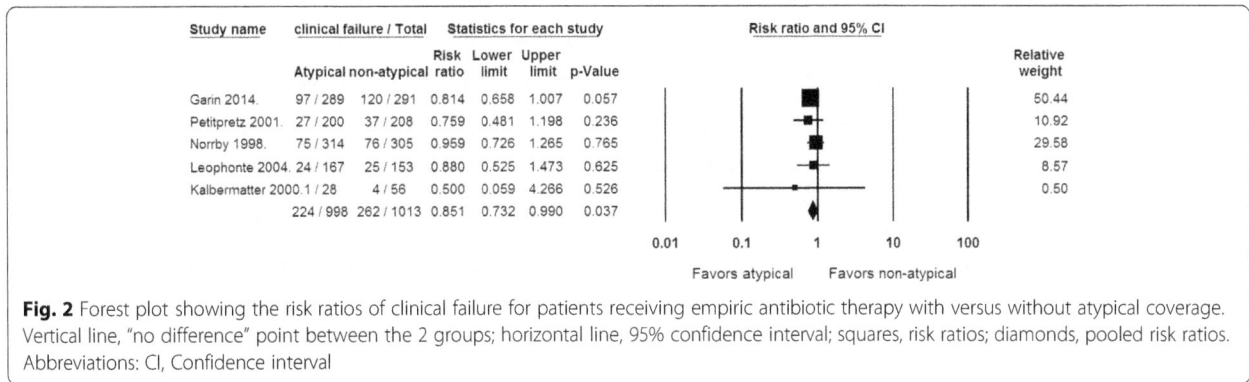

Fig. 2 Forest plot showing the risk ratios of clinical failure for patients receiving empiric antibiotic therapy with versus without atypical coverage. Vertical line, "no difference" point between the 2 groups; horizontal line, 95% confidence interval; squares, risk ratios; diamonds, pooled risk ratios. Abbreviations: CI, Confidence interval

Secondary outcomes: mortality, bacteriologic failure, and adverse events

No statistical significance was identified with regard to any secondary outcomes. Mortality rates were reported in all studies [11–14] but one [14] [Fig. 3]. The rates of mortality, total adverse events, and diarrhea were analyzed using a random-effects model, while bacteriologic failure and adverse events requiring antibiotic discontinuation were analyzed using fixed-effect model. No statistically significant differences between the two regimens were observed in rates of mortality (RR = 0.549 [95% CI, 0.259–1.165, P = 0.118], I^2 = 61.434%; Q = 9.635 [P = 0.022]) bacteriologic failure (RR = 0.816 [95% CI, 0.523–1.272, P = 0.369], I^2 = 0%; Q = 0.47 [P = 0.79]), total adverse events (RR = 0.982 [95% CI, 0.697–1.383, P = 0.918], I^2 = 69.011%; Q = 5.722 [P = 0.057]), diarrhea (RR = 0.746 [95% CI, 0.311–1.790, P = 0.512], I^2 = 65.048%; Q = 6.454 [P = 0.04]), and adverse events requiring antibiotic discontinuation (RR = 0.83 [95% CI, 0.542–1.270, P = 0.39], I^2 = 0%; Q = 0.037 [P = 0.83]).

Discussion

Our meta-analysis of RCTs confirms the benefit of empiric atypical bacteria coverage in hospitalized adult patients with CAP, unlike the other meta-analyses. This meta-analysis provides support for the current major guideline recommendations, including U.S guidelines of Infectious Diseases Society of America as well as European guidelines [1–4], using studies that used regimens recommended by these guidelines. The principal finding of our meta-analysis is that including empiric atypical coverage reduced the rates of clinical failure by approximately 15%. It should be noted that no single trial in our meta-analysis reported a statistically significant difference in the efficacy outcome, though there was a favorable trend in all 5 trials. However, the non-inferiority study by Garin et al., in which the empiric non-atypical bacterial coverage arm failed to meet the pre-specified non-inferiority threshold [14]. It is worth mentioning that a significant difference in clinical cure was found in previous meta-analyses favoring empiric atypical coverage in patients who had *Legionella* pneumonia [5, 6].

Our meta-analysis did not find a significant difference in mortality rates, which is consistent with other meta-analyses of RCTs [5–7]. Regimens that provided atypical coverage did not result in significantly more adverse events; however, adverse events were assessed in the studies involving respiratory fluoroquinolones and not in the macrolide-β-lactam combination study. The individual studies were not powered to detect differences in mortality and were not focused on adverse events. It remains unclear if adding empiric atypical coverage with a macrolide or doxycycline to a β-lactam increases the rate of adverse events. Future RCTs should evaluate benefits

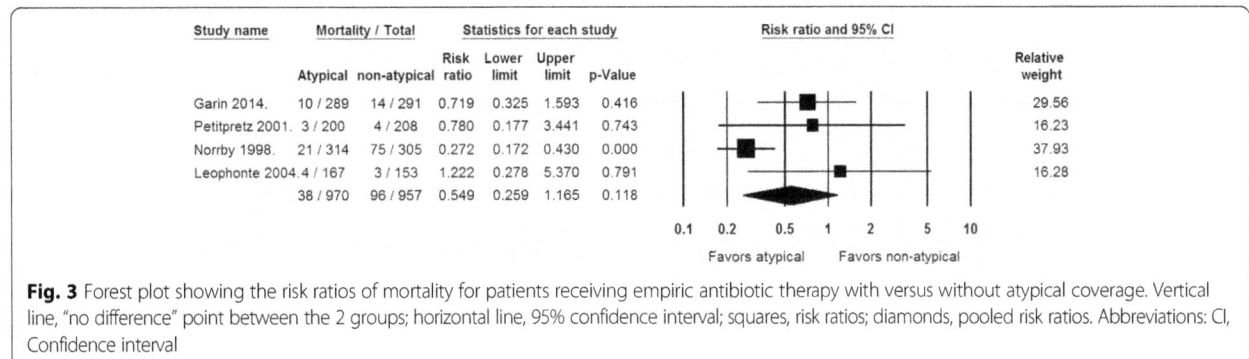

Fig. 3 Forest plot showing the risk ratios of mortality for patients receiving empiric antibiotic therapy with versus without atypical coverage. Vertical line, "no difference" point between the 2 groups; horizontal line, 95% confidence interval; squares, risk ratios; diamonds, pooled risk ratios. Abbreviations: CI, Confidence interval

in terms of efficacy and potential harm in terms of adverse events and increased cost.

Our meta-analysis differs from prior meta-analyses of RCTs [5–7]. These meta-analyses included some studies of non-recommended comparators. For example, the inclusion of ciprofloxacin as monotherapy would be inappropriate due to poor activity against S. pneumoniae. The use of macrolide monotherapy may be inappropriate for the same reason and depending on the selected macrolide, coverage of H. influenzae may be poor. Studies of agents that have been withdrawn from the market, such as temafloxacin, have been included in these meta-analysis. Another limitation of prior meta-analyses is a focus on longer term outcomes (e.g. at 30 day follow up) and, therefore, any observed benefit could be attributed to confounding factors. The inclusion of studies that permitted adding empiric atypical coverage to the arm the should have lacked atypical coverage could bias the results against the benefit of including atypical coverage because it makes the two groups more similar and reduce our ability to assess the true benefit of empiric atypical coverage.

The stringent inclusion criteria make our meta-analysis unique, increases its clinical relevance, and addresses antibiotic regimens recommended in major CAP guidelines. Published studies including non-recommended and withdrawn antibiotics for hospitalized CAP adults were excluded to provide results that are relevant to clinical practice. In addition, we preferred clinical failure rates that were reported earlier rather than at the final assessment at post therapy follow up. Using outcomes collected at around day 30 post treatment allows for accumulation of confounding events including changes in therapy and evolution of underlying illness. For example, clinical failure rates in the Petitpretz et al. study [12] were 46/200 (23%) vs. 44/208 (21.2%) in two meta-analyses [5, 6] because they reported the rates during follow-up; the rates were 27/200 (12.2%) vs 37/208 (17.8%) in one meta-analysis [8] as well as ours when using rates reported at the end of therapy (rates difference, 1.8% vs 5.6%, respectively). RCTs should embrace early clinical outcome as an endpoint since this provides the most direct information about antimicrobial efficacy and improves discrimination of differences between treatments. The Food and Drug Administration's 2014 guidance for developing drugs for treatment of community-acquired bacterial pneumonia stated that the time points at 36–48 h and 48–72 h after starting therapy demonstrate the greatest treatment effect of clinical recovery [17]. The guidance calls for a primary endpoint assessment on day 3 to day 5 of treatment.

Only five RCTs were found that meet our inclusion criteria. Despite the relatively small number of studies, subgroup analyses were performed for completeness and are available in the Additional file 1. Exclusion by language of publication can introduce bias and affects the results. However, only one study was excluded because of language in our meta-analysis [16]. Given the fact that the results of this study were available in an English abstract, we verified that including this study would not have altered the conclusions of our meta-analysis. Unfortunately, most RCTs have not reported detailed information about resistance rates, which is important to consider in studies of infectious diseases. Amoxicillin was used for typical coverage in one of the studies that we included and the coverage that this agent provides coverage that is inferior to that of moxifloxacin against S. pneumoniae, H. influenzae and M. catarrhalis. However, only one study included amoxicillin, in which all patients had their H. influenzae eradicated except three patients [13]. Amoxicillin is one of the recommended antibiotics per major guidelines and it is preferred over other excluded agents such as ciprofloxacin. Since moxifloxacin provides atypical coverage and better typical coverage, the treatment effect is not limited to the additional atypical coverage. Two of the studies included amoxicillin/clavulanate for typical bacterial coverage. The only deficiency here would be in coverage of penicillin non-susceptible S. pneumoniae; however, the incidence of these isolates in CAP studies is typically low [18–20]. In fact, this coverage deficit could be a problem when comparing any beta-lactam other than ceftaroline to a respiratory fluoroquinolone. If the goal is to evaluate impact of atypical coverage, then confounding factors need to be minimized. Therefore, a trial of ceftaroline versus ceftaroline plus a macrolide or respiratory fluoroquinolone would be valuable to sort out the effect of atypical coverage.

Etiologic diagnosis has evolved so that the pathogen can be identified in almost 90% of CAP cases [21]. In one study, atypical pathogens were detected in just over 4% of CAP cases [21]; however, there are outbreaks of Legionella spp. and areas with higher endemic incidence [22]. Given this low incidence, it is unlikely that any single RCT will ever be able to demonstrate the effect of atypical coverage for CAP. A better approach would be to include empiric atypical coverage for hospitalized (sicker) patients with CAP and then streamline therapy if the etiology is identified.

Conclusions

Our restricted but targeted meta-analysis of RCTs was able to define a significant reduction (approximately 15%) in clinical failure with the inclusion of atypical coverage in hospitalized adults with CAP. No significant differences were found in terms of secondary outcomes including mortality, bacteriologic failure and adverse events. Our meta-analysis provides supports for the current recommendations of the major CAP guidelines. However, some of the difference noted may be due to differences in typical coverage between treatment arms.

Abbreviations
CAP: Community-acquired pneumonia; CI: Confidence interval; RCTs: Randomized clinical trials; RR: Risk ratio

Acknowledgements
We thank the librarian, Jennifer Martin, for assistance with formulating the search strategy. The results presented here are part of the M.S. thesis of KE.

Funding
None.

Authors' contributions
KE and DEN formulated the research idea, and were involved with all steps of this meta-analysis. KE performed all statistical analyses and drafted the initial manuscript. SA and AA performed the database searches, helped with data extraction, and critically reviewed the manuscript. MA critically reviewed the manuscript. IA, ACK, and DEN critically reviewed the statistical analyses and revised the manuscript after critical review. All authors have seen and approved the manuscript and contributed significantly to the work.

Competing interests
The authors declare that they have any competing interests.

Consent for publication
Not applicable.

Author details
[1]Department of Clinical Pharmacy, King Abdulaziz University, P.O. Box 80200, Jeddah Postal code 21589, Saudi Arabia. [2]College of Pharmacy, University of Arizona, Drachman Hall – B306, 1295 N Martin Ave, P.O.Box 210202, Tucson, AZ, USA. [3]Division of Infectious Diseases, Department of Medicine, University of Arizona, Tucson, AZ, USA. [4]Department of Internal Medicine, Division of Infectious Diseases, University of Nebraska Medical Center, Omaha, NE, USA.

References
1. Mandell LA, Wunderink RG, Anzueto A, et al. Infectious Diseases Society of America/American Thoracic Society consensus guidelines on the management of community-acquired pneumonia in adults. Clin Infect Dis. 2007;44(Suppl 2): S27–72.
2. Lim WS, Baudouin SV, George RC, et al. BTS guidelines for the management of community acquired pneumonia in adults. Thorax. 2009;64(Suppl 3):1–55.
3. Woodhead M, Blasi F, Ewig S, et al. Guidelines for the management of adult lower respiratory tract infections. Clin Microbiol Infect. 2011;17(6):1–24.
4. National Institute for Health and Care Excellence. Diagnosis and management of community- and hospital-acquired pneumonia in adults. Published 3 Dec 2014. Available at: https://www.nice.org.uk/guidance/cg191. Accessed 25 May 2016.
5. Eliakim-Raz N, Robenshtok E, Shefet D, et al. Empiric antibiotic coverage of atypical pathogens for community-acquired pneumonia in hospitalized adults. Cochrane Database Syst rev. 2012;9:CD004418.
6. Mills GD, Oehley MR, Arrol B. Effectiveness of beta lactam antibiotics compared with antibiotics active against atypical pathogens in non-severe community acquired pneumonia: meta-analysis. BMJ. 2005;330(7489):456.
7. Shefet D, Robenshtok E, Paul M, Leibovici L. Empirical atypical coverage for inpatients with community-acquired pneumonia: systematic review of randomized controlled trials. Arch Intern Med. 2005;165(17):1992–2000.
8. Nie W, Li B, Xiu Q. β-Lactam/macrolide dual therapy versus β-lactam monotherapy for the treatment of community-acquired pneumonia in adults: a systematic review and meta-analysis. J Antimicrob Chemother. 2014;69(6):1441–6.
9. Horita N, Otsuka T, Haranaga S, et al. Beta-Lactam plus macrolides or beta-lactam alone for community-acquired pneumonia: a systematic review and meta-analysis. Respirology. 2016;21(7):1193–200.
10. Higgins JPT, Altman DG, Sterne JAC. Chapter 8: assessing risk of bias in included studies In: Higgins JPT, Green S eds. Cochrane handbook for systematic reviews of interventions version 5.1.0. The Cochrane collaboration, 2011. Available at: http://www.cochrane-handbook.org. Accessed 8 June 2016.
11. Leophonte P, File T, Feldman C. Gemifloxacin once daily for 7 days compared to amoxicillin/clavulanic acid thrice daily for 10 days for the treatment of community-acquired pneumonia of suspected pneumococcal origin. Respir Med. 2004;98(8):708–20.
12. Petitpretz P, Arvis P, Marel M, Moita J, Urueta J. CAP5 Moxifloxacin study group. Oral moxifloxacin vs high-dosage amoxicillin in the treatment of mild-to-moderate, community-acquired, suspected pneumococcal pneumonia in adults. Chest. 2001;119(1):185–95.
13. Norrby SR, Petermann W, Willcox PA, Vetter N, Salewski E. A comparative study of levofloxacin and ceftriaxone in the treatment of hospitalized patients with pneumonia. Scand J Infect Dis. 1998;30(4):397–404.
14. Garin N, Genné D, Carballo S, et al. β-Lactam monotherapy vs β-lactam-macrolide combination treatment in moderately severe community-acquired pneumonia: a randomized noninferiority trial. JAMA Intern Med. 2014;174(12):1894–901.
15. Kalbermatter V, Bagilet D, Diab M, Javkin E. Oral levofloxacin versus intravenous ceftriaxone and amoxicillin/clavulanic acid in the treatment of community-acquired pneumonia that requires hospitalization. Medicina Clinica. 2000; 115(15):561–3.
16. Kohno S, Watanabe A, Aoki N, et al. Clinical phase III comparative study of intravenous levofloxacin and ceftriaxone in community-acquired pneumonia treatment. J. Chemother. 2011;59:32–45.
17. Guidance for Industry. Community-acquired bacterial pneumonia: developing drugs for treatment. Rockville: US Department of Health and Human Services, Food and Drug Administration; 2014.
18. Postma DF, van Werkhoven CH, van Elden LJ, et al. Antibiotic treatment strategies for community-acquired pneumonia in adults. N Engl J Med. 2015;372(14):1312–23.
19. Zhong NS, Sun T, Zhuo C, et al. Ceftaroline fosamil versus ceftriaxone for the treatment of Asian patients with community-acquired pneumonia: a randomised, controlled, double-blind, phase 3, non-inferiority with nested superiority trial. Lancet Infect Dis. 2015;2:161–71.
20. File TM Jr, Low DE, Eckburg PB, et al. Integrated analysis of FOCUS 1 and FOCUS 2: randomized, doubled-blinded, multicenter phase 3 trials of the efficacy and safety of ceftaroline fosamil versus ceftriaxone in patients with community-acquired pneumonia. Clin Infect Dis. 2010;51(12):1395–405.
21. Gadsby NJ, Russell CD, McHugh MP, et al. Comprehensive molecular testing for respiratory pathogens in community-acquired pneumonia. Clin Infect Dis. 2016;62(7):817–23.
22. World Health Organization. Legionellosis. Published June 2016. Available at: http://www.who.int/mediacentre/factsheets/fs285/en/. Accessed 3 Aug 2016.

10

Impact of oral hygiene involving toothbrushing *versus* chlorhexidine in the prevention of ventilator-associated pneumonia

Claudia Fernanda de Lacerda Vidal[1*], Aurora Karla de Lacerda Vidal[2], José Gildo de Moura Monteiro Jr.[3], Aracele Cavalcanti[4], Ana Paula da Costa Henriques[5], Márcia Oliveira[6], Michele Godoy[7], Mirella Coutinho[7], Pollyanna Dutra Sobral[7], Claudia Ângela Vilela[7], Bárbara Gomes[7], Marta Amorim Leandro[8], Ulisses Montarroyos[9], Ricardo de Alencar Ximenes[10] and Heloísa Ramos Lacerda[11]

Abstract

Background: Nosocomial pneumonia has correlated to dental plaque and to oropharynx colonization in patients receiving mechanical ventilation. The interruption of this process, by preventing colonization of pathogenic bacteria, represents a potential procedure for the prevention of ventilator-associated pneumonia (VAP).

Methods: The study design was a prospective, randomized trial to verify if oral hygiene through toothbrushing plus chlorhexidine in gel at 0.12% reduces the incidence of ventilatior-associated pneumonia, the duration of mechanical ventilation, the length of hospital stay and the mortality rate in ICUs, when compared to oral hygiene only with chlorhexidine, solution of 0.12%, without toothbrushing, in adult individuals under mechanical ventilation, hospitalized in Clinical/Surgical and Cardiology Intensive Care Units (ICU). The study protocol was approved by the Ethical Committee of Research of the Health Sciences Center of the Federal University of Pernambuco – Certificate of Ethical Committee Approval (CAAE) 04300012500005208. Because it was a randomized trial, the research used CONSORT 2010 checklist criteria.

Results: Seven hundred sixteen patients were admitted into the ICU; 219 fulfilled the criteria for inclusion and 213 patients were included; 108 were randomized to control group and 105 to intervention group. Toothbrushing plus 0.12% chlorhexidine gel demonstrated a lower incidence of VAP throughout the follow up period, although the difference was not statistically significant ($p = 0.084$). There was a significant reduction of the mean time of mechanical ventilation in the toothbrushing group ($p = 0.018$). Regarding the length of hospital stay in the ICU and mortality rates, the difference was not statistically significant ($p = 0.064$).

Conclusions: The results obtained showed that, among patients undergoing toothbrushing there was a significant reduction in duration of mechanical ventilation, and a tendency to reduce the incidence of VAP and length of ICU stay, although without statistical significance.

Keywords: Pneumonia, Mechanical ventilator, Oral hygiene, Toothbrushing, Chlorhexidine, Intensive care

* Correspondence: vidal.claudia@gmail.com
[1]Tropical Medicine Health Sciences Center, Committee on Infection Control of Hospital das Clinicas, Universidade Federal de Pernambuco, Av. Professor Moraes Rego, 1235 Hospital das Clínicas - Cidade Universitária, Recife, Pernambuco 50670-901, Brazil

Background

Nearly 9% to 40% of infections acquired in the Intensive Care Unit (ICU) are ventilator-associated pneumonia (VAP), and are related to increased length of hospital stay, higher morbidity and mortality, which significantly affects hospital costs [1, 2].

Nosocomial pneumonia has been correlated to dental plaque and to oropharynx colonization in patients receiving mechanical ventilation (MV). The endotracheal tube works as a conductor of the microorganisms of the oropharynx to the lower respiratory tract, and these are frequently identified as etiological agents of the nosocomial pneumonia [3–5].

The interruption of this process, by preventing colonization of pathogenic bacteria, represents a potential procedure for the prevention of VAP [6].

Considering that the microbiota of the oral cavity plays an important role in the development process of VAP, some studies have indicated that the topical application of chlorhexidine, initiated before intubation, reduces nosocomial infections in patients submitted to elective cardiac surgery [7, 8].

However, although the pharmacological control of bacterial plaque, through the use of chlorhexidine is practical and widely accepted among health professionals, the chemical approach against accumulated plaque is marginal, since the plaque acts as a biofilm in which the bacteria is considerably less sensitive to antimicrobial therapy – when compared to the free-moving planktonic form [9]. Therefore, mechanical cleansing, through toothbrushing may be the most effective method of removing all pathogens from the plaque, including anaerobes and multiresistant bacteria such as methicilline-resistant *Staphylococcus aureus*, (MRSA) or *Pseudomonas* [10].

The mechanical removal of microorganisms can increase the efficacy of the effects of chlorhexidine in the remaining bacteria or in bacterial regrowth, according to Kishimoto and Urade [11].

Although many studies suggest a potential relation between deficient oral care and increased incidence of VAP, the available evidence is still limited. This study was designed to verify if oral hygiene through toothbrushing with chlorhexidine in gel at 0.12% reduces the incidence of ventilatior-associated pneumonia, the duration of mechanical ventilation, the length of hospital stay and the mortality rate in ICU, when compared to oral hygiene only with chlorhexidine, solution of 0.12%, without toothbrushing, in adult individuals under mechanical ventilation, hospitalized in Clinical/Surgical and Cardiology Intensive Care Units. The toothbrushing is the basis for the removal of dental plaque and consequently reduction of oral bacterial load, reducing the risk for VAP.

Methods

We conducted a prospective, randomized study of oral hygiene with 0.12% chlorhexidine solution every 12 h (control group) *versus* toothbrushing plus 0.12% chlorhexidine gel every 12 h (intervention group) in three ICU of public hospitals and one ICU of a philanthropic hospital in Recife, Brazil, from July 2013 to January 2014. The study protocol was approved by the Ethical Committee of Research of the Health Sciences Center of the Federal University of Pernambuco – CAAE 04300012500005208 and a written informed consent was obtained from all patients or relative before randomization. A research team was responsible for designing and executing the study, analyzing data, interpreting findings and writing the manuscript. The authors vouch for the accuracy and completeness of the reported data.

The primary endpoint was to assess the impact of introducing toothbrushing as a component of oral care on the incidence of VAP. The secondary endpoints were to identify differences in duration of mechanical ventilation, length of hospital stay and mortality rate in ICU between the studied groups.

Recruitment, randomization and follow up
Study population
Individuals who were consecutive admitted into the four participating Intensive Care Units (total of 46 beds) and that fulfilled the inclusion criteria: age equal or greater than 18 years; submitted to intubation; expected to remain on mechanical ventilation for >48 h; and without evidence of pulmonary infection at admission. Individuals without teeth, suspicion of pneumonia at the time of intubation, pregnancy, tracheostomy and chlorhexidine allergy also were excluded.

The participants also underwent the standard protocol for prevention of VAP, which included maintaining a semirecumbent body position, with head elevation of $\geq 30°$, gastrointestinal bleeding prophylaxis, deep venous thrombosis prophylaxis and daily interruption of sedation with assessing the possibility of extubation.

Among the four Intensive Care Units, three were medical/surgical with total of 36 beds and the other a cardiac ICU with 10 beds. About 65% of hospitalized patients in the ICU were medical care while 35% were surgical patients, and among medical patients, 20% were cardiac.

Randomization

Patients were randomized within 24 h of intubation and initiation of mechanical ventilation for the control group (oral hygiene with 0.12% chlorhexidine solution every 12 h), or the intervention group (toothbrushing plus 0.12% chlorhexidine gel every 12 h) by means of opaque sealed envelopes containing the results from a computer generated random list.

Nurses responsible for assistance in ICU, previously trained by the research team, opened the envelope containing the assigned group within 24 h of intubation and included in the nursing systematized assistance plan the group of oral hygiene for which the patient had been randomized (control group or intervention group). Researchers and physicians did not know to which of both groups the individuals belonged, providing information to blind. The nurses and practical nurses were trained to implement oral hygiene according to the protocols established for both groups.

Treatment regimens

Whereas in most of the studies reviewed, the concentration was more widely used chlorhexidine 0.12%, especially in the few studies comparing with toothbrushing, and the fact of the hospitals participating in the study had only the formulation of chlorhexidine 0.2% for use in the study population and the "kit" for toothbrushing, obtained through donations and own resources of the principal investigator, containing the antiseptic chlorhexidine in concentration 0.12%, the research team defined the use of two study groups, as described below.

Control group

Individuals undergoing oral hygiene every 12 h, through aspiration of oropharyngeal secretion, immediately applying 15 ml of 0.12% chlorhexidine gluconate oral solution using a *swab* on all tooth surfaces, tongue and mucosal surface of the mouth. The whole process was performed by nursing staff and followed the specific standard operating procedure.

Intervention group

Individuals undergoing oral hygiene every 12 h through aspiration of oropharyngeal secretion. Immediately after, toothbrushing was carried out on all tooth surfaces, tongue and mucosal surface of the mouth through the use of toothbrushes with small and soft bristles, and dental gel based on 0.12% chlorhexidine gluconate. After the previous steps proceeded with rinsing and suction through a catheter coupled to own toothbrush for this purpose aspiration. The whole process was performed by nursing staff and followed the specific standard operating procedure.

Clinical dental examination

The Decayed, Missing and Filled Teeth Index (DMF) [12] was also calculated through the oral clinical exam, following the sequence of admission of the individuals in the study, by using a spatula and flat dental mirror

under the light of unit with the examiner the patient's right. Different dental spaces were examined one by one, systematically, including the right and left upper quadrants, and immediately the right and left lower quadrants.

Definitions and data collection

Trainings were conducted by the principal investigator and by a collaborator dentist, to the whole team and all health professionals involved at the four participating institutions, with the aim of standardizing processes to operationalize the study, uniformity of approaches and calibration between participating professionals. This first stage of the study took place from July 2012 to July 2013, which enabled the start of randomization and data collection between July 2013 and January 2014.

After randomization, demographic, clinical and microbiological data was collected by the researchers throughout the follow up period of the individuals.

Based on clinical criteria, suspected VAP was defined as the presence of a new or progressive pulmonary infiltrate on chest radiography, associated to a minimum of two among three clinical criteria: fever (axilar temperature ≥ 37.8 °C), leukocytosis ($>10 \times 10^3/mm^3$) or leukopenia ($<3 \times 10 \times 10^3/mm^3$), and purulent respiratory secretions (American Thoracic Society, 2005) – considering that bronchoscopy with quantitative cultures are not routinely used in the ICU study participants. Pneumonia defined by microbiological criteria included bacterial growth of endotracheal aspirates and bronchoalveolar lavage (bronchoscopic) with values $\geq 10^6$ cfu / ml and $\geq 10^4$ cfu / ml, respectively, associated with clinical criteria of pneumonia described above [13].

The clinical follow up included daily evaluation of the following data: temperature, leukocyte count, PaO_2/FiO_2 ratio, presence or absence of purulent respiratory secretions. Results of chest radiographies were routinely evaluated, as well as microbiological exams when available.

Early VAP defined as ventilator-associated pneumonia that occurs within four days of intubation whereas late-onset VAP as ventilator-associated pneumonia that occurs from the fifth day of intubation [13].

The participation of individuals ended on the 28th day of follow up or upon the occurrence of death, extubation or transfer.

Statistical analysis

The sample size required to achieve a 50% reduction in suspected VAP, based on a VAP rate of 15,8% in the control group, with an 80% power and a error of 5%, was calculated to be 286 patients in each group. VAP incidence was reported as percentage and the incidence density as episodes per 1,000 days of mechanical ventilation. Discrete variables expressed as counts and percentages, and continuous variables as means and standard deviation (SD). The Decayed, Missing and Filled Teeth Index, calculated by the ratio between the total number of permanent teeth that are decayed, missed or filled and the total number of individuals of the sample, expressed as absolute number.

For the clinical and demographic characteristics of patients, differences between groups were assessed using Chi-square test for categorical variables, and Student *t*-test for continuous variables. The associations were expressed as Relative Risk (RR) and *p* values with 95% confidence interval (CI). In the multivariate analysis, logistic regression was applied to adjust potential confusion factors. The significance level of all the analyses was defined as $p < 0,05$. STATA version 12.0 was the software used for the analysis.

Results

In the period from July 2013 to January 2014, were included 213 patients in the study, from which 108 were randomized to control group (oral hygiene with 0.12% chlorhexidine solution every 12 h) and 105 to intervention group (toothbrushing plus 0.12% chlorhexidine gel every 12 h. The patients were recruited from 4 Intensive Therapy Units in Recife, 69 patients (32.4%) being from Hospital 1, 50 patients (23.5%) from Hospital 2, 43 patients (20,2%) from Hospital 3, and 51 patients (23.9%) from Hospital 4. During this period, a total of 716 patients were admitted into the ICU of which 497 were excluded. Among the main causes of exclusion of patients admitted in ICU are suspected pneumonia admission, patients without teeth, tracheostomy, extubated withing 12 h wich resulted in failure to apply the oral hygiene protocol, missing randomization withing 24 h of admission. noninvasive ventilation. However, 219 fulfilled the criteria for inclusion in the study. Of these, 6 were later excluded; 4 had a mechanical ventilation period inferior to 48 h and 2 did not have defined outcomes due to the end of the study period (Fig. 1), in which resources are over.

Comparing the groups regarding clinical characteristics at admission, there was no statistically significant difference (*p* >0.05) (Table 1).

Among the 213 patients, ventilatior-associated pneumonia occurred in 45 (21.1%), 28 being patients from the control group and 17 from the intervention group, with incidence density equal to 14.2 by 1.000 MV/day. The use of toothbrushing plus 0.12% chlorhexidine gel demonstrated a lower incidence of VAP throughout the follow up period, although the difference was not statistically significant (*p* = 0.084). Clinical/radiological criteria defined 95.6% of cases of VAP; only 2 patients had microbiological diagnosis. Most cases of VAP (80%)

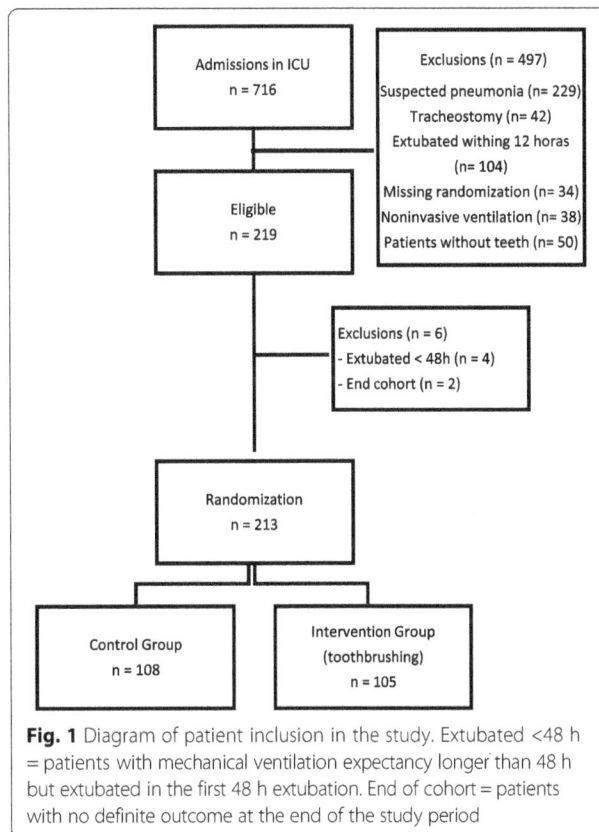

Fig. 1 Diagram of patient inclusion in the study. Extubated <48 h = patients with mechanical ventilation expectancy longer than 48 h but extubated in the first 48 h extubation. End of cohort = patients with no definite outcome at the end of the study period

occurred after the 4th day of mechanical ventilation (late-onset VAP). The relative risk of death was higher in the control group, increasing the risk of death by 41%, although it was not statistically significant (Table 2).

When considering the patients who were discharged from the ICU, there was a significant reduction of the mean time of mechanical ventilation in the group of patients who were submitted to toothbrushing (*p* = 0.018). The categorized analysis on duration of mechanical ventilation, there was a tendency for increased risk of long stay in mechanical ventilation for the control group (Chi-square for trend *p* = 0.073) (Table 2).

Regarding the length of hospital stay in the ICU, the difference was not statistically significant (*p* = 0.064), but there was a tendency to reduce in the length of stay in the ICU for the intervention group (Table 2).

Overall, the results showed a better scenario among patients undergoing toothbrushing. However, regarding the risk of VAP and death, the sample seems insufficient in size to detect a difference.

With respect to oral health status of the population, after stratification of the sample according to age, the DMF was of 24.9, 25.6, 26.4 and 27.0, for ages 45 to 54 years, 55 to 64 years, 65 to 74 years and 75 years of more, respectively. The amount of missing teeth accounted for more than 50% of the index in each of the age groups. Mean number of teeth present in the mouth,

Table 1 Characteristics at ICU admission of patients who received oral hygiene with chlorhexidine 0.12% oral solution (control group) and toothbrushing with chlorhexidine gel 0.12% (intervention group)

Characteristics	Control group (n = 108)	Intervention group (n = 105)	P value
Sex			
Male	54 (50,0%)	51 (48,6%)	0,835
Female	54 (50,0%)	54 (51,4%)	
Age (in years)	63,2 ± 14,5	59,4 ± 14,5	0,059
Causes for intubation			
Acute respiratory failure secondary to pulmonary event	23 (21,3%)	29 (27,6%)	0,610
Acute respiratory failure secondary to cardiovascular event	51 (47,2%)	43 (40,9%)	
Acute respiratory failure secondary to neuromuscular event	6 (5,6%)	8 (7,6%)	
Acute respiratory failure secondary to foreing body aspiration	1 (0,9%)	0 (-)	
Other cause	27 (25,0%)	25 (23,8%)	
Intubation process			
Elective	23 (21,3%)	27 (25,7%)	0,678
Urgent	78 (72,2%)	70 (66,7%)	
Emergency	7 (6,5%)	8 (7,6%)	
Previous antibiotic use			
Yes	21 (19,4%)	26 (24,8%)	0,349
No	87 (80,6%)	79 (75,2%)	
APACHE II	22,2 ± 7,7	21,9 ± 7,5	0,767
Admission diagnosis			
Pulmonary disease	8 (18,6%)	5 (15,2%)	0,586
Cardiovascular disease	25 (58,1%)	23 (69,7%)	
Endocrine disease	2 (4,6%)	2 (6,1%)	
Cerebrovascular disease	0 (-)	1 (3,0%)	
Kidney disease	4 (9,3%)	1 (3,0%)	
Digestive disease	2 (4,6%)	1 (3,0%)	
Other	2 (4,6%)	0 (-)	
Comorbidities			
Pulmonary disease	25 (23,2%)	22 (21,0%)	0,699
Cardiovascular disease	92 (85,2%)	83 (79,1%)	0,242
Endocrine disease	66 (61,1%)	54 (51,4%)	0,154
Cerebrovascular disease	9 (8,3%)	11 (10,5%)	0,592
Kidney disease	22 (20,4%)	27 (25,7%)	0,354
Digestive disease	13 (12,0%)	17 (16,2%)	0,384
Hematologic disease	5 (4,6%)	4 (3,8%)	0,766

with respect to age groups, was 18.5 from 45 to 54 years; 14.8 from 55 to 64 years; 13.7 from 65 to 74 years and 10.3 for 75 years or more.

In the analysis of the clinical signs of periodontal disease, the most common findings were gingivitis and periodontitis, where 72% of the sample showed any sign of periodontal disorder characterized by the presence of tartar; reddened, swollen and bleeding gums; gingival pockets; gingival recession and tooth mobility.

Finally, no adverse events were reported associated with toothbrushing or chlorhexidine use.

Discussion

In the present study, the use of toothbrushing plus 0,12% chlorhexidine gel demonstrated a lower incidence of VAP during the follow up period (28 VAP cases – control group X 17 VAP cases – intervention group), but the difference was not statistically

Table 2 Risk of VAP, duration of mechanical ventilation, length of stay and mortality in hospitalized patients in the ICU undergoing oral hygiene with chlorhexidine 0.12% oral solution (Control group) and toothbrushing with chlorhexidine gel 0.12% (Intervention group)

Events	Control group ($n = 108$)	Intervention group ($n = 105$)	RR	CI(95%)	P value
VAP					
No	80 (47,6%)	88 (52,4%)	1,0	-	-
Yes	28 (62,2%)	17 (37,8%)	1,81	0,93 – 3,57	0,084
Death					
No	81 (48,8%)	85 (51,2%)	1,0	-	-
Yes	27 (57,5%)	20 (42,5%)	1,41	0,73 – 2,70	0,296
Duration of mechanical ventilation[b]					
Mean ± sd	11,1 ± 7,6	8,7 ± 5,0	1,063	1,011 – 1,120	0,018[a]
Categorization[c]					
Up to 5 days	13 (37,1%)	22 (62,9%)	1,0	-	-
6 to 10 days	40 (48,8%)	42 (41,2%)	1,61	0,71 – 3,70	0,249
11 days and more	28 (57,1%)	21 (42,9%)	2,27	0,93 – 5,55	0,073
Length of ICU[b]					
Mean ± sd	13,9 ± 8,6	11,9 ± 7,77	1,032	0,999 – 1,065	0,064
Categorization[d]					
Up to 5 days	11 (39,3%)	17 (60,7%)	1,0	-	-
6 to 10 days	38 (50,0%)	38 (50,0%)	1,54	0,64 – 3,70	0,333
11 days and more	59 (54,1%)	50 (45,9%)	1,82	0,78 – 4,34	0,164

[a]statistically significant association
[b]Among patients who were discharged from the ICU ($n = 166$)
[c]Chi-squared test for trend ($x^2 = 3,205$; $p = 0,073$)
[d]Chi-squared test for trend ($x^2 = 1,801$; $p = 0,179$)

significant ($p = 0.084$). Despite this, there was a significant reduction in the mean time of mechanical ventilation in the group of patients who were submitted to toothbrushing ($p = 0.018$). This study identified a tendency for shorter length of ICU stay and reducing mortality for the toothbrushing group, although without statistical significance. However, there was an increase of 41% in the relative risk of death for the control group, which reinforces the trend toward better clinical outcome for the intervention group.

There are many studies designed to prove the role of mechanical cleansing of dental plaque and its association with the reduction of VAP [14–16], but the results are limited.

Systematic revision and meta-analysis, including four studies with a total of 828 patients submitted to oral hygiene with and without toothbrushing, did not demonstrate benefits regarding reduction of VAP, duration of MV or length stay in ICU, for the toothbrushing group [17].

Alhazzani et al. [18] recently published a systemic revision and meta-analysis, to formulate a critical analysis of the impact of using toothbrushing as part of oral hygiene for individuals under intensive care and mechanical ventilation – analyzing studies published between

1980 and March of 2012. Six randomized studies, involving 1,408 patients – from which five compared toothbrushing with standard oral hygiene, and the sixth compared manual toothbrushing *versus* electric toothbrushing – fulfilled the inclusion criteria. Four studies demonstrated a tendency to lower rates of ventilator-associated pneumonia, although without statistical significance ($p = 0.26$). One only study, which presented low bias risk estimated by the Cochrane method, suggested that toothbrushing significantly reduced VAP occurrence ($p = 0.006$). No difference was observed between manual or electric toothbrushing. Moreover, there were no statistically significant differences regarding length of ICU stay or hospital mortality.

Although our study has demonstrated significant reduction in meantime mechanical ventilation, one limitation was the small sample size through interruption of the study.

The study discontinuation, due to lack of inputs for oral hygiene according to the study protocol, contributed to the failure to achieve the number of patients needed to more appropriate analysis of any difference between the groups. In fact, the sample calculation considered an VAP incidence in our region; however, financial resources ended, hospitals could not comply with the acquisition of materials needed to continue the search, and the data were analyzed with discontinuation of the study, what is meant a limitation of the research. Despite of this, like the studies above cited, tendency for lower incidence of VAP for the intervention group was found in our study.

Unfortunately, we could not work with the ideal number of participants, but even with these difficulties, the results showed trend to better outcomes with the intervention, and significant difference in mean time mechanical ventilation. Thus, operational difficulties relating to financial resources, considering the study in a country with few resources, developing country, and three public hospitals among 04 hospitals, which also involves little financial resources, defined the completion of research ahead of schedule time.

In spite of this, we consider relevant findings, which indicate a significant difference in mean time mechanical ventilation, and show a tendency to lower risk of death and lower absolute number of VAP in the population under the intervention.

Also it chose to work with only to study groups and use of chlorhexidine 0.12%, approved and widely used in various studies, which would allow comparison of the control group with the intervention group, to which the only difference is the use of brushing, since also in this group was the dental gel with 0.12% chlorhexidine. Thus, avoiding bias in relation to different concentrations of chlorhexidine and proceeds with the analysis of the differential component that has been the target of research, the role of brushing. The restriction on the number of treatment arms was importante, since the power would not have been suficiente.

In addition, the high VAP incidence (14.1/1,000 MV-day) pointed out in this study, when compared with data from the National Healthcare Safety Network (2.1 to 10.7 per 1,000 MV-day) [19], denotes the necessity to adopt more effective proven measures to reduce pneumonia in patients who are undergoing mechanical ventilation in our Intensive Care Units.

Although the four participating institutions of the study introduced the "bundle" for VAP prevention [20], the fifth component of the package of measures – oral hygiene – was not contemplated in the units before this study, and the justifications found for this gap point to technical difficulties, lack of knowledge about the importance of the measure by the professional team at the ICU, and lack of a standard protocol and adequate material resources. This gave rise to efforts, by the multiprofessional health team – made up of nurses, physicians, hospital infection control service professionals, physiotherapists and surgeon-dentist – in order to address the technical and material deficiencies, and effective application of a standard protocol for oral

hygiene, including toothbrushing, for planning this randomized study.

In the last two decades, numerous published data has shown that inadequate oral hygiene increases the incidence of pneumonia both in the community and in hospitalized individuals undergoing intensive care [21]. Dental plaque serves as a reservoir for microorganisms associated to pulmonary infections, and these respiratory pathogens quickly colonize the plaque of patients hospitalized in ICU undergoing mechanical ventilation [3, 4]. Thus, care protocols represent an essential component for the reduction of VAP [21]. In order to control vies information in our study, a team of dentists performed the dental evaluation in all patients in the study, and have trained all nursing professionals to oral hygiene with toothbrushing with chlorhexidine 0.12%, through a standard protocol for oral care.

From that oral assessment, another finding was the high DMF index described in this study, despite the limitations of the indicator itself – obtained from the clinical examination restricted to the crown of the tooth and not showing secondary tooth losses to periodontal disease or orthodontic reasons [22] – denotes the level of oral health impairment for this population group. Measures are necessary to better promote oral health, since these critical patients who undergoing to mechanical ventilation present high risk of infection, especially of the inferior respiratory tract.

The following question remains: Why measure as effective for plaque rupture fails to demonstrate proven benefit in this patient population? The results of the different studies must be analyzed cautiously. First, establishing the VAP diagnosis for patients undergoing mechanical ventilation is much more complex when compared with community-acquired pneumonia. In addition, opinions among physicians about the diagnostic criteria also differ. Thus, the few studies included in the meta-analysis of Gu et al. [17], who used the VAP as the main outcome, could present disappointing results in relation to evidence about the expected superiority of toothbrushing as method of pneumonia prevention [21]. In our study, clinical/radiological criteria were used for the diagnosis of VAP, which could result in misdiagnosis, once the gold standard is represented by microbiological diagnosis. To minimize this possible bias in classification, standardization of clinical criteria, training of physicians responsible for diagnosing and *Kappa* test were used, which enabled the standardization of concepts and validate the diagnosis of VAP in this study. With the objective of minimizing possible bias of information and/or classification, different teams of professionals were defined to apply the oral hygiene protocol (nursing) and definition of VAP diagnosis (medical).

Another important point is that more precise criteria for investigation of the role of dental plaque rupture should be used when the design of studies which seeking to validate the role of toothbrushing as a primary measure for VAP prevention. The use of scores to evaluate dental plaque, suggested by Wise and Williams [21], helps to prove the efficacy of toothbrushing and makes possible the analysis of its influence in VAP incidence. Observational study demonstrated an increase in the occurrence of dental bacterial plaque along the length of intubation using dental plaque scores [23].

It is difficult to interpret the studies that do not show a reduction in VAP occurrence. The results of these studies could reflect mistakes during the toothbrushing procedure, that is, no reduction in the plaque score or removal of dental plaque by itself would not affect the incidence of VAP [21]. Moreover, the use of chlorhexidine appears to attenuate the effects of toothbrushing on VAP (p for interaction = 0.02) [18]. According to Labeau [24], the well-conducted meta-analysis by Alhazzani et al. [18] supports toothbrushing as a potential strategy for reducing VAP and oral care without the application of this method should be considered, at least, an improper practice.

Improving mouth hygiene represents one of innumerous interventions that can affect VAP occurrence [25]. The ideal would be to design more studies to define the adequate method for oral hygiene in this population of patients, using more precise measurements to validate the removal of dental plaque (plaque score) by toothbrushing, having as the main outcome the mortality rate. This would implicate a great number of recruits before the planning of studies evaluating VAP incidence, with greater probability of bias because of the diagnostic complexity, which is something that would complicate the interpretation of the results.

Conclusions

In summary, the results obtained showed that, among patients undergoing toothbrushing there was a significant reduction in duration of mechanical ventilation, and a tendency to reduce the incidence of VAP and length of ICU stay, although this last results without statistical significance. Therefore, about the risk of VAP risk and death, the sample no appears to have been large enough to detect differences in this magnitude. More studies are needed in order to define optimal oral hygiene, use of dental plaque score, and observation of the impact of oral hygiene measures, mainly on hospital and ICU mortality rates.

Abbreviations
CAAE: Certificate of ethical committee approval; CI: Confidence interval; DMF: Decayed, missing and filled teeth index; ICU: Intensive care unit; MRSA: Methiciline-resistant *staphylococcus aureus*; MV: Mechanical ventilator; RR: Relative risk; SD: Standard deviation; VAP: Ventilator associated pneumonia

Acknowledgements
The authors thanks the hospitals and multidisciplinary teams who participated and contributed to the feasibility study.

Funding
The study was funded by the lead researcher of the Research Fund Program of Academic Strengthening of University of Pernambuco, and support the four participating hospitals own resources.

Authors' contributions
CFLV conceived of the study, participated in its design and coordination, acquisition, analysis and interpretation of data of the work, and written the manuscript as a part of her doctoral thesis in Tropical Medicine and final approval of the version to be published. AKLV contributed to the conception and acquisition of data. trained for oral hygiene, revised and final approval of the version to be published. JGMMJ contributed to the acquisition of data, critical review and final approval of the version to be published. AC contributed to the acquisition of data, critical review and final approval of the version to be published. APTH contributed to the acquisition of data, critical review and final approval of the version to be published. MO contributed to the acquisition of data, critical review and final approval of the version to be published. MG contributed to the acquisition of data, critical review and final approval of the version to be published. MC contributed to the acquisition of data, critical review and final approval of the version to be published. PDC contributed to the acquisition of data, critical review and final approval of the version to be published. CAV contributed to the acquisition of data, critical review and final approval of the version to be published. BG contributed to the acquisition of data, critical review and final approval of the version to be published. MAL contributed to the acquisition of data, critical review and final approval of the version to be published. UM participated in the conception, analysis of data, revision of the work and final approval of the version to be published. RAAX participated in the design of the work, interpretation of data of the work, critical review for important intellectual content and final approval of the version to be published. HRM participated in the design of the work, interpretation of data of the work, critical review for important intellectual content and final approval of the version to be published.

Competing interests
On behalf of all authors, the corresponding author states that there is no conflict of interest.

Consent for publication
Not applicable.

Author details
[1]Tropical Medicine Health Sciences Center, Committee on Infection Control of Hospital das Clínicas, Universidade Federal de Pernambuco, Av. Professor Moraes Rego, 1235 Hospital das Clínicas - Cidade Universitária, Recife, Pernambuco 50670-901, Brazil. [2]Department of Pathology, Institute of Biological Sciences, Universidade de Pernambuco, Hospital de Câncer de Pernambuco, Real Hospital Português de Beneficência em Pernambuco, Recife, Pernambuco, Brazil. [3]Cardiac Intensive Care Unit, Pronto-Socorro Cardiológico de Pernambuco, Universidade de Pernambuco, Recife, Pernambuco, Brazil. [4]Committee on Infection Control, Pronto-Socorro Cardiológico de Pernambuco, Universidade de Pernambuco, Recife, Pernambuco, Brazil. [5]Committee on Infection Control, Real Hospital Português de Beneficência em Pernambuco, Recife, Pernambuco, Brazil. [6]Intensive Care Unit, Hospital Agamenon Magalhães, Secretaria de Saúde de Pernambuco, Recife, Pernambuco, Brazil. [7]Intensive Care Unit, Hospital das Clínicas, Universidade Federal de Pernambuco, Recife, Pernambuco, Brazil. [8]Committee on Infection Control of Hospital das Clínicas, Universidade Federal de Pernambuco, Recife, Pernambuco, Brazil. [9]Institute of Biological Sciences, Universidade de Pernambuco, Recife, Pernambuco, Brazil. [10]Faculty

of Medical Sciences, Tropical Medicine Health Sciences Center, Universidade Federal de Pernambuco, Recife, Pernambuco, Brazil. [11]Department of Infectious and Parasitic Diseases, Faculty of Medical Sciences, Tropical Medicine Health Sciences Center, Universidade Federal de Pernambuco, Recife, Pernambuco, Brazil.

References

1. Byers JF, Sole ML. Analysis of factors related to the development of ventilator-associated pneumonia: use of existing databases. Am J Crit Care. 2000;9:344–9.
2. Tablan OC, Anderson LJ, Besser R, Bridges C, Hajjeh R; Healthcare Infection Control Practices Advisory Committee. Guidelines for preventing health-care-associated pneumonia, 2003: recommendations of CDC and the Healthcare Infection Control Practices Advisory Committee. http://www.cdc.gov/hicpac/pdf/guidelines/HApneu2003guidelines.pdf. Accessed 10 Dec 2010.
3. Scannapieco FA, Stewart EM, Mylotte JM. Colonization of dental plaque by respiratory pathogens in medical intensive care patients. Crit Care Med. 1992;20:740–5.
4. Fourrier F, Duvivier B, Boutigny H, Koussel-Delvallez M, Chopin C. Colonization of dental plaque: A source of nosocomial infections in intensive care unit patients. Crit Care Med. 1998;26:301–8.
5. Grap MJ, Munro CL, Elswick Jr RK, Sessler CN, Ward KR. Duration of action of a single, early oral application of chlorhexidine on oral microbial flora in mechanically ventilated patients: a pilot study. Heart Lung. 2004;33(2):83–91.
6. Dallas J, Kollef M. Oral Descontamination to prevent ventilator-associated pneumonia: is it a sound strategy? CHEST. 2009;135:1116–18.
7. Houston S, Hougland P, Anderson JJ, LaRocco M, Kennedy V, Gentry LO. Effectiveness of 0.12% chlorhexidine gluconate oral rinse in reducing prevalence of nosocomial pneumonia in patients undergoing heart surgery. Am J Crit Care. 2002;11:567–70.
8. Segers P, Speekenbrink RG, Ubbink DT, van Ogtrop ML, de Mol BA. Prevention of nosocomial infection in cardiac surgery by decontamination of the nasopharynx and oropharynx with chlorhexidine gluconate: a randomized controlled trial. JAMA. 2006;296:2460–6.
9. Cate JM. Biofilms, a new approach to the microbiology of dental plaque. Odontology. 2006;94:1–9.
10. Scannapieco FA. Role of oral bacteria in respiratory infection. J Periodontol. 1999;70:793–802.
11. Kishimoto H, Urade M. Mechanical tooth cleaning before chlorhexidine application. Am J Respir Crit Care Med. 2007;175:418.
12. DMFT index. http://classof2011indexwikisite.wikispaces.com/DMFT+Index. Accessed 05 Feb 2014.
13. American Thoracic Society. Guidelines for the management of adults with hospital-acquired, ventilator-associated, and healthcare-associated pneumonia. american thoracic society documents. Am J Respir Crit Care Med. 2005;171:388–416.
14. Halm MA, Armola R. Effect of oral care on bacterial colonization and ventilator-associated. Am J Crit Care. 2009;18:275–8.
15. Munro CL, Grap MJ, Jones DJ, McClish DK, Sess CN. Chlorhexidine, toothbrushing, and preventing ventilator-associated pneumonia in critically ill adults. Am J Crit Care. 2009;18:428–37.
16. Pobo A, Lisboa T, Rodriguez A, Sole R, Magret M, Trefler S, Gómez F, Rello J, RASPALL Study Investigators. A randomized trial of dental brushing for preventing ventilator-associated pneumonia. Chest. 2009;136:433–39.
17. Gu WJ, Gong YZ, Pan L, Ni YX, Liu JC. Impact of oral care with versus without toothbrushing on the prevention of ventilator-associated pneumonia: A systematic review and meta-analysis of randomized controlled trials. Crit Care. 2012;16:R 190.
18. Alazzani W, Smith O, Muscedere J, Medd J, Cook D. Toothbrushing for critically ill mechanically ventilated patients: a systematic review and meta-analysis of randomized trials evaluating ventilator-associated pneumonia. Crit Care Med. 2013;41(2):646–55.
19. Edwards JR, Peterson KD, Andrus ML, et al. National Healthcare Safety Network (NHSN) Report, data summary for 2006 through 2007, issued November 2008. Am J Infect Control. 2008;36:609–26.
20. Institute for Healthcare Improvement. Getting Started Kit: Prevent Ventilator-Associated Pneumonia. How to Guide.2008; http://www.ihi.org/IHI/Programs/Campaign/Campaign.htm?TabId=2#PreventVentilator-AssociatedPneumonia. Accessed 10 Dec 2010.
21. Wise MP, Williams DW. Oral care and pulmonar infection- the importance of plaque scoring. Crit Care. 2013;17:101.
22. World Health Organization. Oral health surveys: basic methods. 4th ed. Geneva. WHO Library Cataloguing in Publication Data. http://www.paho.org/hq/dmdocuments/2009/OH_st_Esurv.
23. Needleman I, Hyun-Ryu J, Brealey D, Sachdev M, Moskal-Fitzpatrick D, Bercades G, Nagle J, Lewis K, Agudo E, Petrie A, Suvan L, Donos N, Singer M. The impact of hospitalization on dental plaque accumulation: an observational study. J Clin Periodontol. 2012;39:1006–11.
24. Labeau S. Oral care for mechanically ventilated patients involving toothbrushing. Crit care Med. 2013;41(7):e136.
25. Rello J, Lode H, Cornaglia G, Masterton R. VAP care bundle for prevention of ventilator-associated pneumonia. Intensive Care Med. 2010;36:773–80.

11

Proposed risk factors for infection with multidrug-resistant pathogens in hemodialysis patients hospitalized with pneumonia

Jae-Uk Song[1†], Hye Kyeong Park[2†], Hyung Koo Kang[2] and Jonghoo Lee[3*†] (iD)

Abstract

Background: In patients with hemodialysis-associated pneumonia (HDAP), information on both microbiologic features and antimicrobial strategies is limited. The aim of this study is to investigate predictive factors of infection with multidrug-resistant (MDR) pathogens in HDAP patients.

Methods: This was a multicenter, retrospective, and observational study. Enrolled patients were classified into MDR or non-MDR pathogens groups according to culture results. We examined risk factors of infection with MDR pathogens and created a decision support tool using these risk factors.

Results: MDR pathogens were identified in 24 (22.8%) out of a total of 105 HDAP patients. The most common MDR pathogens were methicillin-resistant *Staphylococcus aureus* (10 patients, 9.5%) and the isolation rate of *Pseudomonas aeruginosa* was 6.6%. Logistic regression showed two variables were associated with the isolation of MDR pathogens: recent hospitalization (adjusted odds ratio [OR]: 2.951, 95% confidence interval [CI]: 1.022–8.518) and PSI (Pneumonia Severity Index) score (adjusted OR: 1.023, 95% CI: 1.005–1.041). The optimal cut-off value for PSI score using a receiver operating characteristic curve analysis was 147. According to the presence of 0, 1, or 2 of the identified risk factors, the prevalence of MDR pathogens was 7.6, 28.2 and 64.2%, respectively ($p < 0.001$ for trend). The area under the curve of the prediction tool was 0.764 (95% CI: 0.652–0.875).

Conclusions: We demonstrated that recent hospitalization and PSI > 147 are risk factors of infection with MDR pathogens in HDAP patients. This simple proposed tool would facilitate more accurate identification of MDR pathogens in these patients.

Keywords: Pneumonia, Hemodialysis, End-stage renal disease, Multidrug resistance, Pathogen

Background

In hemodialysis (HD) populations, pneumonia is common and a leading cause of death [1, 2]. Because of the uremic internal milieu and the very frequent coexistence of serious comorbid medical conditions, these patients can be considered chronically immunosuppressed [3]. According to the United States Renal Dada System (USRDS) registry, approximately 20% of patients developed pneumonia in the 1-year period following initiation of dialysis therapy [1]. The mortality rates from pneumonia in hemodialysis (HD) patients were higher than those from pneumonia in the general population [2]. Therefore, early proper management is important to reduce mortality in HD patients with pneumonia.

Until now, there are no guidelines focused primarily on hemodialysis-associated pneumonia (HDAP). Because the 2005 American Thoracic Society (ATS)/Infectious Diseases Society of America (IDSA) guidelines included HDAP as a category of HCAP, HDAP patients could receive broad-spectrum antibiotics targeted against multidrug-resistant (MDR) pathogens [4]. But, several studies demonstrated

* Correspondence: lovlet@paran.com
†Equal contributors
3Department of Internal Medicine, Jeju National University Hospital, Jeju National University School of Medicine, Aran 13 gil 15, Jeju-si, Jeju Special Self-Governing Province 690-767, South Korea

that HCAP does not always identify MDR pathogens [5]. The 2016 ATS/IDSA guidelines removed the concept of HCAP among a category of nosocomial pneumonia [6].

The clinical epidemiology of HDAP has received little attention to date [7]. A previous study including some data used in the present study revealed that the HDAP group was clinically more similar to the CAP group than to the HCAP other than HDAP (O-HCAP) [7]. Accordingly, whether MDR pathogens-targeted antibiotics should be selected in patients with HDAP is unclear. Because of the uncertainty surrounding the actual risks of infection with MDR pathogens in HDAP patients and the increasing burden of end-stage renal disease worldwide [8], more data are required for a better distinct targeted therapeutic approach. Therefore, we investigated microbiologic characteristics and novel predictive factors of infection with MDR pathogens in patients hospitalized with HDAP. We also developed a prediction tool using these risk factors to identify subjects infected with MDR pathogens.

Methods
Study design, populations, and recorded parameters
We retrospectively conducted observational cohort studies at three institutions (Jeju National University Hospital, Kangbuk Samsung Hospital, and Ilsan Paik Hospital) between January 2011 and December 2015. Some of the clinical data for patients enrolled at Jeju National University Hospital were included in an article published in 2016 [7].

Patients were screened by the Korean Standard Classification of Diseases-7 codes of the followings; J18.0–18.9 as representative codes of pneumonia in the primary discharge diagnosis and N18.5, N18.9, or Z49.1 as codes of HD [9]. The medical records and radiological findings were reviewed to confirm the diagnosis of pneumonia by the following criteria: the presence of a new infiltrate on chest radiography with symptoms and signs of a lower respiratory tract infection. And patients on regular intermittent HD 3 times a week were included in the analysis. We excluded the following types of patients: (1) those who did not receive dialysis at the time of admission, (2) those who underwent continuous renal replacement therapy after organ failure developed by pneumonia, (3) those who had hospital-acquired pneumonia (HAP) developed at least 48 h after hospital admission, (4) those who did receive continuous ambulatory peritoneal dialysis, (5) those who re-visited within 10 days of discharging, and (6) those who transferred from other hospitals after hospitalization for >48 h.

According to culture results, enrolled patients were classified as MDR or non-MDR pathogens groups. We compared clinical characteristics, severity of pneumonia, identified pathogens, antibiotics, and clinical outcomes between the two groups. The severity of pneumonia was assessed by the CURB-65 (confusion, urea, respiratory rate, blood pressure, age more than 65 years) and Pneumonia Severity Index (PSI) scores [10, 11].

Definitions
HDAP was defined as pneumonia developing in patients receiving chronic HD within 30 days. O-HCAP was defined using the criteria of the 2005 ATS/IDSA guidelines as follows: recent history of hospitalization in an acute care hospital for ≥2 days in the past 90 days; residence in a nursing home or long-term care facility (NHAP, nursing home-acquired pneumonia); or recent outpatient intravenous therapy or wound care within the past 30 days [4]. Severe pneumonia was defined according to ATS/IDSA 2007 criteria [12].

In accordance with the 2005 ATS/IDSA guidelines [4], methicillin-resistant *Staphylococcus aureus* (MRSA), *Pseudomonas aeruginosa*, extended-spectrum beta-lactamase (ESBL)-producing or carbapenem-resistant *Klebsiella pneumoniae* and *Escherichia coli*, *Acinetobacter baumanii*, and *Stenotrophomonas maltophilia* were considered to be MDR pathogens. According to susceptibility test criteria for lower respiratory tract pathogens, the appropriateness of antibiotic therapy was analyzed for all cases with an etiological diagnosis. Inappropriate antibiotic therapy was defined if the empirical antibiotics were not effective or unnecessarily broad against the identified pathogens based on in vitro susceptibility testing [13]. Failure of initial antibiotics therapy was defined as death during initial treatment or change of antibiotics from initial agents to others after 48 h due to clinical instability [14].

Microbiology
Sputum, tracheal aspirate, bronchial alveolar lavage fluid or blood samples were investigated for microbial analysis. Respiratory samples were cultured in a semi-quantitative manner, and pathogens were identified when a predominant microorganism was detected from group 4 or 5 sputum, according to Geckler's grading system [15]. Blood cultures were considered as pathogens if there was no other infection source for a positive blood culture. Paired serology for *Mycoplasma pneumoniae* or *Chlamydia pneumoniae* and urinary antigen tests for *Streptococcus pneumoniae* and *Legionella pneumophila* serogroup 1 were also recorded if these exams were checked. The antibiotic sensitivity of all isolates was determined using a disc diffusion method, according to the Clinical and Laboratory Standards Institute guidelines [16].

Statistical analyses
Data are presented as medians and interquartile ranges (IQRs; 25th and 75th percentiles) for continuous variables and as numbers and percentages for categorical variables. For comparison of continuous variables, the Mann-Whitney U-test between two

groups and the Kruskal-Wallis test among three groups were used to compare the median values. Categorical variables were compared using the Pearson χ^2 test, and the Fisher's exact test was used when any cell contained fewer than five data points.

To identify independent predictive factors associated with occurrence of MDR pathogens, we performed multivariate logistic regression analyses, as measured by the estimated odds ratio (OR) with 95% confidence interval (CI). Potential candidate variables with a P-value less than 0.05 in univariate analysis were entered into the regression model. From logistic regression results, we created predictive tool to identify patients with HDAP due to MDR pathogens. We classified patients based on the presence of risk factors for MDR pathogens. Then, we evaluated the predictive value of the proposed support tool for correctly indicating the presence of infection with MDR pathogens via a receiver operating characteristic (ROC) curve. The estimated area under the ROC curve (AUC) values were compared using the Hanley-McNeil test [17]. The cut-off point that showed the highest Youden Index was considered the optimal cut-off value [18]. All tests were two-sided, and P-values <0.05 were considered statistically significant. All analyses were performed using the Statistical Package for the Social Sciences (SPSS) network version 18.0 (SPSS; Chicago, IL, USA).

Results

Baseline characteristics and clinical outcomes

A total of 887 patients were initially identified through medical records. Of these patients, 703 were excluded for the reasons in the followings; 536 did not meet pneumonia definitions, 111 did not receive dialysis at the time of admission, and 56 underwent CCRT after organ failure developed by pneumonia (Fig. 1). A total of 184 patients (21.1%) were enrolled as the dialysis related to pneumonia. Seventy-nine patients were excluded for the reasons presented in Fig. 1. Finally, a total of 105 patients were included in the present study.

There were 68 males and 37 females, with a median age of 71 years. MDR pathogens were identified in 24 patients (22.8%). The baseline clinical characteristics and clinical outcomes of the total 105 HDAP patients are summarized in Table 1.

Microbiological etiology

Table 2 shows the distribution of causative organisms. Of the total 105 HDAP patients, the responsible pathogens were determined only in 53 patients (50.4%). The most common pathogen was S. aureus (17, 16.1%), which consisted of methicillin-sensitive S. aureus (7, 6.6%) and MRSA (10, 9.5%), followed by K. pneumoniae (11, 10.4%) and S. pneumoniae (10, 9.5%). The isolation rates of drug-resistant gram-

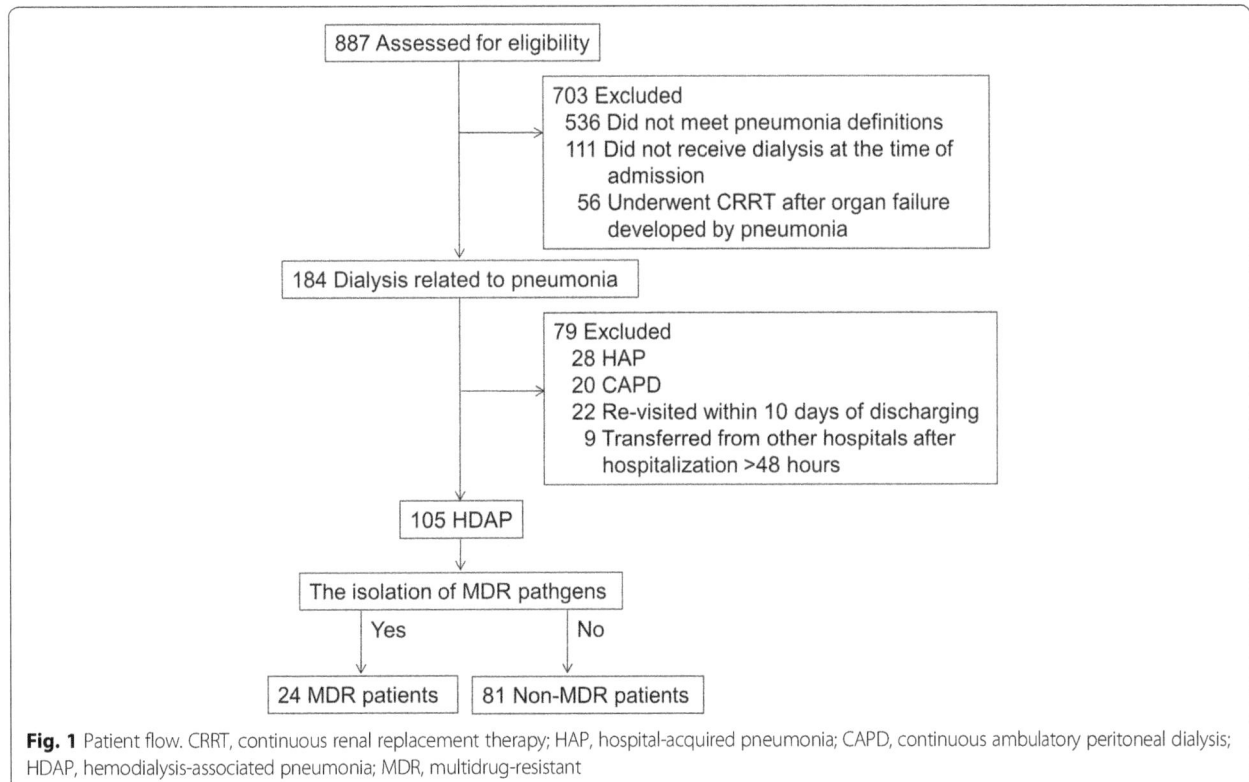

Fig. 1 Patient flow. CRRT, continuous renal replacement therapy; HAP, hospital-acquired pneumonia; CAPD, continuous ambulatory peritoneal dialysis; HDAP, hemodialysis-associated pneumonia; MDR, multidrug-resistant

Table 1 Baseline clinical characteristics and treatment outcomes of patients admitted with hemodialysis-associated pneumonia

Characteristics	Overall patients (n = 105)	MDR pathogens group (n = 24)	Non-MDR pathogens group (n = 81)	P Value
Age (years)	71 (61–76)	73 (62–79)	71 (61–76)	0.199
Male	68 (64.8%)	15 (62.5%)	53 (65.4%)	0.792
Female	37 (35.2%)	9 (37.5)	28 (34.6%)	0.792
Time interval between dialysis and pneumonia (months)	30 (11–69)	21 (10–74)	34 (12–69)	0.541
Etiology of dialysis[a]				
Diabetes mellitus	60 (57.1%)	14 (58.3%)	46 (56.7%)	0.344
Hypertension	57 (54.2%)	11 (45.8%)	46 (56.7%)	0.893
Glomerulonephropathy	6 (5.7%)	1 (4.1%)	5 (6.1%)	1.000
Idiopathic	7 (6.6%)	2 (8.3%)	5 (6.1%)	0.658
Others	13 (12.3%)	1 (4.1%)	12 (14.8%)	0.289
Tube feeding	9 (8.5%)	5 (20.8%)	4 (4.9%)	0.028
HCAP criteria other than HDAP		17 (70.8%)	27 (33.3%)	0.001
Recent hospitalization	42 (40.0%)	16 (66.6%)	26 (32.0%)	0.002
NHAP	10 (9.5%)	5 (20.8%)	5 (6.1%)	0.047
Recent intravenous therapy	10 (9.5%)	3 (12.5%)	7 (8.6%)	0.692
Clinical parameters				
Severe pneumonia	37 (35.2%)	13 (54.1%)	24 (29.6%)	0.027
Confusion	15 (14.2%)	6 (25.0%)	9 (11.1%)	0.103
Respiratory failure	47 (44.7%)	14 (58.3%)	33 (40.7%)	0.128
Sepsis or septic shock at onset	15 (14.2%)	7 (29.1%)	8 (9.8%)	0.040
ICU admission	22 (20.9%)	10 (41.6%)	12 (14.8%)	0.005
Need for ventilator	6 (5.7%)	3 (12.5%)	3 (3.7%)	0.131
Radiological findings				
Multi-lobar involvement	73 (69.5%)	20 (83.3%)	53 (65.4%)	0.094
Pleural effusion	33 (31.4%)	6 (25.0%)	27 (33.3%)	0.440
Laboratory findings				
WBC (/mm^3)	11,200 (7400–15,015)	13,210 (8200–18,600)	10,680 (7150–14,960)	0.104
CRP (mg/dl)	8.5 (3.7–15.1)	9.4 (4.8–16.0)	7.1 (3.7–14.7)	0.364
Procalcitonin, n = 62, (mg/dl)	1.1 (0.4–5.9)	1.7 (0.5–6.8)	0.9 (0.3–5.6)	0.571
Indices for disease severity				
CURB-65 score	2 (1–2)	2 (1–3)	2 (1–2)	0.095
CURB-65 score ≥ 3	19 (18.0%)	7 (29.1%)	12 (14.8%)	0.133
PSI score	123 (105–145)	148 (120–181)	118 (99–139)	0.001
PSI class IV or V	91 (86.6%)	23 (95.8%)	68 (83.9%)	0.181
Initial antibiotic therapy				
as CAP	47 (44.7%)	4 (16.6%)	43 (53.0%)	0.002
as HAP	58 (55.2%)	20 (83.3%)	38 (46.9%)	0.002
Use of Anti-MRSA agents	7 (6.6%)	4 (16.6%)	3 (3.7%)	0.046
Clinical outcomes				
Use of inappropriate antibiotics	21 (20.0%)	15 (62.5%)	6 (7.4%)	<0.001
Change of initial antibiotics	40 (38.0%)	13 (54.1%)	27 (33.3%)	0.065
Failure of initial antibiotics therapy	29 (27.6%)	11 (45.8%)	18 (22.2%)	0.254
Duration of antibiotic therapy (days)	12 (10–15)	12 (9–22)	12 (10–15)	0.401

Table 1 Baseline clinical characteristics and treatment outcomes of patients admitted with hemodialysis-associated pneumonia (*Continued*)

Characteristics	Overall patients (*n* = 105)	MDR pathogens group (*n* = 24)	Non-MDR pathogens group (*n* = 81)	*P* Value
Length of hospital stay (days)	11 (7–17)	14 (9–25)	11 (7–16)	0.093
Pneumonia-related mortality rate	8 (7.6%)	6 (25.0%)	2 (2.4%)	0.002
Hospital mortality rate	11 (10.4%)	6 (25.0%)	5 (6.1%)	0.016

Data are presented as median (interquartile range) or number (%)
MDR multidrug-resistant, *HCAP* healthcare-associated pneumonia, *HDAP* hemodialysis-associated pneumonia, *NHAP* nursing home-acquired pneumonia, *ICU* intensive care unit, *WBC* white blood cell, *CRP* C-reactive protein, *CAP* community-acquired pneumonia, *MRSA* methicillin-resistant *Staphylococcus aureus*, *CURB-65* Confusion, Urea, Respiratory rate, Blood pressure, Age ≥ 65, *PSI* Pneumonia Severity Index
[a]allowed for overlap

negative bacteria *P. aeruginosa, A. baumanii*, ESBL-producing *K. pneumoniae* were 6.6, 5.7, and 2.8%, respectively.

Predictive factors associated with occurrence of MDR pathogens

Table 3 shows multivariate logistic regression analyses of the four risk factors for MDR pathogens: tube feeding, recent hospitalization, NHAP, and PSI score. Recent

Table 2 Microorganisms identified in patients admitted with hemodialysis-associated pneumonia

Microorganisms[a]	No. of patients (%)
Identified microorganisms[b] Gram-positive bacteria	53 (50.4%)
Streptococcus pneumoniae	10 (9.5%)
Staphylococcus aureus	17 (16.1%)
MSSA	7 (6.6%)
MRSA	10 (9.5%)
Gram-negative bacteria	
Pseudomonas aeruginosa	7 (6.6%)
Haemophilus influenza	0 (0%)
Klebsiella pneumoniae	11 (10.4%)
ESBL (+)	3 (2.8%)
ESBL (−)	8 (7.6%)
Acinetobacter baumannii	6 (5.7%)
Stenotrophomonas maltophilia	1 (0.9%)
Mycoplasma pneumonia	2 (1.9%)
Other gram-negative species[c]	5 (4.7%)
Polymicrobial pathogens	8 (7.6%)
Multidrug-resistant pathogens[d]	24 (22.8%)

Data are presented as number (%)
HDAP: hemodialysis-associated pneumonia; MSSA: methicillin-sensitive *Staphylococcus aureus*; MRSA: methicillin-resistant *Staphylococcus aureus*
[a]Allowed for overlap
[b]One or more pathogens may be listed
[c]Other gram-negative species include *Escherichia coli, Enterobacter species, Serratia marcescens*, and *Legionella pneumophilia*
[d]Multidrug-resistant pathogens include Methicillin-resistant *Staphylococcus aureus* (MRSA), *Pseudomonas* species, *Acinetobacter* species, *Stenotrophomonas maltophilia*, and extended-spectrum β-lactamase (ESBL)-producing Enterobacteriaceae

hospitalization and PSI score was independently associated with the isolation of MDR pathogens in HDAP patients (adjusted OR: 2.951, 95% CI: 1.022–8.518, *p* = 0.045 and adjusted OR: 1.023, 95% CI: 1.005–1.041, *p* = 0.011, respectively). ROC curve analysis was used to assess optimal cutoff values for PSI score. The maximum sum of sensitivity and specificity was 147 for PSI (sensitivity 54.1%, specificity 85.1%, positive predictive value 52.0%, and negative predictive value 86.2%, Fig. 2).

Proposed decision support tool for prediction of MDR pathogens

Based on the multivariate logistic regression analysis of the association with occurrence of MDR pathogens in patients with HDAP, PSI score > 147 and recent hospitalization were considered as predictive MDR risk factors. We created a decision support tool to predict MDR pathogens. Patients divided into low (without any risk factors)-, intermediate (with only one risk factor)-, and high (with both two risk factors)-risk strata based on two predictive MDR risk factors.

The ROC curves for prediction tool and PSI score are shown in Fig. 2 The prediction tool had a higher discriminatory power to identify MDR pathogen infection than PSI score, although there was no statistically significant difference (*p* = 0.228). The area under the curve (AUC) of the prediction tool (AUC: 0.764, 95% CI: 0.652–0.875, *p* < 0.001) tended to be greater than that of the PSI score (AUC: 0.718, 95% CI: 0.593–0.842, *p* = 0.001) (*p* = 0.236). The optimal cutoff for the prediction tool was 1 (sensitivity 83.3%, specificity 59.3%,

Table 3 Multivariate logistic regression analysis for predictive factors associated with multidrug-resistant pathogens in patients admitted with hemodialysis-associated pneumonia

Risk factors	Odds ratio (95% confidence interval)	*P* Value
Tube feeding	2.229 (0.459–10.819)	0.320
Recent hospitalization	2.951 (1.022–8.518)	0.045
NHAP	3.535 (0.823–15.183)	0.090
PSI score	1.023 (1.005–1.041)	0.011

NHAP nursing home-acquired pneumonia, *PSI* Pneumonia Severity Index

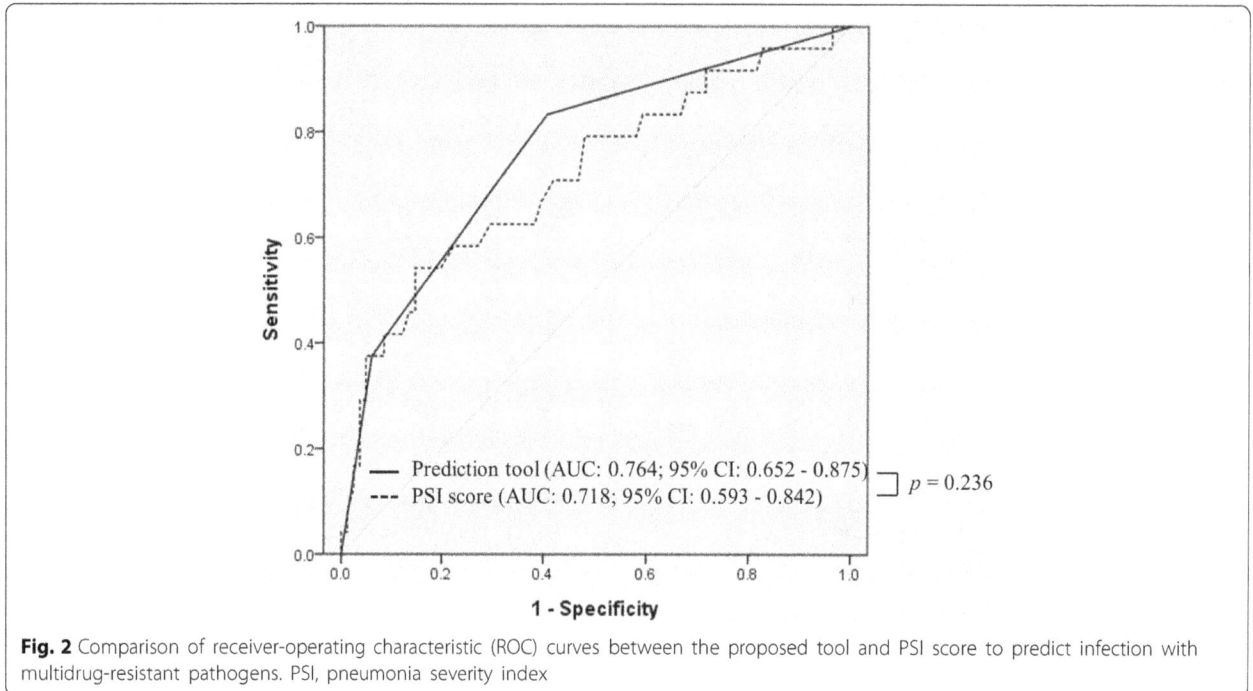

Fig. 2 Comparison of receiver-operating characteristic (ROC) curves between the proposed tool and PSI score to predict infection with multidrug-resistant pathogens. PSI, pneumonia severity index

positive predictive value 37.7%, and negative predictive value 92.3%). According to the risk stratification based on number of MDR risk variables, the prevalence of MDR pathogens was 7.6, 28.2 and 64.2%, respectively (p < 0.001 for trend, Table 4 and Fig. 3).

Discussion

The current study revealed that 22.8% of hospitalized patients with HDAP had MDR pathogens. We also demonstrated that the occurrence of MDR pathogens was significantly associated with recent hospitalization within 3 months and PSI score more than 147. On the basis of these findings, we proposed a simple predictive tool to determine the risk of infection with MDR pathogens in HDAP using the number of risk factors. As the number of risk factors increased, the prevalence of infection with MDR pathogens also increased (low - 7.6%, intermediate - 28.2% and high - 64.2%, respectively; $p < 0.001$ for trend). Overall, this model had moderate predictive value, as demonstrated by the ROC curve (AUC: 0.764, 95% CI: 0.652–0.875). To our knowledge, this is the first study that proposes evidence based tool to predict infection with MDR pathogens among HDAP patients.

Previous studies have demonstrated that the isolation rate of MDR pathogens shows interregional differences in HCAP patients [5]. Also, HCAP consists of very heterogeneous subgroups [4], and there is little evidence that all criteria for HCAP convey similar risks for infection with MDR pathogens. This contributed to the removal of the concept of HCAP in the new 2016 ATS/IDSA guidelines for management of HAP and ventilator-associated pneumonia [6]. But, the concept of HCAP as a separate clinical entity would be still valid, because frequent interactions with the healthcare system can have potential risk for MDR pathogens [6]. Discordant results about the isolated rate of MDR pathogens among previous studies may be caused by the fact that the concept of HCAP includes various criteria for heterogeneous conditions [4], which did not have similar risks for infection with MDR pathogens [19]. Among the category of HCAP, only NHAP have been studied considerably, and MDR pathogens were not frequently isolated in these patients [20–25]. In contrast, the previous studies on HCAP included a relatively small proportion of 2.5~10.4% of HDAP patients [7, 13, 26–29]. Therefore, it is not known whether it is desirable to actively apply the guideline-concordant treatment to all patients with HDAP [4].

Table 4 Proposed prediction tools for multidrug-resistant pathogens in patients admitted with hemodialysis-associated pneumonia

Risk of MDR pathogens	Predictive factors	No. of patients	No. (%) of patients isolated with MDR pathogens
Low	PSI score ≤ 147 and no recent hospitalization	52	4 (7.6%)
Moderate	PSI score > 147 or recent hospitalization	39	11 (28.2%)
High	PSI score > 147 and recent hospitalization	14	9 (64.2%)

MDR multidrug-resistant, *PSI* Pneumonia: Severity Index

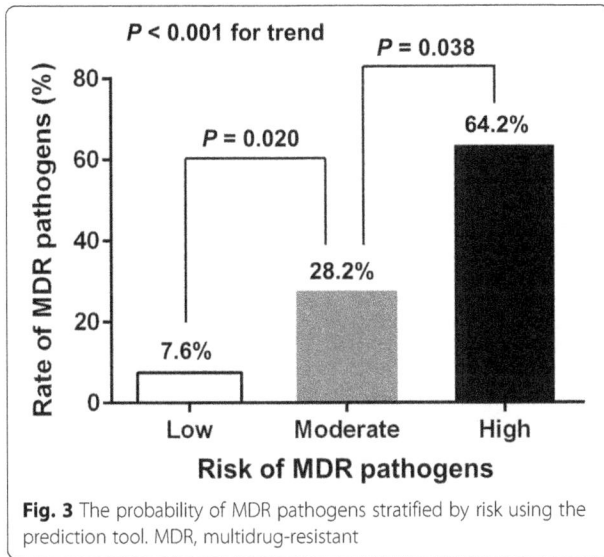

Fig. 3 The probability of MDR pathogens stratified by risk using the prediction tool. MDR, multidrug-resistant

There are few studies focusing on the actual risk of MDR pneumonia in HDAP patients, resulting in a lack of microbiologic data on HDAP as a different category of HCAP. Although most HD patients live outside of hospitals, they manifest various degrees of immunodeficiency, regularly visit the hospital, and receive ongoing healthcare more often than non-HD patients. Compared to the general population, these characteristics of HD patients may contribute to the high incidence of MDR pathogens, which is not related to HD itself. Therefore, there is a question regarding whether all patients with HDAP should receive antibiotic therapy against MDR pathogens [30, 31].

We found two large cohort studies using the USRDS registry for clinical epidemiology of HDAP patients and four retrospective studies applying to the concept of HDAP [1, 2, 7, 30–32]. Unfortunately, in large cohort studies, the microorganisms in more than 80% of the patients hospitalized with HDAP could not be identified [1, 2]. The detection rate of *P. aeruginosa* was about 2%, but the rate of total isolated MDR pathogens was not mentioned in either study [1, 2]. In addition, four retrospective studies have demonstrated inconsistent MDR pathogen distributions in HDAP patients [7, 30–32]. In line with previous HDAP studies, the rate of isolated MDR pathogens was 5.6 to 35.4%, although microorganisms could not be identified in most patients. The detection rates of MRSA, *P. aeruginosa*, and *A. baumanii* were 0%~27.5%, 1.6%~16.7%, and 0%~4.2%, respectively [7, 30–32]. In the present study, MDR pathogens were identified in 22.8% of cases; of these, the most frequent microorganisms were MRSA (9.5%), followed by *P. aeruginosa* (6.6%), *A. baumanii* (5.7%). However, the rates of isolated MDR pathogens in previous studies and this study revealed a variable incidence range [7, 30–32].

Although we cannot offer satisfactory explanations for these various incidence rates of MDR pathogen distribution, these discordant results may be related to whether the selected populations included the other criteria for HCAP. The studies demonstrating relatively low MDR pathogen infections included patients who only met HDAP criterion without O-HCAP components for HCAP classification [7, 31]. On the contrary, the remaining studies enrolled patients who included the other criteria for HCAP, and reported relatively high incidence of MDR pathogens [30, 32]. In line with this concept, among 61 patients who only met HDAP criterion without the other criteria for HCAP in our study, the isolated rate of MDR pathogens was relatively low (7 patients, 11.4%). We also demonstrated that presence of O-HCAP components exhibited higher occurrence of MDR pathogens in patients with HDAP. Among the O-HCAP category, recent hospitalization and NHAP were more frequently observed in the MDR pathogens group. Especially, recent hospitalization was independently associated with the isolation of MDR pathogens in multivariable analysis. Therefore, our study found that MDR pathogen infection in HDAP could be associated with recent hospitalization, rather than HD status itself, similar to previous studies [19, 26]. The present study revealed that PSI score than 147 was also significantly associated with HDAP caused by MDR pathogens. Furthermore, the proposed prediction tool using these two risk factors showed a moderate discriminatory power for risk stratification for an infection with MDR pathogens in HDAP patients. Therefore, our findings could be helpful in physicians' decisions to select HDAP patients who need to be treated for MDR pathogens.

The present study has several limitations. Firstly, the main limitation of this study is retrospective design. Because the effect of missing data in the results is unknown, our study may be vulnerable to selection bias. And a small sample size did not allow us to draw a robust conclusion. We were unable to enroll a large number of HDAP patients despite the fact that they were collected from three centers over 5 years. Larger studies are needed to validate our results and to strengthen the power to identify risk factors of MDR pathogens. Secondly, the microbiological etiology could be identified in only about 50% of enrolled patients. Possible reasons for low detections would include an inability to collect lower respiratory tract specimens, prior antibiotic use before specimen collection, insensitive diagnostic tests for known pathogens, a lack of testing for other recognized pathogens such as *coxiella*, unknown pathogens, and possible noninfectious causes such as aspiration pneumonitis [33]. Thirdly, median age of the patients is 71 years in the present study. Aging is associated with declines in adaptive and innate immunity [34]. Infections occur more frequently in the elderly, and the age-related remodeling of the immune system plays any role in the development of HDAP or HDAP with MDR pathogens [34]. Although age was not associated with the isolation of MDR pathogens among HDAP patients in our study, the results might be biased towards the old age population. Finally, the analysis for distribution of MDR pathogens included entire study populations with culture-negative pneumonia. Thus, we may have skewed our findings in that the true incidence of MDR pathogens could have been underestimated. In this study, we founded two independent risk factors for occurrence of MDR pathogens in patients with HDAP. And the prevalence of MDR pathogens was <10% in patients without one of these risk factors. If validated in subsequent multicenter studies, this prediction rule could potentially assist clinicians who are deciding on whether to administer anti-MRSA or anti-pseudomonal therapy to patients with HDAP.

Conclusion

This multicenter, retrospective, observational study offers the findings of the clinical epidemiology, microbiology, and predictive factors of MDR pathogens in patients with HDAP. The HDAP concept itself as an HCAP has limited value in selecting patients harboring MDR pathogens. It could be necessary to stratify the patients with regard to risk factors in order to properly identify infection with MDR pathogens. Although large-scale prospective studies are needed to confirm our results, our findings would be helpful for physicians' decisions to select HDAP patients harboring MDR pathogens.

Abbreviations
A. baumannii: *Acinetobacter baumannii*; ATS/IDSA: American Thoracic Society/ Infectious Diseases Society of America; CAP: community-acquired pneumonia; CRP: C-reactive protein; CURB-65: Confusion, Urea, Respiratory rate, Blood pressure, Age ≥ 65; ESBL: Extended-spectrum b-lactamase; HAP: Hospital-acquired pneumonia; HCAP: Healthcare-associated pneumonia; HD: Hemodialysis; HDAP: Hemodialysis-associated pneumonia; ICU: Intensive care unit; *K. pneumoniae*: *Klebsiella pneumoniae*; MDR: Multidrug-resistant; MRSA: Methicillin-resistant *Staphylococcus aureus*; NHAP: Nursing home-acquired pneumonia; O-HCAP: The HCAP other than HDAP; *P. aeruginosa*: *Pseudomonas aeruginosa*; PSI: Pneumonia Severity Index; *S. aureus*: *Staphylococcus aureus*; *S. pneumoniae*: *Streptococcus pneumoniae*; USRDS: The United States Renal Dada System; WBC: White blood cell

Acknowledgements
Nil.

Funding
This study was funded by a research grant from Chong Kun Dang Corp.

Authors' contributions
J-US and HKP contributed to the study design, data acquisition, and writing of the manuscript. HKK contributed to data acquisition, and data interpretation. JL contributed to the study design, data acquisition, data interpretation, statistical analysis, writing of the manuscript, and is responsible for the study. All authors read and approved the final manuscript.

Consent for publication
Not applicable.

Competing interests
The authors declare that they have no competing interests.

Author details
[1]Division of Pulmonary and Critical Care Medicine, Department of Internal Medicine, Kangbuk Samsung Hospital, Sungkyunkwan University School of Medicine, Seoul, South Korea. [2]Division of Pulmonary and Critical Care Medicine, Department of Internal Medicine, Ilsan Paik Hospital, Inje University College of Medicine, Goyang-si, South Korea. [3]Department of Internal Medicine, Jeju National University Hospital, Jeju National University School of Medicine, Aran 13 gil 15, Jeju-si, Jeju Special Self-Governing Province 690-767, South Korea.

References
1. Guo H, Liu J, Collins AJ, Foley RN. Pneumonia in incident dialysis patients–the United States renal data system. Nephrol Dial Transplant. 2008;23:680–6.
2. Slinin Y, Foley RN, Collins AJ. Clinical epidemiology of pneumonia in hemodialysis patients: the USRDS waves 1, 3, and 4 study. Kidney Int. 2006; 70:1135–41.
3. Vanholder R, Ringoir S. Infectious morbidity and defects of phagocytic function in end-stage renal disease: a review. J Am Soc Nephrol. 1993;3: 1541–54.
4. American Thoracic Society. Infectious Diseases Society of America. Guidelines for the management of adults with hospital-acquired, ventilator-associated, and healthcare-associated pneumonia. Am J Respir Crit Care Med. 2005;171:388–416.
5. Chalmers JD, Rother C, Salih W, Ewig S. Healthcare-associated pneumonia does not accurately identify potentially resistant pathogens: a systematic review and meta-analysis. Clin Infect Dis. 2014;58:330–9.
6. Kalil AC, Metersky ML, Klompas M, Muscedere J, Sweeney DA, Palmer LB, et al. Management of Adults with Hospital-Acquired and Ventilator-Associated Pneumonia: 2016 clinical practice guidelines by the Infectious Diseases Society of America and the American Thoracic Society. Clin Infect Dis. 2016;63:e61–e111.
7. Lee JH, Moon JC. Clinical characteristics of patients with hemodialysis-associated pneumonia compared to patients with non-hemodialysis community-onset pneumonia. Respir Med. 2016;111:84–90.
8. Lee YK, Kim K, Kim DJ. Current status and standards for establishment of hemodialysis units in Korea. Korean J Intern Med. 2013;28:274–84.
9. Korean Standard Statistical Classification. The standard of classification of disease and cause of death [Internet]. Daejeon, Korea; Korean Standard Statistical Classification; 2016 [cited at 2017 Aug 11]. Available from: https://kssc.kostat.go.kr:8443/ksscNew_web/link.do?gubun=AQ5004.
10. Lim WS, van der Eerden MM, Laing R, Boersma WG, Karalus N, Town GI, et al. Defining community acquired pneumonia severity on presentation to hospital: an international derivation and validation study. Thorax. 2003;58:377–82.
11. Fine MJ, Auble TE, Yealy DM, Hanusa BH, Weissfeld LA, Singer DE, et al. A prediction rule to identify low-risk patients with community-acquired pneumonia. New Engl J Med. 1997;336:243–50.
12. Mandell LA, Wunderink RG, Anzueto A, Bartlett JG, Campbell GD, Dean NC, et al. Infectious Diseases Society of America/American Thoracic Society consensus guidelines on the management of community-acquired pneumonia in adults. Clin Infect Dis. 2007;44(Suppl 2):S27–72.
13. Micek ST, Kollef KE, Reichley RM, Roubinian N, Kollef MH. Health care-associated pneumonia and community-acquired pneumonia: a single-center experience. Antimicrob Agents Chemother. 2007;51:3568–73.
14. Maruyama T, Fujisawa T, Okuno M, Toyoshima H, Tsutsui K, Maeda H, et al. A new strategy for healthcare-associated pneumonia: a 2-year prospective multicenter cohort study using risk factors for multidrug-resistant pathogens to select initial empiric therapy. Clin Infect Dis. 2013;57:1373–83.
15. Geckler RW, Gremillion DH, McAllister CK, Ellenbogen C. Microscopic and bacteriological comparison of paired sputa and transtracheal aspirates. J Clin Microbiol. 1977;6:396–9.

16. Clinical and Laboratory Standards Institute: Methods for Dilution Antimicrobial Susceptiblity Tests for Bacteria That Grow Aerobically; Approved Standard-Eighth Edition. Clin Lab Stand Inst 2008;29:M07-A08.
17. Hanley JA, McNeil BJ. The meaning and use of the area under a receiver operating characteristic (ROC) curve. Radiology. 1982;143:29–36.
18. Bewick V, Cheek L, Ball J. Statistics review 13: receiver operating characteristic curves. Crit Care. 2004;8:508–12.
19. Shorr AF, Zilberberg MD, Micek ST, Kollef MH. Prediction of infection due to antibiotic-resistant bacteria by select risk factors for health care-associated pneumonia. Arch Intern Med. 2008;168:2205–10.
20. Ewig S, Klapdor B, Pletz MW, Rohde G, Schutte H, Schaberg T, et al. Nursing home-acquired pneumonia in Germany: an 8-year prospective multicentre study. Thorax. 2012;67:132–8.
21. Ma HM, Wah JL, Woo J. Should nursing home-acquired pneumonia be treated as nosocomial pneumonia? J Am Med Dir Assoc. 2012;13:727–31.
22. Polverino E, Dambrava P, Cilloniz C, Balasso V, Marcos MA, Esquinas C, et al. Nursing home-acquired pneumonia: a 10 year single-centre experience. Thorax. 2010;65:354–9.
23. Nakagawa N, Saito Y, Sasaki M, Tsuda Y, Mochizuki H, Takahashi H. Comparison of clinical profile in elderly patients with nursing and healthcare-associated pneumonia, and those with community-acquired pneumonia. Geriatr Gerontol Int. 2014;14:362–71.
24. Liapikou A, Polverino E, Cilloniz C, Peyrani P, Ramirez J, Menendez R, et al. A worldwide perspective of nursing home-acquired pneumonia compared with community-acquired pneumonia. Respir Care. 2014;59:1078–85.
25. Koh SJ, Lee JH. Clinical characteristics of nursing home-acquired pneumonia in elderly patients admitted to a Korean teaching hospital. Korean J Intern Med. 2015;30:638–47.
26. Jung JY, Park MS, Kim YS, Park BH, Kim SK, Chang J, et al. Healthcare-associated pneumonia among hospitalized patients in a Korean tertiary hospital. BMC Infect Dis. 2011;11:61.
27. Chalmers JD, Taylor JK, Singanayagam A, Fleming GB, Akram AR, Mandal P, et al. Epidemiology, antibiotic therapy, and clinical outcomes in health care-associated pneumonia: a UK cohort study. Clin Infect Dis. 2011;53:107–13.
28. Shindo Y, Sato S, Maruyama E, Ohashi T, Ogawa M, Hashimoto N, et al. Health-care-associated pneumonia among hospitalized patients in a Japanese community hospital. Chest. 2009;135:633–40.
29. Zilberberg MD, Shorr AF, Micek ST, Mody SH, Kollef MH. Antimicrobial therapy escalation and hospital mortality among patients with health-care-associated pneumonia: a single-center experience. Chest. 2008;134:963–8.
30. Kawasaki S, Aoki N, Kikuchi H, Nakayama H, Saito N, Shimada H, et al. Clinical and microbiological evaluation of hemodialysis-associated pneumonia (HDAP): should HDAP be included in healthcare-associated pneumonia? J Infect Chemother. 2011;17:640–5.
31. Taylor SP, Taylor BT. Health care-associated pneumonia in haemodialysis patients: clinical outcomes in patients treated with narrow versus broad spectrum antibiotic therapy. Respirology. 2013;18:364–8.
32. Wang PH, Wang HC. Risk factors to predict drug-resistant pathogens in hemodialysis-associated pneumonia. BMC Infect Dis. 2016;16:377.
33. Jain S, Self WH, Wunderink RG, Fakhran S, Balk R, Bramley AM, et al. Community-acquired pneumonia requiring hospitalization among U.S. adults. N Engl J Med. 2015;373:415–27.
34. Fuentes E, Fuentes M, Alarcón M, Palomo I. Immune system dysfunction in the elderly. An Acad Bras Cienc. 2017;89:285–99.

12

Radiologic findings as a determinant and no effect of macrolide resistance on clinical course of *Mycoplasma pneumoniae* pneumonia

In Ae Yoon[1†], Ki Bae Hong[1†], Hoan Jong Lee[1,2], Ki Wook Yun[1,2], Ji Young Park[1], Young Hoon Choi[3], Woo Sun Kim[3], Hyunju Lee[2,4], Byung Wook Eun[5], Young Min Ahn[5], Eun Young Cho[6], Hwa Jin Cho[7] and Eun Hwa Choi[1,2*]

Abstract

Background: With the emergence of macrolide resistance, concerns about the efficacy of macrolides for the treatment of *Mycoplasma pneumoniae* (MP) pneumonia in children have been raised. This study aimed to determine the effect of macrolide resistance on the outcome of children who were hospitalized with MP pneumonia.

Methods: Between 2010 and 2015, we performed culture of MP from nasopharyngeal samples obtained from children who were hospitalized with pneumonia at five hospitals in Korea. Macrolide resistance was determined by the analysis of 23S rRNA gene transition and the minimal inhibitory concentrations of four macrolides. Medical records were reviewed to analyze the clinical response to treatment with macrolides.

Results: MP was detected in 116 (4.8%) of the 2436 children with pneumonia. MP pneumonia was prevalent in 2011 and 2015. Of the 116 patients with MP pneumonia, 82 (70.7%) were macrolide-resistant. There were no differences in the age distribution, total duration of fever, and chest x-ray patterns between the macrolide-susceptible and macrolide-resistant groups. After macrolide initiation, mean days to defervescence were longer in the macrolide-resistant group than in macrolide-susceptible group (5.7 days vs. 4.1 days, $P = 0.021$). However, logistic regression analysis revealed that the presence of extrapulmonary signs ($P = 0.039$), homogeneous lobar consolidation ($P = 0.004$), or parapneumonic effusion ($P < 0.001$) were associated with fever duration of ≥ 7 days after the initiation of macrolides, regardless of macrolide resistance.

Conclusions: This study demonstrated that fever duration in MP pneumonia was determined by the radiologic findings of chest x-ray, not by the presence of macrolide resistance. The results highlight the need for future studies to assess therapeutic benefit from macrolides in the treatment of children with MP pneumonia.

Keywords: *Mycoplasma pneumoniae*, Pneumonia, Macrolides, Resistance, Radiologic findings

Background

Mycoplasma pneumoniae (MP) is one of the most common causes of community-acquired pneumonia in children and young adults, accounting for approximately 10–30% of all cases of community-acquired pneumonia [1, 2]. Outbreaks have been occurring in cycles every 3–4 years in Korea, mostly during the late summer through the early autumn [3–5]. Emerging resistance to macrolides among MP is of great concern since a macrolide-resistant MP strain was first reported in 1997 [6, 7]. The macrolide resistance rate in Japan increased from 30% in 2006 to 93% in 2011 [7]. Recent reports showed that the resistant rate was as high as 97% among children with MP pneumonia in China in 2012 [8–10]. In Korea, the macrolide resistance rate among children with MP pneumonia increased from 0% in 2000 to 62.9% in 2011 [4].

* Correspondence: eunchoi@snu.ac.kr
†Equal contributors
[1]Department of Pediatrics, Seoul National University Children's Hospital, Seoul, South Korea
[2]Department of Pediatrics, Seoul National University College of Medicine, Seoul, South Korea

Although macrolides are recommended for the first-line treatment for MP pneumonia, the efficacy of macrolides in the treatment of *M. pneumoniae* infection remains unclear. In addition, with the increase in macrolide resistance, concerns about the efficacy of macrolides for the treatment of MP pneumonia in children have been raised [11]. In contrast, previous studies also show clinical improvement with macrolides in patients with macrolide-resistant MP infection [12]. Overall, data are limited on the clinical response to macrolides in macrolide-resistant MP pneumonia. The aim of this study was to compare the clinical response of the children hospitalized with macrolide-resistant vs. macrolide-susceptible MP pneumonia to macrolide treatment. In addition, this study sought risk factors for pronged fever in the children with MP pneumonia.

Methods

Subjects

Between September 2010 and December 2015, five hospitals participated in this study, including Seoul National University Children's Hospital (Seoul), Seoul National University Bundang Hospital (Seongnam), Eulji Hospital (Seoul), Chungnam University Hospital (Daejeon), and Chonnam University Hospital (Gwangju). Cases from three hospitals were included from June 2014 to December 2015 to collect pneumonia cases from three different regions distant from Seoul, while those from Seoul National University Children's Hospital and Eulji Hospital were enrolled throughout the study period.

This study enrolled the children who were hospitalized with a confirmed diagnosis of MP pneumonia and also were treated with macrolides without introducing or changing with tetracyclines or fluoroquinolones. Nasopharyngeal aspirates or swabs were obtained from children hospitalized with acute lower respiratory tract infections (LRTIs) as a strategy of routine patient care. Diagnosis of MP pneumonia was based on 1) the presence of infiltration in chest radiography together with clinical symptoms and signs such as fever (defined as ≥38 °C by axillary temperature), cough, or sputum and 2) MP detected by culture or positive test results for the MP *P1* gene by PCR. MP-specific antibody was measured using a microparticle agglutination test Serodia-MycoII kit (Fujirebio, Tokyo, Japan). A 4-fold or greater rise in titers or a single titer of ≥1: 640 were considered to indicate current MP infection [5]. The following conditions were excluding criteria: underlying diseases that can modify the clinical course of MP pneumonia, hospital-acquired pneumonia, bacterial co-infection, and treatment with other anti-mycoplasmal antibiotics such as levofloxacin or tetracycline.

Nasopharyngeal samples were kept at 4 °C and sent to the laboratory of the Seoul National University Children's Hospital for the culture of MP and analysis of macrolide resistance within 24 h from the collection of the samples.

Mycoplasma pneumoniae detection

Cultivation of MP was performed at the Seoul National University Children's Hospital. Reference strain M129 (ATCC 29342) was cultured in parallel with the clinical samples using pleuropneumonia-like organism (PPLO) broth and agar. Two hundred microliters of the nasopharyngeal specimen were serially diluted 64-fold. The broth medium was composed of 70 mL of PPLO broth, 20 mL of horse serum, 10 mL of 25% yeast extract, 2.5 mL of 20% glucose, 200 μL of 1% phenol red, 1 mL of 2.5% thallium acetate, 0.5 mL of 200,000 units/mL penicillin G potassium, and 0.5 mL of 20,000 μg/mL cefotaxime. The agar was prepared with the same components as the broth medium except that cefotaxime was omitted and 1.2% agar powder was added instead of broth powder. The broth and the agar media were incubated aerobically at 37 °C for 6 weeks.

The plates were observed daily to identify color changes in the broth medium from red to transparent orange. Upon color change, 10 μL were sub-cultured onto agar plates. Spherical MP colonies were observed under a microscope at 100X magnification. In addition, *P1* gene was amplified by PCR for the confirmation of MP. DNA was also extracted directly from the nasopharyngeal samples and subsequently amplified for *P1* gene. Each reaction mixture was prepared with the following: 2 μL of template, 2 μL of 10X reaction buffer, 2.0 mM of MgCl$_2$, 0.2 mM of dNTP mix, 4 pmoL of each forward and reverse primer, 1 U of Taq DNA polymerase (Takara Bio Inc., Shiga, Japan), and distilled water to a final volume of 20 μL. Reaction conditions were set as follows: denaturation at 95 °C for 30 s, 35 cycles of annealing at 58 °C, and elongation at 72 °C for 40 s. Cases were included when cultures grew MP that was subsequently confirmed to be positive for the *P1* gene by PCR. Cases with positive MP PCR of the nasopharyngeal aspirates were also included.

Determination of macrolide resistance

PCR to amplify domain V of the 23S rRNA gene was performed on cultured MP isolates or DNA extracted from nasopharyngeal samples. The primers used were MP23SV-F (5′-TAA CTA TAA CGG TCC TAA GG) and MP23SV-R (5′-ACA CTT AGA TGC TTT CAG CG). DNA from the reference strain M129 (ATCC 29342), was used as a positive control, and distilled water was used as a negative control. The 851- bp PCR products were purified using an AccuPrep® PCR Purification Kit (Bioneer, Inc., Daejeon, Korea), and samples were sequenced to identify the transitions in domain V of the 23S rRNA gene that have been associated with macrolide resistance [13]. The presence of 23S rRNA gene transitions were regarded as resistant to macrolides. For 56 cultured strains, the minimal inhibitory concentrations (MICs) were determined by use of a microdilution method. Briefly, frozen stocks were thawed and diluted in a broth media to a concentration of 10^4 color change units (CCU)/mL. The MICs of MP strains were then measured using microdilution method in triplicate for the following 4 antimicrobial agents: azithromycin, clarithromycin, erythromycin, and roxithromycin. Each antimicrobial was serially diluted 2-fold, with a range from 0.0008 μg/mL to 128 μg/mL. MIC was defined as the lowest antibiotic concentration at which color did not change at the time when the color of positive control (media containing MP strains only) changed [14]. If negative control (media only) showed color change, the test was discarded. MIC of the reference strain M129 was determined as a control.

Clinical data collection and assessment of clinical outcome

The patients' demographics, clinical manifestations, number of febrile days, duration of macrolide treatment, and the laboratory results were collected on a standardized form through review of the medical records by a pediatrician in each hospital. A febrile day was defined as a day on which the body temperature exceeded 38 °C at least once. Clinical parameters such as oxygen requirement, mechanical ventilator support were reviewed. Chest x-rays at the time of admission were reviewed independently by two radiologists. Chest x-ray findings were categorized into homogeneous dense lobar consolidation, patchy consolidation, nodular opacities, and bilateral parahilar infiltration (Fig. 1). Parapneumonic effusion, defined as ≥1 cm width on the decubitus view, was also included in the analysis. The pediatricians and radiologists were all blinded to the results of the macrolide susceptibility of MP. In the five participating hospitals, macrolide agents were initially chosen for the treatment of MP pneumonia. All physicians were unware of the results of 23S rRNA mutation during the treatment. The results from the susceptibility test did not have any impact on the choice of antibiotics because the susceptibility results take up to 6 weeks.

Statistical analyses

The data were analyzed using SPSS software version 19.0 (SPSS Inc., Chicago, IL, USA). For all of the statistical tests, a p-value of <0.05 was considered statistically significant. Differences between categorical variables were tested using the chi-squared or Fisher's exact test with univariate and multivariate logistic regression analysis. The Mann-Whitney U test or t-test were used to

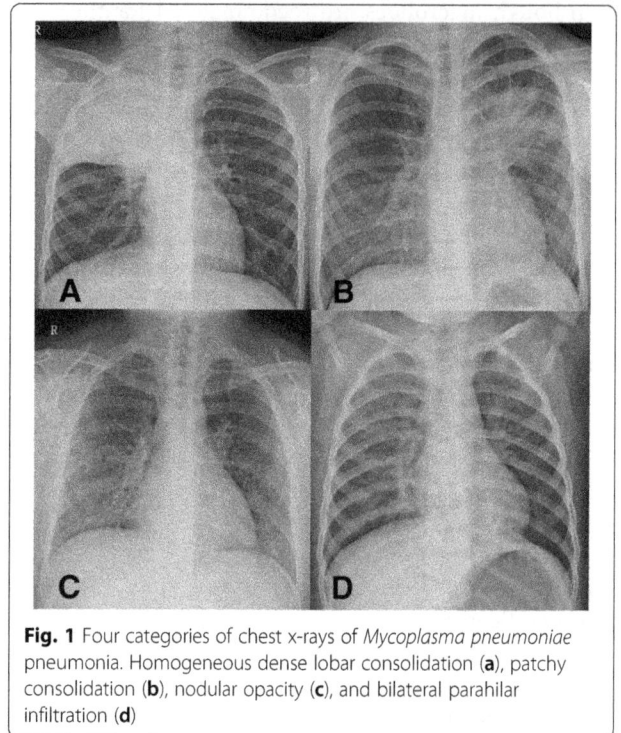

Fig. 1 Four categories of chest x-rays of *Mycoplasma pneumoniae* pneumonia. Homogeneous dense lobar consolidation (**a**), patchy consolidation (**b**), nodular opacity (**c**), and bilateral parahilar infiltration (**d**)

compare the age and duration of febrile days between the groups as appropriate.

Results

Demographics of patients with MP pneumonia

Between September 2010 and December 2015, a total of 2436 nasopharyngeal samples were obtained from children hospitalized with acute LRTIs. Of those, MP was detected in 250 samples (10.3%). A total of 116 children who were hospitalized with MP pneumonia were included after excluding cases that had any of the exclusion criteria such as underlying diseases, hospital-acquired pneumonia, bacterial coinfection, use of quinolone or tetracycline. Overall, 50.9% of the patients were male, and the mean age was 6.0 years; 9.5% were <2 years old, 31.9% were 2–4 years old, and 58.6% were ≥5 years old. The mean duration of fever was nine days (range 1–30 days), and the mean days of admission were 9 days. MP-specific antibody titers were ≥4-fold or greater in 52 (44.8%) patients and single antibody titers ≥1:640 in 49 (42.2%) patients. Remaining 15 patients did not have paired serum samples.

Prevalence of macrolide resistance

The annual distribution of 116 MP-positive samples over 6 years is shown in Fig. 2. During the study period, MP pneumonia was prevalent in 2011 and in 2015. Overall, 82 samples (70.7%) carried transitions in the 23S rRNA gene. The transition observed in the 23S rRNA gene was exclusively the A2063G transition. The macrolide

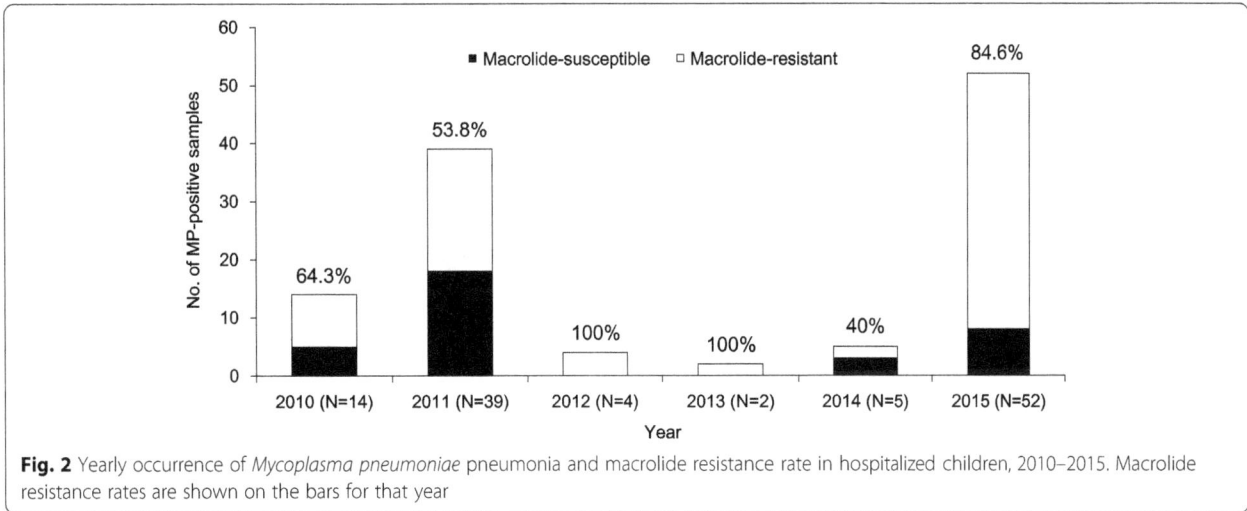

Fig. 2 Yearly occurrence of *Mycoplasma pneumoniae* pneumonia and macrolide resistance rate in hospitalized children, 2010–2015. Macrolide resistance rates are shown on the bars for that year

resistance rates during the two outbreaks were 53.8% (21/39) in 2011 and 84.6% (44/52) in 2015. Of the 59 MP isolates that underwent MIC testing for four macrolides (azithromycin, clarithromycin, erythromycin, and roxithromycin), the MICs of 23 MP isolates that lacked the transition in the 23S rRNA gene ranged from 0.001 to 0.008 µg/mL. In contrast, the MICs of the 36 MP isolates that had a transition in the 23S rRNA gene were significantly higher, ranging from 2 to >128 µg/mL (Table 1).

Clinical features of MP pneumonia

The clinical parameters and demographics of the children hospitalized with MP pneumonia were compared according to the presence of macrolide resistance (Table 2). Of the macrolides used, roxithromycin was predominantly used ($n = 56$), followed by clarithromycin ($n = 30$). One patient used azithromycin only, and 29 cases used two different macrolides during their course of treatment. There were no differences in the type of macrolides used or the mean days of treatment duration (12 days vs. 11 days) between the macrolide-susceptible and macrolide-resistant groups. The mean ages were not different between the macrolide-susceptible and macrolide-resistant groups (5.7 years vs. 6.1 years, $P = 0.574$).

Overall, the mean days of fever were nine days. There was no significant difference in the total duration of fever between the macrolide-susceptible and macrolide-resistant groups (9.4 days vs. 8.9 days, $P = 0.322$). Most patients were tested for the detection of MP no later than 7 days except 14 (12%) patients who presented after 7 days of fever. While the number of febrile days before macrolide treatment did not differ between the groups (4.9 days vs. 4.3 days, $P = 0.315$), the mean days to defervescence after macrolide initiation were longer in the macrolide-resistant group than in macrolide-susceptible group (5.7 days vs. 4.1 days, $P = 0.021$). After the initiation of macrolide treatment, more cases had a fever for more than 7 days in the macrolide-resistant group compared with those in the macrolide-susceptible group (37.8% vs. 17.6%, $P = 0.034$). There were no differences in oxygen requirement, mechanical ventilator support between the groups. Significant differences were not observed between the two groups in the presence of extrapulmonary signs.

Relationship between clinical course and findings of chest x-ray

In comparing the findings of chest x-rays at the time of admission, the patients exhibited bilateral parahilar

Table 1 Minimal inhibitory concentrations (MICs) to macrolides for *Mycoplasma pneumoniae* strains

Macrolides	MICs (µg/mL) for strains					
	With 23S rRNA transition ($n = 36$)			Without 23S rRNA transition ($n = 23$)		
	Range	MIC_{50}	MIC_{90}	Range	MIC_{50}	MIC_{90}
Azithromycin	1 ~ 64	8	16	0.001 ~ 0.001	0.001	0.001
Clarithromycin	8~ > 128	64	128	0.001 ~ 0.002	0.001	0.002
Erythromycin	2~ > 128	16	128	0.001 ~ 0.004	0.001	0.002
Roxithromycin	0.032 ~ 128	8	32	0.001 ~ 0.008	0.001	0.004

MIC_{50} and MIC_{90} are MICs at which 50% and 90% of the isolates were inhibited by the antimicrobials, respectively

Table 2 Demographics and clinical characteristics of *Mycoplasma pneumoniae* pneumonia to the presence of macrolide resistance

Parameters	Macrolide-susceptible (N = 34)	Macrolide-resistant (N = 82)	P
Male gender	22 (64.7)	37 (45.1)	0.055
Age			
Mean, years ± SD	5.7 ± 3.9	6.1 ± 3.3	0.574
< 2 years	6 (17.6)	6 (7.3)	0.104
≥ 2–4 years	12 (35.3)	25 (30.5)	
≥ 5 years	16 (47.1)	51 (62.2)	
Mean febrile days, SD	8.9 ± 3.9	9.4 ± 5.3	0.322
Fever days before initiation of macrolides			
Mean ± SD, days	4.9 ± 3.5	4.3 ± 2.6	0.315
Fever days after initiation of macrolides			
Mean ± SD, days	4.1 ± 2.9	5.7 ± 4.7	0.021
≥ 7 days	6 (17.6)	31 (37.8)	0.034
Oxygen requirement	5 (14.7)	15 (18.3)	0.217
Mechanical ventilator	0 (0)	2 (2.4)	1.0
Extrapulmonary signs	6 (17.6)	9 (11.0)	0.798
Skin rash	4 (11.8)	8 (9.8)	0.745
Hematology	1 (2.9)	1 (1.2)	0.502
Neurologic	1 (2.9)	0 (0)	0.293
Radiology findings			
Homogeneous dense lobar consolidation	9 (26.5)	35 (42.7)	0.101
Patchy consolidation	13 (38.2)	24 (29.3)	0.346
Nodular opacities	7 (20.6)	12 (14.6)	0.430
Bilateral parahilar infiltration	5 (14.7)	11 (13.4)	0.855
Parapneumonic effusion	4 (11.8)	18 (22.0)	0.298

Data are no. (%) of patients, unless otherwise indicated

infiltration (*n* = 16), nodular opacity (*n* = 19), patchy consolidation (*n* = 37), and homogeneous dense lobar consolidation (*n* = 44). Parapneumonic effusion was observed in 22 patients. Overall, there was no significant difference in the proportions of specific chest x-ray patterns according to the presence of macrolide resistance (Table 2).

Mean days to defervescence following macrolide initiation were longer in children with MP pneumonia when they showed homogeneous dense consolidation (7.27 days vs. 4.01 days, *P* < 0.001) and parapneumonic effusion (9.73 days vs. 4.20 days, *P* < 0.001) than those who did not. In contrast, children with parahilar infiltration showed shorter duration of fever (1.63 days vs. 5.83 days, *P* < 0.001). Parapneumonic effusion was frequently accompanied by homogeneous dense lobar consolidation (*n* = 18) and patchy consolidation (*n* = 4). It is also notable that patients with parapneumonic effusion tended to show extrapulmonary signs more frequently than those without (77.3% vs.11.7%, *P* < 0.001).

Risk factors associated with prolonged fever in MP pneumonia

To evaluate the factors associated with a longer fever duration, the patients were grouped by fever duration into groups of <7 days or ≥7 days (Table 3). Univariate analysis revealed that macrolide resistance (*P* = 0.034), extrapulmonary signs (*P* = 0.006), homogeneous lobar consolidation (*P* < 0.001), and parapneumonic effusion (*P* < 0.001) were significantly associated with the children with fever of 7 days or longer. In contrast, parahilar infiltration was associated with shorter fever days (*P* = 0.003).

Multivariate analysis showed that extrapulmonary signs (aOR; 3.037, 95% CI; 1.057–8.726), homogeneous lobar consolidation (aOR; 3.610, 95% CI; 1.519–8.580), and parapneumonic effusion (aOR; 9.705, 95% CI; 3.031–31.075) were responsible for prolonged fever ≥7 days following macrolide treatment regardless of macrolide resistance.

Discussion

Due to increasing recognition of macrolide-resistant MP worldwide, there is a growing concern over the efficacy

Table 3 Risk factors for prolonged fever following macrolide treatment

Parameters	Fever duration following macrolide treatment		Univariate model	Multivariate model		
	<7 days (N = 79)	≥7 days (N = 37)	P	aOR[a]	P	95% CI
Male gender	40 (50.6)	19 (51.4)	0.942			
Age in years, mean ± SD	5.8 ± 3.2	6.3 ± 3.9	0.499			
Macrolide resistance	51 (64.6)	31 (83.8)	0.034	2.687	0.072	0.917–7.878
Extrapulmonary signs	9 (11.4)	12 (32.4)	0.006	3.037	0.039	1.057–8.726
Radiology findings						
Lobar consolidation	21 (26.6)	23 (62.2)	0.000	3.610	0.004	1.519–8.580
Patchy consolidation	27 (34.2)	10 (27.0)	0.441			
Nodular opacities	15 (19.0)	4 (10.8)	0.420			
Parahilar infiltration	16 (20.3)	0 (0)	0.003			
Parapneumonic effusion	5 (6.3)	17 (45.9)	0.000	9.705	0.000	3.031–31.075

Data are no. (%) of patients, unless otherwise indicated
[a]Adjusted odds ratio

of macrolide treatment for children with macrolide-resistant MP pneumonia. Given the versatile features of MP pneumonia, which are determined by the patient's age, the immunologic response of the host, and extrapulmonary manifestations [2], a more comprehensive approach must be established to analyze the clinical outcome of MP pneumonia according to the presence of macrolide resistance. In this study, we compared fever duration following macrolide treatment between the macrolide-susceptible and macrolide-resistant groups for the children hospitalized with MP pneumonia who had fever and radiological abnormalities on chest x-rays. The main findings from this study were that children with MP pneumonia tended to have prolonged fever when they accompanied extrapulmonary signs, homogeneous lobar consolidation, or parapneumonic effusion. It is important to note that macrolide resistance alone did not contribute to fever duration after the initiation of macrolide treatment.

MP containing transitions in the 23S rRNA gene has been reported worldwide since 2000. Japan reported more than 40% MP resistance during 2008–2010 [13, 15]. For China, more than 80% of MP infections are caused by macrolide-resistant strains [8, 16, 17]. Studies in the United States, Israel and Italy reported an approximately 26–30% prevalence of macrolide resistance [18–20]. Studies have demonstrated that the A2063G and A2064G transitions in domain V of 23S rRNA confer high-level resistance to 14-, 15-, 16-membered ring macrolides [21–23]. In our study, 70.7% of the patients with MP pneumonia had a 23S rRNA gene transition. Because a previous study reported that the macrolide resistance rate among children with MP pneumonia has been increasing and was 62.9% in 2011 [4], some physicians often change their treatment to levofloxacin when patients are not responding to macrolides. Thus, 34

patients (39.5%) of the 86 patients with MP pneumonia in 2015 received levofloxacin for their treatment and had to be excluded from the current study.

Most MP infections in children are known as mild and self-limiting, while only a small portion of the patients need hospitalization. The duration of symptoms can be shortened by the early administration of macrolides [11]. Initially, treatment of MP pneumonia with antimicrobials was supported by a randomized trial of 290 marine recruits that showed a shortening of fever duration, alleviation of cough, and improvement of chest x-rays [24]. An in vitro study also favored antimicrobials for the eradication of MP [25]. Before the emergence of macrolide-resistant MP, a retrospective study found that empirical therapy with macrolides decreased the duration of hospital stays, but this study had a major limitation in that microbiologic diagnosis was not adequately performed [26]. A recent systematic review that evaluated the effect of treating MP pneumonia demonstrated that there was no significant clinical benefit of antimicrobial therapy in children with MP pneumonia [27].

However, some studies have reported that patients infected with MP-resistant strains had more febrile days and a longer duration of persistent cough than those infected with MP-susceptible strains [28–30]. One study found that 15 out of 21 patients with macrolide-resistant MP pneumonia remained febrile for more than 48 h after the initiation of macrolide, but when treatment was changed to minocycline, fever disappeared within 48 h in all patients [28]. A study performed in Japan concluded that 5- to 7-day treatment with minocycline or doxycycline was effective for macrolide-resistant MP infection, as shown by the reduced number of MP DNA copies 3 days after treatment [31]. In this study, the authors also found that tosufloxacin, a fluoroquinolone, was superior to azithromycin or clarithromycin in reducing fever within 48 h after antibiotic administration for macrolide-resistant MP pneumonia. According to these studies, macrolide resistance contributes to clinical severity, and macrolides are considered as inappropriate first-choice drugs; thus, alternative treatment seem to be necessary for macrolide-resistant MP infections. In the meanwhile, a recent systematic review raised a question about benefit from macrolide treatment for MP pneumonia [32].

Our study found that macrolide resistance alone did not contribute to fever duration after macrolide treatment in children who were hospitalized for MP pneumonia. The findings may further suggest that macrolide treatment for macrolide-susceptible MP pneumonia may not contribute to significant clinical improvement compared to no antimicrobial treatment. Focal reticulonodular infiltration or perihilar interstitial infiltration are considered to be common findings of MP pneumonia [2, 33]. However, children who did not respond to macrolides more likely to show homogeneous dense lobar consolidation, extrapulmonary manifestations, and parapneumonic effusion.

This study has several limitations. Retrospective nature of the study may be subject to the possibility of incomplete clinical information. However, this study used fever as an objective parameter for clinical outcome that was measured and recorded by hospital staff. In addition, because this study assessed the clinical efficacy of macrolide for the children who were hospitalized with MP pneumonia, it may represent severe cases of MP pneumonia and cannot be generalized to overall pictures of MP pneumonia. In this study, roxithromycin was the frequently prescribed macrolide. Because high antibiotic resistance rate has been a major problem among children in Korea, there is a consensus to avoid macrolides with a long half-life such as azithromycin and clarithromycin. Despite these limitations, clinical information was gathered by those who were blinded to the results of macrolide resistance. We applied strict diagnostic criteria for MP infection, positive culture or PCR along with MP-specific antibody response, to avoid variability in diagnostic criteria. This study enrolled previously healthy children to minimize confounding factors that can contribute to clinical outcome. By excluding mild cases with MP pneumonia for whom the efficacy of antimicrobial treatment cannot often be distinguished from spontaneous resolution, clinical benefits of macrolide treatment were better assessed for those with severe manifestations. In addition, this study was first to use four distinct patterns of chest x-rays as a tool to measure severity of MP pneumonia.

Conclusions

Given the current trend of the increasing prevalence of macrolide resistance, our study suggests that lobar consolidation with or without parapneumonic effusion and extrapulmonary manifestations were associated with severe clinical outcome of MP pneumonia while macrolide resistance was not a determinant of clinical course of MP pneumonia.

Acknowledgements
We are grateful to Seong Yeon Lee for her excellent technical assistance.

Funding
This research was supported by the Basic Science Research Program through the National Research Foundation of Korea, which is funded by the Ministry of Education, Science and Technology (NRF-2015R1D1A1A09059589).

Authors' contributions
EHC and HJL conceived the original research idea and were the lead authors for this paper. Drs. IAY and KBH performed laboratory work including culture of MP and DNA extraction, sequencing analysis, and antimicrobial susceptibility test to determine macrolide resistance. Drs. IAY and KBH wrote the first draft and analyzed the clinical data which were collected from five different hospitals. Drs. KWY, JYP, HL, BWE, YMA, EYC, and HJC participated in enrolling patients, collecting nasopharyngeal samples and clinical data at five different hospitals. Drs YHC and WSK were key authors who defined four radiologic patterns of chest x-rays and reviewed chest x-rays. All authors read and approved the final manuscript.

Competing interests
The authors declare that they have no competing interests.

Consent for publication
Not applicable.

Author details
[1]Department of Pediatrics, Seoul National University Children's Hospital, Seoul, South Korea. [2]Department of Pediatrics, Seoul National University College of Medicine, Seoul, South Korea. [3]Department of Radiology, Seoul National University Hospital, Seoul, South Korea. [4]Department of Pediatrics, Seoul National University Bundang Hospital, Seongnam, South Korea. [5]Department of Pediatrics, Eulji Hospital, Seoul, South Korea. [6]Department of Pediatrics, Chungnam National University Hospital, Daejeon, South Korea. [7]Department of Pediatrics, Chonnam National University Hospital, Gwangju, South Korea.

References
1. Matsuoka M, Narita M, Okazaki N, Ohya H, Yamazaki T, Ouchi K, et al. Characterization and molecular analysis of macrolide-resistant *Mycoplasma pneumoniae* clinical isolates obtained in Japan. Antimicrob Agents Chemother. 2004;48:4624–30.
2. Atkinson TP, Balish MF, Waites KB. Epidemiology, clinical manifestations, pathogenesis and laboratory detection of *Mycoplasma pneumoniae* infections. FEMS Microbiol Rev. 2008;32:956–73.
3. Eun BW, Kim NH, Choi EH, Lee HJ. *Mycoplasma pneumoniae* in Korean children: the epidemiology of pneumonia over an 18-year period. J Inf Secur. 2008;56:326–31.
4. Hong KB, Choi EH, Lee HJ, Lee SY, Cho EY, Choi JH, et al. Macrolide resistance of *Mycoplasma pneumoniae*, South Korea, 2000-2011. Emerg Infect Dis. 2013;19:1281–4.

5. Kim NH, Lee JA, Eun BW, Shin SH, Chung EH, Park KW, et al. Comparison of polymerase chain reaction and the indirect particle agglutination antibody test for the diagnosis of *Mycoplasma pneumoniae* pneumonia in children during two outbreaks. Pediatr Infect Dis J. 2007;26:897–903.

6. Miyashita N, Kawai Y, Akaike H, Ouchi K, Hayashi T, Kurihara T, et al. Macrolide-resistant *Mycoplasma pneumoniae* in adolescents with community-acquired pneumonia. BMC Infect Dis. 2012;12:126.

7. Takei T, Morozumi M, Ozaki H, Fujita H, Ubukata K, Kobayashi I, et al. Clinical features of *Mycoplasma pneumoniae* infections in the 2010 epidemic season: report of two cases with unusual presentations. Pediatr Neonatol. 2013;54:402–5.

8. Liu Y, Ye X, Zhang H, Xu X, Li W, Zhu D, et al. Antimicrobial susceptibility of *Mycoplasma pneumoniae* isolates and molecular analysis of macrolide-resistant strains from shanghai, China. Antimicrob Agents Chemother. 2009; 53:2160–2.

9. Zhao F, Liu G, Wu J, Cao B, Tao X, He L, et al. Surveillance of macrolide-resistant *Mycoplasma pneumoniae* in Beijing, China, from 2008 to 2012. Antimicrob Agents Chemother. 2013;57:1521–3.

10. Ho PL, Law PY, Chan BW, Wong CW, To KK, Chiu SS, et al. Emergence of macrolide-resistant *Mycoplasma pneumoniae* in Hong Kong is linked to increasing macrolide resistance in multilocus variable-number tandem-repeat analysis type 4-5-7-2. J Clin Microbiol. 2015;53:3560–4.

11. Ferwerda A, Moll HA. Groot Rd. respiratory tract infections by *Mycoplasma peumoniae* in childrne: a revies of diagnostic and therapeutic measures. Eur J Pediatr. 2001;160:483–91.

12. Gardiner SJ, Gavranich JB, Chang AB. Antibiotics for community-acquired lower respiratory tract infections secondary to *Mycoplasma pneumoniae* in children. Cochrane Database Syst Rev. 2015;1:CD004875.

13. Okazaki N, Narita M, Yamada S, Izumikawa K, Umetsu M, Kenri T, et al. Characteristics of macrolide-resistant *Mycoplasma pneumoniae* strains isolated from patients and induced with erythromycin in vitro. Microbiol Immunol. 2001;45:617–20.

14. Clinical and Laboratory Standards Institute. Performance standards for antimicrobial susceptibility testing-twenty-first information Spplement: approved standard M100-S21. Wayne, PA: CLSI; 2011.

15. Morozumi M, Ubukata K, Takahashi T. Macrolide-resistant *Mycoplasma pneumoniae*: characteristics of isolates and clinical aspects of community-acquired pneumonia. J Infect Chemother. 2010;16:78–86.

16. Liu Y, Ye X, Zhang H, Xu X, Li W, Zhu D, et al. Characterization of macrolide resistance in *Mycoplasma pneumoniae* isolated from children in shanghai. China Diagn Microbiol Infect Dis. 2010;67:355–8.

17. Xin D, Mi Z, Han X, Qin L, Li J, Wei T, et al. Molecular mechanisms of macrolide resistance in clinical isolates of *Mycoplasma pneumoniae* from China. Antimicrob Agents Chemother. 2009;53:2158–9.

18. Averbuch D, Hidalgo-Grass C, Moses AE, Engelhard D, Nir-Paz R. Macrolide resistance in *Mycoplasma pneumoniae*, Israel, 2010. Emerg Infect Dis. 2011; 17:1079–82.

19. Chironna M, Sallustio A, Esposito S, Perulli M, Chinellato I, Di Bari C, et al. Emergence of macrolide-resistant strains during an outbreak of *Mycoplasma pneumoniae* infections in children. J Antimicrob Chemother. 2011;66:734–7.

20. Wolff BJ, Thacker WL, Schwartz SB, Winchell JM. Detection of macrolide resistance in *Mycoplasma pneumoniae* by real-time PCR and high-resolution melt analysis. Antimicrob Agents Chemother. 2008;52:3542–9.

21. Morozumi M, Hasegawa K, Kobayashi R, Inoue N, Iwata S, Kuroki H, et al. Emergence of macrolide-resistant *Mycoplasma pneumoniae* with a 23S rRNA gene mutation. Antimicrob Agents Chemother. 2005;49:2302–6.

22. Bebear CM, Pereyre S. Mechanisms of drug resistance in *Mycoplasma pneumoniae*. Curr Drug Targets Infect Disord. 2005;5:263–71.

23. Morozumi M, Iwata S, Hasegawa K, Chiba N, Takayanagi R, Matsubara K, et al. Increased macrolide resistance of *Mycoplasma pneumoniae* in pediatric patients with community-acquired pneumonia. Antimicrob Agents Chemother. 2008;52:348–50.

24. Kinston JR, Chanock RM, Mufson MA, Hellman LP, James WD, Fox HH, et al. Eaton agent pneumonia. JAMA. 1961;176:118–23.

25. Critchley IA, Jones ME, Heinze PD, Hubbard D, Engler HD, Evangelista AT, et al. In vitro activity of levofloxacin against contemporary clinical isolates of *Legionella pneumophila*, *Mycoplasma pneumoniae* and *Chlamydia pneumoniae* from North America and Europe. Clin Microbiol Infect. 2002;8:214–21.

26. Shah SS, Test M, Sheffler-Collins S, Weiss AK, Hall M. Macrolide therapy and outcomes in a multicenter cohort of children hospitalized with *Mycoplasma pneumoniae* pneumonia. J Hosp Med. 2012;7:311–7.

27. Biondi E, McCulloh R, Alverson B, Klein A, Dixon A, Ralston S. Treatment of mycoplasma pneumonia: a systematic review. Pediatrics. 2014;133:1081–90.

28. Kawai Y, Miyashita N, Yamaguchi T, Saitoh A, Kondoh E, Fujimoto H, et al. Clinical efficacy of macrolide antibiotics against genetically determined macrolide-resistant *Mycoplasma pneumoniae* pneumonia in paediatric patients. Respirology. 2012;17:354–62.

29. Matsubara K, Morozumi M, Okada T, Matsushima T, Komiyama O, Shoji M, et al. A comparative clinical study of macrolide-sensitive and macrolide-resistant *Mycoplasma pneumoniae* infections in pediatric patients. J Infect Chemother. 2009;15:380–3.

30. Suzuki S, Yamazaki T, Narita M, Okazaki N, Suzuki I, Andoh T, et al. Clinical evaluation of macrolide-resistant *Mycoplasma pneumoniae*. Antimicrob Agents Chemother. 2006;50:709–12.

31. Okada T, Morozumi M, Tajima T, Hasegawa M, Sakata H, Ohnari S, et al. Rapid effectiveness of minocycline or doxycycline against macrolide-resistant *Mycoplasma pneumoniae* infection in a 2011 outbreak among Japanese children. Clin Infect Dis. 2012;55:1642–9.

32. Spuesens EB, Meyer Sauteur PM, Vink C, van Rossum AM. *Mycoplasma pneumoniae* infections-does treatment help? J Inf Secur. 2014;69:S42–6.

33. Othman N, Isaacs D, Daley AJ, Kesson AM. *Mycoplasma pneumoniae* infection in a clinical setting. Pediatr Int. 2008;50:662–6.

13

The impact of community-acquired pneumonia on the health-related quality-of-life in elderly

Marie-Josée J. Mangen[1]*⊙, Susanne M. Huijts[1,2], Marc J. M. Bonten[1,3] and G. Ardine de Wit[1]

Abstract

Background: The sustained health-related quality-of-life of patients surviving community-acquired pneumonia has not been accurately quantified. The aim of the current study was to quantify differences in health-related quality-of-life of community-dwelling elderly with and without community-acquired pneumonia during a 12-month follow-up period.

Methods: In a matched cohort study design, nested in a prospective randomized double-blind placebo-controlled trial on the efficacy of the 13-valent pneumococcal vaccine in community-dwelling persons of ≥65 years, health-related quality-of-life was assessed in 562 subjects hospitalized with suspected community-acquired pneumonia (i.e. diseased cohort) and 1145 unaffected persons (i.e. non-diseased cohort) matched to pneumonia cases on age, sex, and health status (EQ-5D-3L-index). Health-related quality-of-life was determined 1–2 weeks after hospital discharge/inclusion and 1, 6 and 12 months thereafter, using Euroqol EQ-5D-3L and Short Form-36 Health survey questionnaires. One-year quality-adjusted life years (QALY) were estimated for both diseased and non-diseased cohorts. Separate analyses were performed for pneumonia cases with and without radiologically confirmed community-acquired pneumonia.

Results: The one-year excess QALY loss attributed to community-acquired pneumonia was 0.13. Mortality in the post-discharge follow-up year was 8.4% in community-acquired pneumonia patients and 1.2% in non-diseased persons ($p < 0.001$). During follow-up health-related quality-of-life was persistently lower in community-acquired pneumonia patients, compared to non-diseased persons, but differences in health-related quality-of-life between radiologically confirmed and non-confirmed community-acquired pneumonia cases were not statistically significant.

Conclusions: Community-acquired pneumonia was associated with a six-fold increased mortality and 16% lower quality-of-life in the post-discharge year among patients surviving hospitalization for community-acquired pneumonia, compared to non-diseased persons.

Keywords: Quality-of-life, Community-acquired pneumonia, Elderly, Follow-up, Mortality

Background

Community-acquired pneumonia (CAP) causes considerable disease and economic burden. In the Netherlands, the overall incidence of CAP was estimated to be 295 per 100,000 inhabitants, yielding approximately 50,000 episodes per year, with considerable variation between age-groups [1]. Approximately 45% of all CAP episodes occur in persons aged ≥65 years [1]. In the period after recovery, CAP is associated with higher risks on e.g. stroke and other cardiovascular events [2, 3]. Both CAP and the occurrence of these other diseases in the post-discharge period may impact on the health-related quality-of-life (HrQol). However, only limited data are available on HrQol after a CAP episode [4]. In only two of six studies that focused on HrQol after CAP [5–10] patient follow-up exceeded 6 weeks. El Moussaoui et al. [7] followed patients for 18 months using the Short-

* Correspondence: m.j.j.mangen@umcutrecht.nl
[1]Julius Center for Health Sciences and Primary Care, University Medical Center Utrecht, Heidelberglaan 100, 3584 CX Utrecht, The Netherlands

Form (36) Health survey [11] (referred hereafter as SF36), and Honselmann et al. [10] determined the HrQol at one-year post-discharge using the Euroqol EQ-5D-3L instrument [12] (referred hereafter as EQ5D) in patients that had survived an episode of pneumonia and/or sepsis for which admission to intensive care was needed. These studies were all descriptive, and none of these studies quantified the excess quality-adjusted life-years (QALY) lost due to CAP in comparison with non-diseased persons (i.e. no pneumonia). The aim of the current study was to quantify differences in HrQol of community-dwelling elderly with and without CAP during a 12-month follow-up period. In addition, possible HrQol differences between radiologically confirmed and radiologically non-confirmed CAP cases were investigated.

Methods

Study design, setting and participants

The current study, "Costs, Health status and Outcomes of CAP (Community-Acquired Pneumonia)" (CHO-CAP), was executed in parallel to the "Community-Acquired Pneumonia Immunization trial in Adults" (CAPiTA) trial, a placebo-controlled double-blinded RCT evaluating the effectiveness of a 13-valent pneumococcal conjugate vaccine in 84,496 community-dwelling elderly in the Netherlands [13, 14]. The CHO-CAP-study used a nested matched-cohort study design when recruiting patients hospitalized with a clinical suspicion of a pneumonia episode from the CAPITA-study population and prospectively followed them, along with non-diseased subjects (i.e. no pneumonia), for a one-year post-discharge period (Fig. 1) [15]. CAPiTA-participants were approached for study participation in CHO-CAP at the time of vaccination (November-2008-January-2010). Overall, 72,074 CAPiTA-participants[1] received the invitation to return the CHO-CAP-baseline questionnaire together with a signed informed consent form. Those who returned both questionnaire and informed consent formed the CHO-CAP source population (n = 47,476[2]). This source population was a priori eligible for the nested matched-cohort study. Within the CAPiTA-trial, 3225 patients with a suspected pneumonia were identified in 56 Dutch sentinel hospitals. Potential cases for the "diseased"-cohort were subjects with a first-time suspected pneumonia episode, participating in the CHO-CAP source population, without recently diagnosed malignancy and able to complete questionnaires. After hospital discharge, these subjects were invited for participation in the diseased cohort. For feasibility reasons, we included all patients hospitalized with a clinical suspicion, which were later stratified upon either or not receiving a radiological confirmation of CAP by the blinded chest X-ray adjudication committee. Those who consented were visited at home within 2 weeks of

hospital discharge by trained interviewers. They were asked to complete self-administered questionnaires during the home visit (day 0), and at 1, 6 and 12 months after the home visit through postal questionnaires. For each subject in the diseased cohort, two matched non-diseased subjects (i.e. no pneumonia) were identified from the CHO-CAP source population (referred hereafter as non-diseased subjects). Matching was based on age, sex, and EQ-5D-3L-index collected at vaccination, implying that health status of people with suspected pneumonia and their matched non-diseased subjects was similar at the time of vaccination. Non-diseased subjects adhered to the same inclusion criteria as suspected pneumonia patients. They were asked to complete self-administered questionnaires during the home visit (day 0). Further questionnaires were sent by regular mail 1, 6 and 12 months after the home visit. For full details see Mangen et al. [15].

Definitions of subgroups

Additionally, we did distinguish between "radiologically confirmed" CAP cases and the matched non-diseased subjects and "radiologically non-confirmed" CAP cases and their matched non-diseased subjects. A "radiologically confirmed" CAP was defined as the presence of two or more clinical signs of pneumonia together with a chest x-ray consistent with pneumonia, identical to the definition used within the CAPiTA-trial [13].

Data collection

Date of birth, sex, place of residence, loss-to-follow-up due to death during the follow-up period and causes of death were extracted from the CAPiTA-study files [14]. Health status (EQ5D) and socio-demographic status (living situation and education) were collected at the time of vaccination with the CHO-CAP-baseline questionnaire. Full details of data collection of nested matched-cohort study are provided in Mangen et al. [15]. In short, comorbidity details were collected during the home visit. Current living situation was collected at all four contact moments. Health status (EQ5D) was collected thrice for suspected pneumonia cases during the home-visit interview, reflecting health status (1) at day of interview, (2) at the worst moment during the recent pneumonia episode, and (3) previous to the recent pneumonia episode. Health status was also collected at month 1, month 6 and month 12 after initial visit using both EQ5D and SF-36. For non-diseased subjects, both EQ5D and SF-36 were administered at all four contact moments. For suspected pneumonia cases, clinical information on hospital admission (e.g. X-ray result; clinical symptoms; length of stay) was extracted from the CAPiTA-study files [14].

Health status questionnaires

The SF-36 is composed of 36-items measuring health across eight domains (physical functioning, social

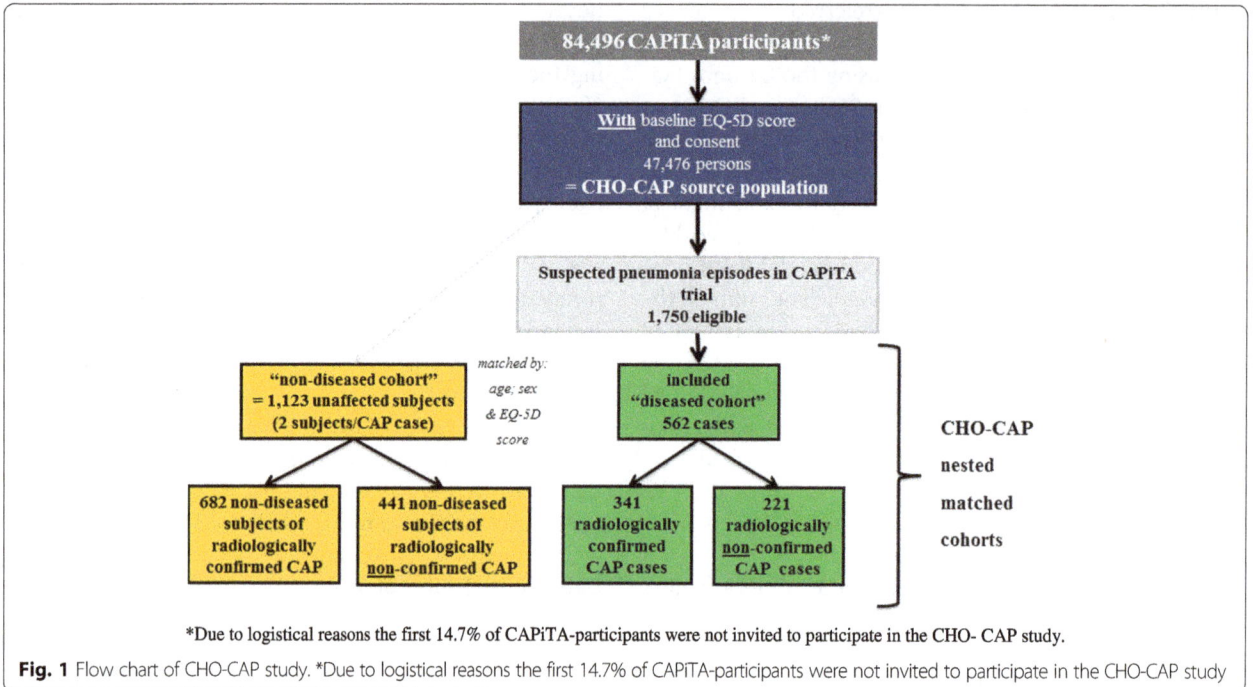

Fig. 1 Flow chart of CHO-CAP study. *Due to logistical reasons the first 14.7% of CAPiTA-participants were not invited to participate in the CHO-CAP study

functioning, role limitations with respect to physical activities, role limitations with respect to emotional activities, pain, mental health, vitality and general health perception). Responses to each item within a domain are combined to generate a score from 0 to 100, where 100 indicates best health [11]. Because of the elderly population - some potentially in poor health - the usual order of items in question 3 was inversed [16]. Applying the scoring-method developed by Brazier et al. [17], we further derived the SF-6D health-index from the SF-36 survey, a numerical index between 0 ("death") and 1 ("full health") [17]. The EQ5D consists of two parts, the EQ-5D-descriptive system and the EQ-visual analogue scale (VAS) [18]. The EQ-VAS records the participants' self-reported health on a VAS from 0 ("Worst imaginable health state") to 100 ("Best imaginable health state") [18]. The EQ5D-descriptive system consists of five domains (mobility, self-care, usual activities, pain/discomfort and anxiety/depression) and three functioning levels (no problems, some problems or severe problems) [12, 18]. The EQ5D health states were scored with the Dutch value-set [19], to obtain EQ-5D-3L summary indexes (EQ-index) ranging from 0 ("death") to 1 ("full health") [12, 19].

QALY estimations
Quality Adjusted Life Years (QALY) is a concept used to reflect a year in full quality of life. Hence, QALYs combine both length of life and quality of life. Quality of life is represented in a value between 0 (death) and 1

(optimal quality of life). QALYs are estimated by multiplying length of life with the indicator value for quality of life. One-year QALY estimates, with and without pneumonia episode included, were calculated for both cohorts, using the self-reported EQ5D health states and its associated index values at the different contact moments based on recorded date of contact moment. An area under the curve approach was followed by interpolating between the observations provided by the patients. For patients who died, we calculated QALY by using the date of death and a utility score of 0 from that date onwards. For missing EQ-indexes, ten imputations were performed. QALYs were calculated in each imputed dataset and averaged over the ten imputed datasets. The observed utility difference between both cohorts was attributed to the CAP episode. Excess QALY loss was calculated for the one-year post-discharge period, excluding and including the CAP episode, respectively (see Additional file 1: Figure S1A for illustration). Additionally, we estimated the QALY and the excess QALY loss for one-year survivors. Pairs of pneumonia cases and non-diseased subjects in which one of the three died during the follow-up were excluded from these estimates.

Data analysis
Health status and QALY estimates in the suspected pneumonia cases and non-diseased subjects are presented for the different follow-up moments, in a decomposed manner (i.e. at the level of the different domains of quality of life) and as summary index. Causes of death

were categorized into five categories: (1) infectious diseases; (2) chronic lung diseases; (3) cancer; (4) cardiovascular events and stroke and (5) others. Depending on the nature and distribution of data, we used Chi-square test for categorical variables (e.g. sex, education) and non-parametric tests for non-normally distributed variables (e.g. scores) to test for differences between both cohorts (i.e. diseased and non-diseased cohort) and for differences between patients with and without confirmed CAP. Correlation between the different instruments was studied using Spearman's rank correlation coefficient. All analyses were performed using IBM SPSS Statistics version 21.

Results

Study participants

Of the 3225 identified suspected pneumonia episodes in the CAPiTA-trial, 1750 (54%) belonged to the CHO-CAP source population, of which 562 (32%) participated; 341 (61%) had radiologically confirmed CAP and 221 (39%) had radiologically non-confirmed CAP (Fig. 1). Reasons for non-participation/exclusion are provided in in the Additional file 1: Table S1A.

Suspected pneumonia cases

Baseline characteristics of the suspected pneumonia cases and their non-diseased subjects are summarized in Table 1. Despite adequate matching on three criteria, non-diseased subjects had fewer comorbidities, were higher educated and were more often from the south of the Netherlands than pneumonia cases (Table 1).

Compared to the non-diseased subjects, suspected pneumonia cases more frequently died during the one-year follow-up period (8.4% vs 1.2%;$p < 0.001$ (in the Additional file 1: Figure S2A.); attributable risk:0.059(95% CI:0.058–0.060)) or withdrew from the study (16.7% vs 9.9%; $p < 0.001$), mainly because of bad health (in the Additional file 1: Table S2A). Chronic lung diseases, cardiovascular events and stroke were more frequently reported as being the cause of death for suspected pneumonia cases than for non-diseased subjects ($p = 0.054$; in the Additional file 1: Table S2A)).

Figure 2 shows the distribution of suspected pneumonia cases and non-diseased subjects reporting problems in the five domains of the EQ5D-instrument at all observation moments. By definition, non-diseased subjects and suspected pneumonia cases had a similar health status at the moment of vaccination. However, during follow-up suspected pneumonia cases more frequently reported problems in the five domains of the EQ5D-instrument than non-diseased subjects at all contact moments and for all domains (Fig. 2). This finding was confirmed by the SF36-questionnaire. Suspected pneumonia cases had persistently lower SF-36 mean scale

scores on all domains and during all contact moments, compared to their non-diseased subjects (Fig. 3). Furthermore, HrQol, as expressed in EQ5D and SF-6D index value and EQ-VAS score of suspected pneumonia cases was constantly lower than HrQol of non-diseased subjects during the one-year follow-up (Table 2, in the Additional file 1: Figure S3A). At month-12, HrQol-scores were significantly lower for survivors in the suspected pneumonia cohort compared to the non-diseased cohort (EQ5D-index:0.74 vs 0.82($p < 0.001$) and SF6D-index:0.68 vs 0.75($p < 0.001$)).

One-year QALY estimates, excluding the CAP episode and using the self-reported EQ5D health status and its associated-index values, were 0.68 and 0.81 for suspected pneumonia cases and non-diseased subjects ($p < 0.001$), yielding a utility difference between both cohorts of –0.13 attributable to suspected pneumonia. One-year QALY estimates, including the CAP episode, were 0.67 and 0.81 for suspected pneumonia cases and non-diseased subjects ($p < 0.001$), yielding an excess QALY loss of 0.15. Slightly smaller QALY differences were obtained when considering only survivors (Table 3), resulting in excess QALY loss of 0.10, if excluding the CAP episode, and 0.11, if including the CAP episode, respectively.

EQ5D-index, EQ-VAS and SF6D-index were positively correlated at all contact moments for suspected pneumonia cases and non-diseased subjects (rho > 0.45), in the Additional file 1: Table S3A and Table S4A. The highest correlation was found between EQ5D-index and SF6D-index for both suspected pneumonia cases and non-diseased subjects (rho >0.67 for all contact moments).

Radiologically confirmed and non-confirmed CAP cases

There were apparent differences between patients with radiologically confirmed and non-confirmed CAP, but when repeating analyses in a stratified manner interpretation did not change. Radiologically confirmed and non-confirmed CAP cases did not differ in baseline characteristics and were adequately matched to their non-diseased subjects (in the Additional file 1: Table S5A). Radiologically confirmed CAP cases stayed significantly longer in hospital than radiologically non-confirmed CAP cases, but had comparable median numbers of clinical symptoms, pneumonia severity index (PSI) scores [20], admissions to ICU and readmissions within 30 days, Table 4. Mortality was higher for patients with radiologically confirmed CAP (10.3%) compared to non-confirmed CAP (5.4%; $p = 0.043$), but the causes of death were comparable (in the Additional file 1: Table S6A). The attributable risks of dying, compared to non-diseased subjects, were 0.083 (95%CI:0.082–0.084) for those with radiologically confirmed CAP and 0.047 (95%CI:0.047–0.048) for those with non-confirmed CAP. As compared to their non-diseased subjects, both

Table 1 Baseline characteristics of suspected pneumonia cases and their non-diseased subjects

	Suspected pneumonia cases (i.e. "diseased" cohort[b])	Non-diseased subjects	p-value
Episodes/subjects	562	1123	
Matching criteria			
Male, in %	71.0	71.1	ns
Age at inclusion[a], median (IQR)	76 (72–82)	76 (72–81)	ns
EQ5D-index (at vaccination), median (IQR)	0.89 (0.78–1.00)	0.89 (0.78–1.00)	ns
Other characteristics			
Number of self-reported comorbidities at inclusion[a], median (IQR)	2 (1–4)	2 (1–3)	<0.001
Educational level, in %			<0.001
Low	53.6	36.3	
Medium	28.3	36.4	
High	17.4	27.0	
Missing	0.7	0.3	
Region, in %			<0.001
North	3.4	4.0	
East	27.4	18.4	
West	32.2	24.1	
South	37.0	53.4	
Living situation at vaccination, in %			ns
Single household	27.6	26.8	
Two or more person/household	71.5	72.8	
Elderly home	0.7	0.4	
Missing	0.2	0.1	
Vaccinated, in %	48.4	51.6	ns

Abbreviations: SD, Standard deviation, *ns* not significant
[a]At inclusion in cohort (= day of home visit). [b]Composed of radiologically confirmed CAP cases (i.e. having a positive X-rays and at least 2 clinical criteria) and radiologically non-confirmed CAP cases

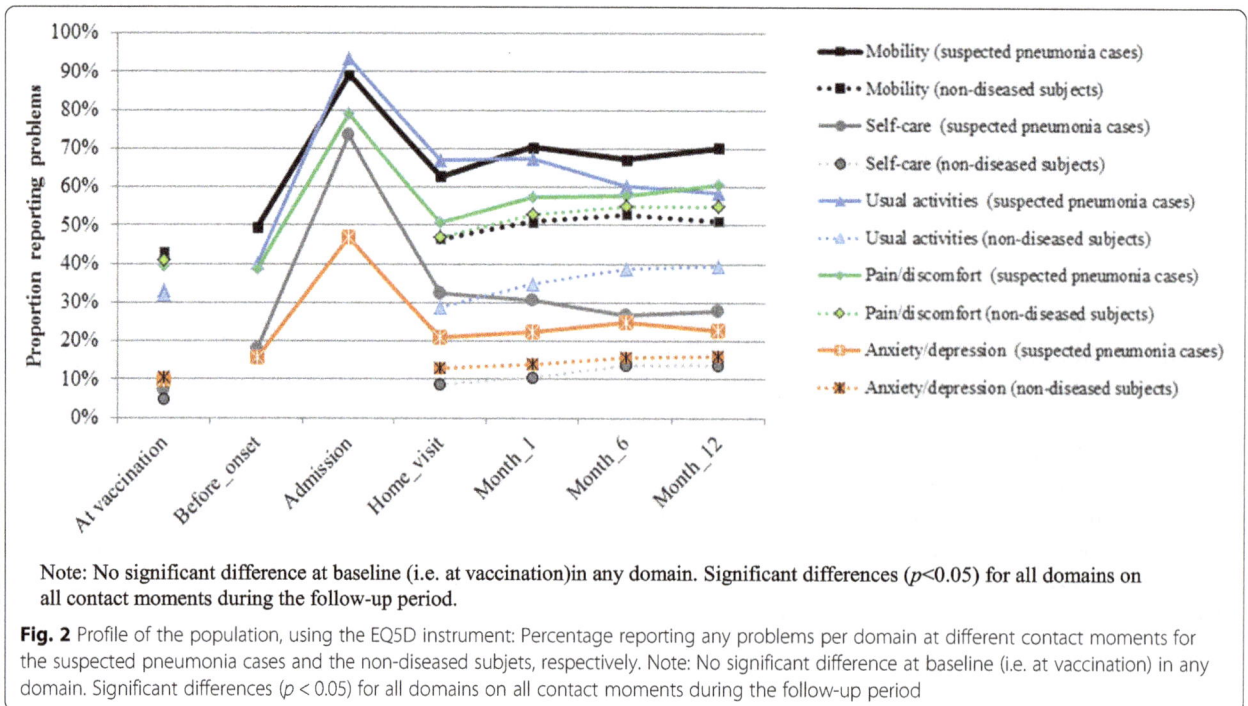

Note: No significant difference at baseline (i.e. at vaccination) in any domain. Significant differences (*p*<0.05) for all domains on all contact moments during the follow-up period.

Fig. 2 Profile of the population, using the EQ5D instrument: Percentage reporting any problems per domain at different contact moments for the suspected pneumonia cases and the non-diseased subjets, respectively. Note: No significant difference at baseline (i.e. at vaccination) in any domain. Significant differences (*p* < 0.05) for all domains on all contact moments during the follow-up period

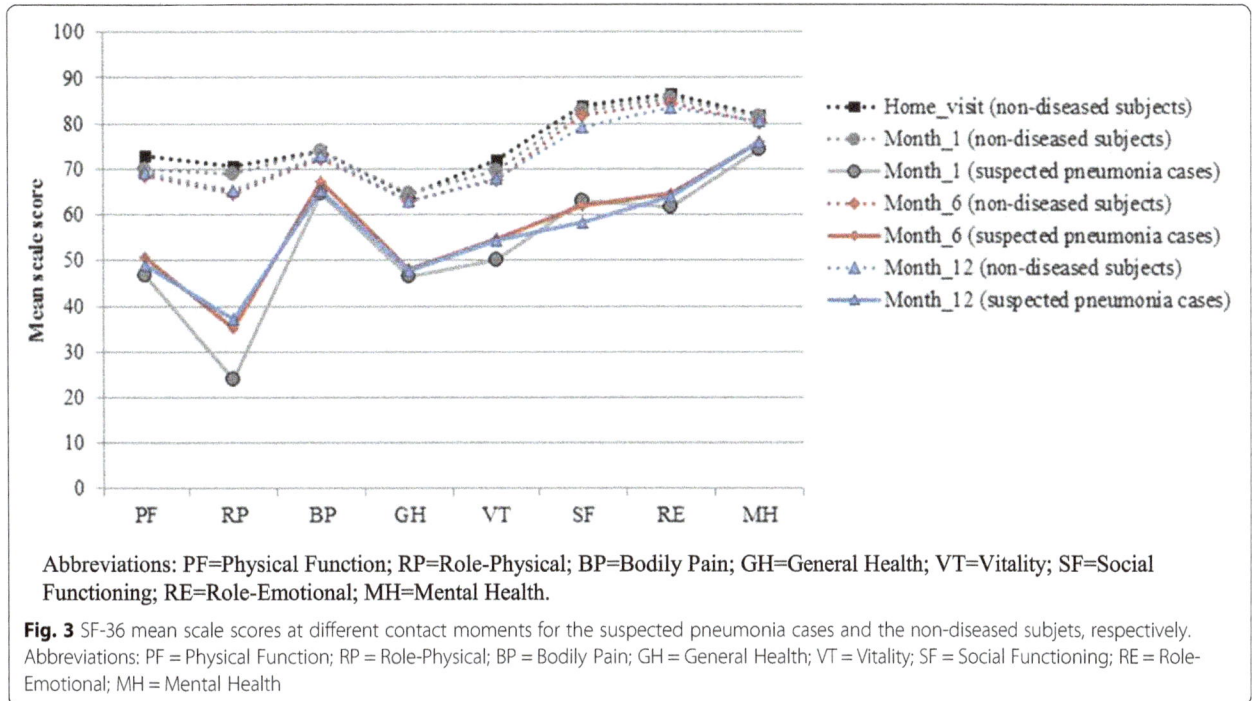

Abbreviations: PF=Physical Function; RP=Role-Physical; BP=Bodily Pain; GH=General Health; VT=Vitality; SF=Social Functioning; RE=Role-Emotional; MH=Mental Health.

Fig. 3 SF-36 mean scale scores at different contact moments for the suspected pneumonia cases and the non-diseased subjets, respectively. Abbreviations: PF = Physical Function; RP = Role-Physical; BP = Bodily Pain; GH = General Health; VT = Vitality; SF = Social Functioning; RE = Role-Emotional; MH = Mental Health

Table 2 EQ5D-index, EQ-VAS and SF6D-index for suspected pneumonia and the non-diseased subjects

	Suspected pneumonia cases		Non-diseased subjects		p-value
	Mean (SD)/Median (IQR)	Missing/died	Mean (SD)/Median (IQR)	Missing/died	
EQ5D-index					
At vaccination[a]	0.87 (0.16)/0.89 (0.78–1.00)	0/0	0.87 (0.16)/0.89 (0.78–1.00)	0/0	ns
Prior to illness onset	0.81 (0.23)/0.86 (0.78–1.00)	0/0	-	-	-
At admission	0.23 (0.32)/0.24 (−0.00–0.43)	0/0	-	-	-
During home visit	0.70 (0.26)/0.78 (0.52–0.89)	0/0	0.84 (0.18)/0.84 (0.78–1.00)	0/0	<0.001
Month 1	0.72 (0.24)/0.78 (0.65–0.89)	60/4	0.83 (0.17)/0.84 (0.78–1.00)	44/2	<0.001
Month 6	0.74 (0.23)/0.78 (0.66–0.89)	85/29	0.82 (0.18)/0.84 (0.78–1.00)	76/4	<0.001
Month 12	0.74 (0.23)/0.78 (0.67–0.89)	104/49	0.82 (0.18)/0.84 (0.78–1.00)	124/14	<0.001
EQ5D-VAS					
Prior to illness onset	71 (15.3)/70 (60–80)	0/0	-	-	-
At admission	33 (16.0)/30 (20–41)	1/0	-	-	-
During home visit	62 (16.7)/65 (50–70)	0/0	76 (13.2)/80 (70–85)	3/0	<0.001
Month 1	64 (16.3)/65 (50–75)	62/4	76 (13.9)/79 (70–85)	37/2	<0.001
Month 6	65 (16.4)/70 (55–78)	86/29	74 (15.2)/75 (65–84)	73/4	<0.001
Month 12	64 (17.5)/69 (50–78)	98/49	75 (14.6)/75 (68–85)	122/14	<0.001
SF6D-index					
During home visit	-	-	0.77 (0.13)/0.79 (0.66–0.88)	9/0	-
Month 1	0.65 (0.13)/0.63 (0.58–0.73)	81/4	0.76 (0.13)/0.77 (0.65–0.88)	69/2	<0.001
Month 6	0.68 (0.14)/0.66 (0.59–0.79)	99/29	0.75 (0.14)/0.75 (0.63–0.88)	116/4	<0.001
Month 12	0.68 (0.14)/0.66 (0.58–0.77)	122/49	0.75 (0.13)/0.75 (0.63–0.87)	149/14	<0.001

Abbreviations: SD Standard deviation, ns not significant
[a]matching criterion

Table 3 Utility difference attributable to suspected pneumonia

	QALY suspected pneumonia case (SE)	QALY non-diseased subjects (SE)	Utility difference attributable to suspected pneumonia
All cases			
One-year post-discharge	0.68 (0.01)	0.81 (0.01)	−0.13
Pneumonia episode & one-year post-discharge	0.67 (0.01)	0.81 (0.01)	−0.15
Only survivors			
One-year post-discharge	0.72 (0.01)	0.82 (0.01)	−0.10
Pneumonia episode & one-year post-discharge	0.71 (0.01)	0.82 (0.01)	−0.11

Abbreviations: QALY quality-adjusted life years, SE standard error

radiologically confirmed and non-confirmed CAP cases had a significantly persistent lower HrQol, independent of the instrument used (see in the Additional file 1: Figure S4A-S6A and Table S7A.). The excess QALY loss attributable to CAP was with 0.14 for radiologically confirmed CAP cases and 0.12 for radiologically non-confirmed CAP cases, of the same magnitude, independent of radiological confirmation of CAP (in the Additional file 1: Table S8A.).

Discussion

In immunocompetent elderly, hospitalization for suspected pneumonia was associated with a six-fold higher risk of mortality and an average loss of QALYs attributable to pneumonia of 0.13 after 1 year, compared to non-diseased subjects. Patients with radiologically confirmed CAP had a two-fold higher mortality risk than those with radiologically non-confirmed CAP, but the average loss of QALYs attributable to CAP among survivors was comparable. The one-year QALY loss associated with a CAP episode (0.13, excluding the CAP episode, and 0.15, including the CAP episode) is twofold higher than the QALY loss that we used [21] in a cost-effectiveness analysis of pneumococcal vaccination (0.071) and is more than tenfold higher than the QALY loss used by Melegaro and Emunds [22] in 2004 and in

most cost-effectiveness studies conducted thereafter in Western European countries (e.g. [23–26]), namely 0.004 for inpatient CAP and 0.0079 for bacteraemia. These estimates of QALY loss were based on expert opinion and not real-life data. Preventing a higher QALY loss through pneumococcal vaccination by definition contributes to more favourable cost-effectiveness of vaccination. For example using a QALY loss of 0.15 rather than 0.07 would have resulted in a somewhat more favourable incremental cost-effectiveness ratio of 8,200 €/QALY versus the 8,650 €/QALY presented in our recently published cost-effectiveness analysis [21]. Although the difference in QALYs is relatively large, the impact on the cost-effectiveness ratio is relatively limited, as mortality has a much higher impact on the cost per QALY gained than quality-of-life.

Strengths of this study include the rigid prospective study design nested within a randomized double-blinded placebo-controlled trial that created the possibility to quantify the excess QALY lost due to CAP in community-dwelling elderly using a one-year follow-up period. We also conducted separate analyses for patients with radiographically confirmed CAP and those without confirmation.

To control for potential biases between pneumonia cases and non-diseased subjects, subjects in both cohorts were matched on age, sex and EQ5D-index as

Table 4 Clinical data of radiologically confirmed and radiologically non-confirmed CAP cases

	Radiologically confirmed CAP cases	Radiologically non-confirmed CAP cases	p-value
Episodes/subjects	341	221	
Positive chest X-ray, in %	100	0	a
Number of clinical criteria, median (IQR)	4 (3–5)	4 (3–5)	ns
PSI score, median (IQR)	93 (80–111)	90 (78–108)	ns
Admitted to ICU, in %	9.7	5.2	ns
Readmitted within 30 days, in %	5.0	3.6	ns
LOS in days, median (IQR)			
At 1st admission,	8 (6–12)	7 (5–11)	0.006
Including readmission	8 (6–11)	7 (5–10)	0.011

Abbreviations: IQR interquartile range, ns not significant
[a]According to definition radiologically confirmed CAP cases had to have a positive X-rays

collected at the time of vaccination. CAP patients had slightly more comorbidities and a lower educational level, factors known to be negatively associated with health status [27–29]. The calculated excess QALY loss might therefore be a slight overestimation of the attributable QALY loss. Furthermore, our study may have suffered from a healthy participant effect, as the study population consisted of subjects that were willing-to-participate in a one-year follow-up study who may have been healthier than the non-responding CAP patients. Indeed, one of the major arguments to refuse participation was self-perceived bad health, and patients with a recent cancer diagnosis were excluded as well. In a sicker population, mortality attributable to CAP would most likely have been higher. As a result, the observed QALY loss attributable to CAP and the mortality risk within the first year post-discharge may have been underestimated.

Conclusion

The current study is the first that provides detailed HrQol during the recovery process of hospitalized elderly suspected pneumonia patients for a one-year post-discharge period using the EQ5D and SF36 questionnaires. It further provides a QALY loss attributable to CAP for community-dwelling elderly, which is a necessity for economic analyses targeted at preventing pneumonia infections and as such contributes to more realistic future estimates of cost-effectiveness of preventive interventions for this infection. The CAP episode is the onset of sustained loss of quality-of-life, with an estimated difference in QALY of 16–18% between CAP patients and their non-diseased subjects.

Endnotes

[1]Due to logistical reasons the first 14.7% of CAPiTA-participants were not invited to participate in the CHO-CAP-study.

[2]48,634 participants returned the questionnaire with signed informed consent. For 47,476 participants (97%) an EQ5D-score could be estimated.

Additional file

Additional file 1: Figure S1A. Observed EQ-5D indexes for suspected pneumonia cases and non-diseased subjects during the one-year post-discharge period, excluding the CAP episode. **Figure S2A.** Survivors (%) in the diseased cohort (i.e. suspected pneumonia cases) and the non-diseased cohort during the one-year follow-up. **Figure S3A.** Mean EQ-5D-3 L-index, EQ-VAS and SF6D-index at different contact moments for the suspected CAP cases and the non-diseased subjects, respectively. **Figure S4A.** Profile of the population using EQ5D-instrument: Percentage reporting any problems per domain at different contact moments for A) the radiologically confirmed CAP cases and their non-diseased subjects, and B) the radiologically non-confirmed CAP cases and their non-diseased subjects, respectively. **Figure S5A.** SF-36 mean scale scores at

different contact moments for A) the radiologically confirmed CAP cases and their non-diseased subjects, and B) the radiologically non-confirmed CAP cases and their non-diseased subjects, respectively. **Figure S6A.** Mean EQ-5D-3 L-index, EQ-VAS and SF6D-index at different contact moments for the radiologically confirmed CAP cases and their non-diseased subjects (A), and for the radiologically non-confirmed CAP cases and their non-diseased subjects (B). **Table S1A.** Exclusion criteria and reasons for nonparticipation in the "diseased" cohort of eligible suspected pneumonia episodes. **Table S2A.** Living situation, loss-to-follow up and deaths of suspected pneumonia cases and non-diseased subjects during the one-year follow-up. **Table S3A.** Spearman's rho for EQ-VAS, EQ5D-index and SF6D-index at the different contact moments for suspected pneumonia cases. **Table S4A.** Spearman's rho for EQ-VAS, EQ5D-index and SF6D-index at the different contact moments for non-diseased subjects. **Table S5A.** Baseline characteristics of radiologically confirmed and non-confirmed CAP cases and their non-diseased subjects. **Table S6A.** Living situation, loss-to-follow up and mortality of radiologically confirmed and non-confirmed CAP cases and their non-diseased subjects during the one-year follow-up. **Table S7A.** EQ5D-index, EQ-VAS and SF6D-index for the radiologically confirmed and non-confirmed CAP cases and their non-diseased subjects. **Table S8A.** Utility differences attributable to radiologically confirmed CAP and radiologically non-confirmed CAP, respectively.

Abbreviations
CAP: Community-acquired pneumonia; CAPiTA: Community-acquired pneumonia immunization trial in adults; CHO-CAP: Costs, health status and outcomes of CAP (Community-Acquired Pneumonia) - study; EQ5D: Euroqol EQ-5D-3L instrument; HrQol: Health-related quality-of-life; QALY: Quality-adjusted life years; SD: Standard deviation; SF36: Short form-36 health survey questionnaire; VAS: Euroqol visual analogue scale

Acknowledgments
The authors would like to thank all "Costs, Health status and Outcomes of community-acquired pneumonia (CAP)" (CHO-CAP) participants for their participation. The "Community-Acquired Pneumonia immunization Trial in Adults" (CAPiTA) team and the CHO-CAP-team from Julius Clinical B.V. in Zeist are acknowledged for their logistic support during the data collection. The CHO-CAP study is made possible by an unrestricted grant from Wyeth Pharmaceuticals, which was acquired by Pfizer Inc. in October 2009, to the University Medical Centre Utrecht.

Funding
The CHO-CAP study is made possible by an unrestricted grant from Wyeth Pharmaceuticals, which was acquired by Pfizer Inc. in October 2009, to the University of Medical Centre of Utrecht.

Authors' contributions
Study concept and design: M-JJM, MJMB, GAdW. Acquisition, analysis, or interpretation of data: M-JJM, SMH, MJMB, GAdW. Drafting of the manuscript: M-JJM. Critical revision of the manuscript for important intellectual content: All authors. Study supervision: MJMB and GAdW. All authors read and approved the final manuscript.

Competing interests
Bonten reports receipt of research funding from Pfizer, and service on the CAPiTA European Expert Meeting. Huijts reports receipt of financial support for printing her PhD thesis from Pfizer. De Wit reports receipt of unrestricted research grant from Pfizer paid to UMCU. Huijts and Mangen's research funding is partially supported by these grants provided to UMCU by Pfizer. Bonten, Huijts, Mangen, and de Wit are UMCU employees. No other disclosures were reported.

Consent for publication
Not applicable.

Role of the sponsor

Pfizer Inc. had no role in the design, analysis, interpretation of the data, or the writing of the manuscript. Pfizer Inc. did review a penultimate version of the manuscript.

Author details

[1]Julius Center for Health Sciences and Primary Care, University Medical Center Utrecht, Heidelberglaan 100, 3584 CX Utrecht, The Netherlands. [2]Department Respiratory Medicine, University Medical Center Utrecht, Utrecht, The Netherlands. [3]Department of Medical Microbiology, University Medical Center Utrecht, Utrecht, The Netherlands.

References

1. Rozenbaum MH, Mangen MJ, Huijts SM, van der Werf TS, Postma MJ. Incidence, direct costs and duration of hospitalization of patients hospitalized with community acquired pneumonia: a nationwide retrospective claims database analysis. Vaccine. 2015;33(28):3193–9.
2. Eurich DT, Johnstone JJ, Minhas-Sandhu JK, Marrie TJ, Majumdar SR. Pneumococcal vaccination and risk of acute coronary syndromes in patients with pneumonia: population-based cohort study. Heart. 2012;98(14):1072–7.
3. Reyes S, Martinez R, Valles JM, Cases E, Menendez R. Determinants of hospital costs in community-acquired pneumonia. Eur Respir J. 2008;31(5):1061–7.
4. Jacob C, Mittendorf T, von der Schulenburg JM G. Costs of illness and health-related quality of life for community-acquired pneumonia–a systematic review. Pneumologie. 2011;65(8):498–502.
5. Torres A, Muir JF, Corris P, Kubin R, Duprat-Lomon I, Sagnier PP, Hoffken G. Effectiveness of oral moxifloxacin in standard first-line therapy in community-acquired pneumonia. Eur Respir J. 2003;21(1):135–43.
6. Gleason PP, Kapoor WN, Stone RA, Lave JR, Obrosky DS, Schulz R, Singer DE, Coley CM, Marrie TJ, Fine MJ. Medical outcomes and antimicrobial costs with the use of the american thoracic society guidelines for outpatients with community-acquired pneumonia. JAMA. 1997;278(1):32–9.
7. El Moussaoui R, Opmeer BC, de Borgie CA, Nieuwkerk P, Bossuyt PM, Speelman P, Prins JM. Long-term symptom recovery and health-related quality of life in patients with mild-to-moderate-severe community-acquired pneumonia. Chest. 2006;130(4):1165–72.
8. Carratala J, Fernandez-Sabe N, Ortega L, Castellsague X, Roson B, Dorca J, Fernandez-Aguera A, Verdaguer R, Martinez J, Manresa F, et al. Outpatient care compared with hospitalization for community-acquired pneumonia: a randomized trial in low-risk patients. Ann Intern Med. 2005;142(3):165–72.
9. Marrie TJ, Lau CY, Wheeler SL, Wong CJ, Vandervoort MK, Feagan BG. A controlled trial of a critical pathway for treatment of community-acquired pneumonia. CAPITAL Study Investigators. Community-Acquired Pneumonia Intervention Trial Assessing Levofloxacin. JAMA 2000; 283(6):749–755
10. Honselmann KC, Buthut F, Heuwer B, Karadag S, Sayk F, Kurowski V, Thiele H, Droemann D, Wolfrum S. Long-term mortality and quality of life in intensive care patients treated for pneumonia and/or sepsis: Predictors of mortality and quality of life in patients with sepsis/pneumonia. J Crit Care. 2015;30(4):721–6.
11. McHorney CA, Ware Jr JE, The RAE, MOS. 36-item short-form health survey (SF-36): II. Psychometric and clinical tests of validity in measuring physical and mental health constructs. Med Care. 1993;31(3):247–63.
12. Dolan P. Modeling valuations for EuroQol health states. Med Care. 1997; 35(11):1095–108.
13. Hak E, Grobbee DE, Sanders EA, Verheij TJ, Bolkenbaas M, Huijts SM, Gruber WC, Tansey S, McDonough A, Thoma B, et al. Rationale and design of CAPITA: a RCT of 13-valent conjugated pneumococcal vaccine efficacy among older adults. Neth J Med. 2008;66(9):378–83.
14. Bonten MJM, Huijts SM, Bolkenbaas M, Webber C, Patterson S, Gault S, van Werkhoven CH, van Deursen AM, Sanders EA, Verheij TJM, et al. 13-valent pneumococcal vaccine in prevention of vaccine-serotype disease. N Engl J Med. 2015;372(12):1114–25.
15. Mangen MJ, Bonten MJ, de Wit GA. Rationale and design of the costs, health status and outcomes in community-acquired pneumonia (CHO-CAP) study in elderly persons hospitalized with CAP. BMC Inf Dis. 2013;13:597.
16. Walters SJ, Munro JF, Brazier JE. Using the SF-36 with older adults: a cross-sectional community-based survey. Age Ageing. 2001;30(4):337–43.
17. Brazier J, Roberts J, Deverill M. The estimation of a preference-based measure of health from the SF-36. J Health Econ. 2002;21(2):271–92.
18. Oppe M, Rabin R, de Charo F, on behalf of the EuroQol Group. EQ-5D user guide. Version 1. Rotterdam: Euroqol; 2008.
19. Lamers LM, McDonnell J, Stalmeier PF, Krabbe PF, Busschbach JJ. The Dutch tariff: results and arguments for an effective design for national EQ-5D valuation studies. Health Econ. 2006;15(10):1121–32.
20. Fine MJ, Auble TE, Yealy DM, Hanusa BH, Weissfeld LA, Singer DE, Coley CM, Marrie TJ, Kapoor WN. A prediction rule to identify low-risk patients with community-acquired pneumonia. N Engl J Med. 1997;336(4):243–50.
21. Mangen MJ, Rozenbaum MH, Huijts SM, van Werkhoven CH, Postma DF, Atwood M, van Deursen AM, van der Ende A, Grobbee DE, Sanders EA, et al. Cost-effectiveness of adult pneumococcal conjugate vaccination in the Netherlands. Eur Respir J. 2015;46(5):1407–16. doi:10.1183/13993003.00325-2015.
22. Melegaro A, Edmunds WJ. Cost-effectiveness analysis of pneumococcal conjugate vaccination in England and Wales. Vaccine. 2004;22(31–32):4203–14.
23. Rozenbaum MH, Hak E, van der Werf TS, Postma MJ. Results of a cohort model analysis of the cost-effectiveness of routine immunization with 13-valent pneumococcal conjugate vaccine of those aged > or =65 years in the Netherlands. Clin Ther. 2010;32(8):1517–32.
24. Rozenbaum MH, van Hoek AJ, Fleming D, Trotter CL, Miller E, Edmunds WJ. Vaccination of risk groups in England using the 13 valent pneumococcal conjugate vaccine: economic analysis. BMJ. 2012;345:e6879.
25. Blommaert A, Bilcke J, Willem L, Verhaegen J, Goossens H, Beutels P. The cost-effectiveness of pneumococcal vaccination in healthy adults over 50: an exploration of influential factors for Belgium. Vaccine. 2016;34(18):2106–12.
26. van Hoek AJ, Miller E. Cost-effectiveness of vaccinating immunocompetent >/=65 year olds with the 13-valent pneumococcal conjugate vaccine in England. Plos One. 2016;11(2):e0149540. doi:10.1371/journal.pone.0149540.
27. Szende A, Janssen B, Cabases's J. Self-Reported Population Health: An International Perspective based on EQ-5D. Springer Dordrecht Heidelberg New York London: Springer Open; 2014. http://download.springer.com/static/pdf/471/bok%253A978-94-007-7596-1.pdf?originUrl=http%3A%2F%2Flink.springer.com%2Fbook%2F10.1007%2F978-94-007-7596-1&token2=exp=1488541001~acl=%2Fstatic%2Fpdf%2F471%2Fbok%25253A978-94-007-7596-1.pdf%3ForiginUrl%3Dhttp%253A%252F%252Flink.springer.com%252Fbook%252F10.1007%252F978-94-007-7596-1*~hmac=81a5af2dd69a3647d40b6dd40b53a63af248614fe9cfbaffb8e462870e2d2ce9. Accessed 3 Mar 2017.
28. Konig HH, Bernert S, Angermeyer MC, Matschinger H, Martinez M, Vilagut G, Haro JM, de Girolamo G, de Graaf R, Kovess V, et al. Comparison of population health status in six european countries: results of a representative survey using the EQ-5D questionnaire. Med Care. 2009;47(2):255–61.
29. Konig H-H, Heider D, Lehnert T, Riedel-Heller SG, Angermeyer MC, Matschinger H, Vilagut G, Bruffaerts R, Haro JM, de Girolamo G, et al. Health status of the advanced elderly in six European countries: results from a representative survey using EQ-5D and SF-12. Health Qual Life Outcomes. 2010;8:143. doi:10.1186/1477-7525-8-143.

14

Exiguobacterium sp. A1b/GX59 isolated from a patient with community-acquired pneumonia and bacteremia

Xingchun Chen[1†], Lijun Wang[2†], Jiali Zhou[3†], Honglong Wu[3], Dong Li[4], Yanchao Cui[4] and Binghuai Lu[4*]

Abstract

Background: Bacterial species belonging to the genus *Exiguobacterium* are facultative anaerobic, non-spore-forming, Gram-positive bacilli, and rarely associated with human infections. Herein, we reported the first case of community-acquired pneumonia (CAP) and bacteremia due to *Exiguobacterium* spp. in China.

Case presentation: An adult male with severe CAP was hospitalized. The pathogen was isolated from his bloodstream and broncho-alveolar lavage fluid. The correct identification of the micro-organism was achieved using 16S rRNA sequencing, and its antibiotic susceptibility test was performed by microdilution method. The Whole Genome Sequencing (WGS) was used to characterize its genetic features and to elucidate its potential pathogenic mechanisms. Furthermore, its genome sequence was also compared with those of 3 publicly-available *Exiguobacterium* strains. A PubMed search was performed for further understanding the features of *Exiguobacterium* infections. Phylogenetic analysis of the 16S rRNA gene sequence showed that the strain GX59 was most closely related to *Exiguobacterium* AT1b (99.7%). The genome of GX59 was 2,727,929 bp in size, harbouring 2855 putative protein-coding genes, 5 rRNA operons, 37 tRNA genes and 1 tmRNA. The multiple genome comparison of 4 *Exiguobacterium* strains demonstrated that *Exiguobacterium* contained 37 genes of secretion systems, including *sec*, *tat*, *FEA*, Type IV Pili and competence-related DNA transformation transporter (*Com*). Virulence factors of the micro-organism included *tlyC*, *NprR*, *MCP*, *Dam*, which might play a critical role in causing lethal infection.

Conclusions: The study highlighted the potential pathogenicity of the genus *Exiguobacterium* for its unique genes encoding various virulence factors and those associated with antibiotic resistance, therefore, its clinical significance should be valued.

Keywords: *Exiguobacterium* spp., Whole genome sequencing, Virulence factors, Antibiotics, Bacteremia, Community-acquired pneumonia

Background

The genus *Exiguobacterium* belongs to the group of *coryneform* bacteria, firstly described in 1983 by *Collins* et al. [1]. It is a facultative anaerobic, Gram-positive bacillus. The pathogenic potential of *Exiguobacterium* spp. seems rather low. To date, only a few cases of bacteremia and skin infection were documented in English literature [2–6]. However, the clinical infection due to the micro-organism might be probably underdiagnosed or unreported, for it tended to be misidentified by routine commercial methods [2–6]. As an emerging pathogen, its pathogenesis should be clarified.

Here, we present a case of community-acquired pneumonia (CAP) and bacteremia due to *Exiguobacterium* sp. strain AT1b/GX59 in a type 2 diabetes mellitus (T2DM) patient. To the best of our knowledge, this is the first fatal case of CAP and bacteremia due to the micro-organism in a healthy male without serious underlying diseases. In order

* Correspondence: zs25041@126.com
†Equal contributors
4Department of Laboratory Medicine, Civil Aviation General Hospital, Peking University Civil Aviation School of Clinical Medicine, No1. Gaojing Street, Chaoyang District, Beijing 100123, China

to generate significant insights into pathogenicity of the micro-organism, its genome was sequenced and compared with 3 *Exiguobacterium* genomes available in NCBI Genbank database.

Case presentation
Medical history
On July 28th, 2014, a 51-year-old male with severe pneumonia, acute respiratory distress syndrome was admitted to People's Hospital of Guangxi Zhuang Autonomous Region at Guangxi, China. He is a farmer living on planting sugarcane and had a history of 8-year T2DM.

At admission, he was febrile (37.8 °C), with a respiratory rate of 60 breaths/min, a pulse rate of 126 beats/min and blood pressure of 165/80 mmHg. He also complained chill, headache, cough, hemoptysis and dyspnea for one day. Physical examination showed that he was in respiratory distress due to chest pain and tightness. Chest CT scan indicated diffuse pulmonary lesions and consolidation. His peripheral leukocyte count was 1.54×10^9/L with 53.9% neutrophils. His blood glucose was badly controlled at 18.0 mmol/L. Results of initial arterial blood gas analyses were: pH 7.42, carbon dioxide pressure (PCO_2) 27 mmHg, and oxygen pressure (PO_2) 31 mmHg. His liver function tests were within reference ranges; however, his creatinine was 183 µmol/L (reference range 54–106 µmol/L) and urea was 12.7 mmol/L (3.2–7.1 mmol/L). Afterwards, broncho-alveolar lavage fluid (BALF) and 3 sets of blood sample were collected for culture. Furthermore, imipenem combined with voriconazol was empirically administered in an attempt to relieve infection.

Two days after our empirical therapy, his blood pressure dropped to 108/55 mmHg, and arterial blood gas analysis showed: pH 7.26, PCO_2 55 mmHg, and PO_2 53 mmHg. The marked changes in lung stroma were detected on CT screening. Poor lung compliance, and following alveolar rupture and subcutaneous emphysema brought the patient into a critical condition. On August 1st, the patient fell into a coma and was brought back home by his family members. He died two days later.

Microbiologic test
Microbial growth was detected in 3 aerobic blood culture bottles obtained through separate needle puncture sites. Direct gram-stain demonstrated Gram-positive, short, and straight rods. Positive blood culture broths were subcultured at 37 °C under 5.0% CO_2. The non-hemolytic, gray colonies were observed on blood agar from both blood and BALF cultures, but turned yellow after 48 h, and there was no growth on MacConkey agar, as shown in Fig. 1. The isolate was catalase positive and oxidase negative. Phenotypic identification of the bacteria by the ANC (BioMerieux, France) card yielded poor identification of *unidentified organism* (isolate Bionumber:

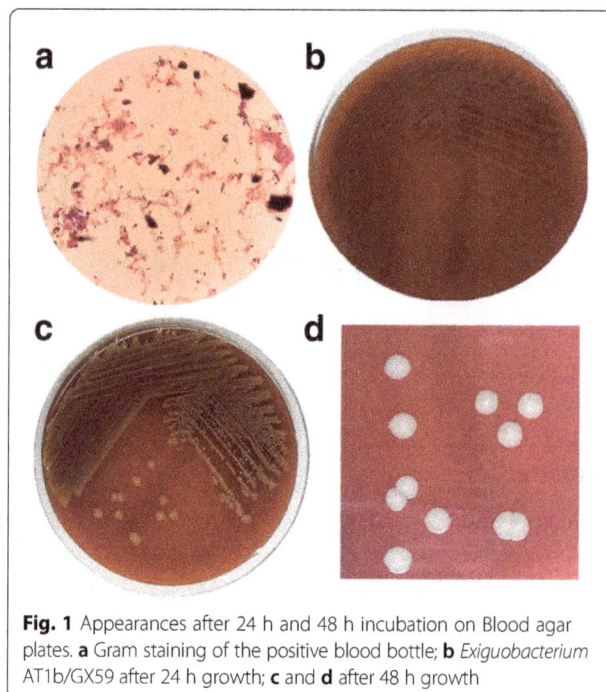

Fig. 1 Appearances after 24 h and 48 h incubation on Blood agar plates. **a** Gram staining of the positive blood bottle; **b** *Exiguobacterium* AT1b/GX59 after 24 h growth; **c** and **d** after 48 h growth

6,521,100,600,035). Antimicrobial susceptibility testing was performed by using micro dilution and E-test method. The MIC results were as follows: susceptible to penicillin (0.064 µg/ml), meropenem (0.064 µg/ml), gentamicin (0.25 µg/ml), ciprofloxacin (0.25 µg/ml), rifampin (0.125 µg/ml), and vancomycin (0.125 µg/ml), but resistant to tetracycline (16 µg/ml), erythromycin (4 µg/ml) and clindamycin (1 µg/ml).

16S rRNA sequencing and phylogenetic analyses
The 16S rRNA sequencing was conducted to identify the pathogen. Other 7 related members of the genus *Exiguobacterium* available in NCBI Genebank database were included for phylogenetic analyses. The sequence analysis of a 1433 bp segment of the 16S rRNA genes of the organism demonstrated an identity of 99.7% with *Exiguobacterium. AT1b* (GenBank accession no. NR_074970.1) (Fig. 2).

Whole genome sequencing (WGS)
To elucidate the potential pathogenicity of the micro-organism in current study, we sequenced its whole genome using a whole-genome shotgun strategy based on the Illumina HiSeq platform. The high-quality reads were generated after filtering low-quality ones, adapter contamination and PCR primers by using the software Trimmomatic (version 0.32). De novo assembly was performed with SOAP denovo (version 2.0.1), an empirically-improved memory-efficient short-read de novo assembler, and gaps were closed by Gap Closer (version 1.12). Furthermore, Gene prediction and annotation were carried out by PROKKA pipeline for rapid prokaryotic genome annotation.

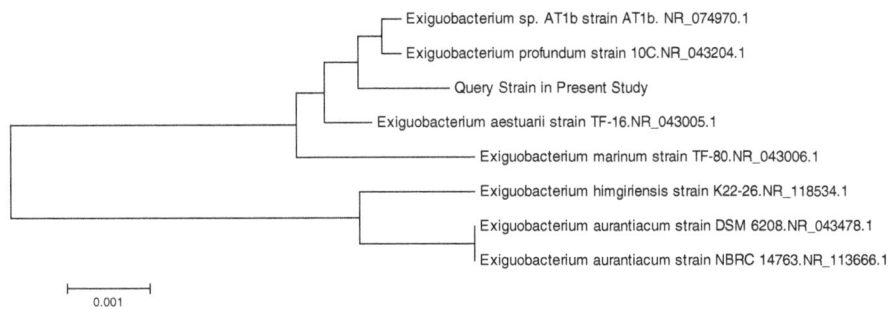

Fig. 2 Phylogenetic relatedness of query isolate to closest neighbors based on 16S rRNA homology. Neighbor-joining tree based on 16S rRNA (1,443 bases) sequences, showing the phylogenetic relationship between query strain in present study and other related members of the genus *Exiguobacterium*

This whole-genome shotgun sequencing project has been deposited at DDBJ/ENA/GenBank under the accession GenBank accession no. GCA_001908175.1. WGS generated 6,916,887 bp pair-end reads with read length of 150 bp. A total of 21 scaffolds were assembled, with an N50 size of 539,676 bp, an N90 size of 103,057 bp and the largest scaffold size of 632,933 bp. The GC content of GX59 was 47.49%, similar to that of other *Exiguobacterium* species. The size of GX59 genome was 2,727,929 bp, containing 2855 putative protein-coding genes, 5 rRNA operons, 37 tRNA genes and 1 tmRNA. The KEGG annotation of the GX59 genome was performed by BlastKOALA, and 52.9% of 2812 entries were annotated (Table 1). The majority of metabolism genes in the genus *Exiguobacterium* enabled it to survive in

Table 1 Summary of *Exiguobacterium* AT1b/GX59 strain KEGG annotation

KEGG (functional category)	GX59 (n)
Genetic Information Processing	418
Environmental Information Processing	351
Amino acid metabolism	161
Carbohydrate metabolism	161
Cellular Processes	172
Metabolism of cofactors and vitamins	103
Nucleotide metabolism	88
Energy metabolism	80
Human Diseases	75
Enzyme families	58
Lipid metabolism	47
Metabolism of other amino acids	35
Metabolism of terpenoids and polyketides	32
Glycan biosynthesis and metabolism	30
Organismal systems	31
Xenobiotics biodegradation and metabolism	25
Biosynthesis of other secondary metabolites	17
Unclassified	231

various environments. BRITE reconstruction result demonstrated that GX59 strain contained 13 antimicrobial resistance genes, including tetracycline resistance genes (*tetB*, and efflux pump *Tet38*), macrolide resistance genes (*msrA*, *vmlR*, *mef*, and *vat*), aminoglycoside resistance genes (*aacC*, *aac6-I*, *aacA7*, *aadA*, and *aadK*), phenicol resistance genes (*catA*), cationic antimicrobial peptide (CAMP) resistance genes (*mprF* and *fmtC*), multidrug resistance efflux pump (*abcA* and *bmrA*), and vancomycin resistance modules (*vanY* and *vanW*).

Ortholog analysis

The genome sequences of *Exiguobacterium* sp. AT1b (GenBank accession no. NR_074970.1), *E. aurantiacum* DSM 6208 (GenBank accession no. NZ_JNIQ01000001.1), and *E. acetylicum* DSM 20416 (GenBank accession no. NZ_JNIR01000001.1) were collected from NCBI Nucleotide database. The protein sequences of above genomes and that of AT1b/GX59 in current study were collected together and searched against itself via multiparanoid program, based on the Blastp algorithm with the following criteria: identity ≥ 50%, coverage ≥ 50%, BLAST score ≥ 50, and confidence score = 1. Afterwards, unique genes of AT1b/GX59 and those shared by all 4 strains were parsed out from the blast results and annotated by KEGG orthology (KO) identifiers in the web-based server called KAAS (KEGG Automatic Annotation Server: http://www.genome.jp/kegg/kaas/).

Virulence factors related to pathogenicity in *Exiguobacterium* strain GX59 by WGS

A total of 261 specific genes of *Exiguobacterium* sp. A1b/GX59 were identified. Moreover, the comparison of general genome features within the 4 *Exiguobacterium* strains indicated that they shared 1919 core genes, which participated in metabolic, cellular, and genetic information processing, respectively (Fig. 3 and Table 2). Of the 1919 shared genes, 65.5% were annotated with KEGG. A variety of secretion system genes involved in pathogenicity mechanism were also identified. The 4 *Exiguobacterium* strains

Discussion

The clinical characterizations of *Exiguobacterium* species isolated previously from different infectious samples were listed in Table 3 [2–6]. As documented, most infections due to *Exiguobacterium* spp. had underlying diseases, such as liver cirrhosis [2], intravenous drug abuse and multiple myeloma [6]. However, the patient in present study was in a generally healthy condition, though he suffered from T2DM. Although a male patient infected by the micro-organism was previously healthy, different from our patient, he had only an ulcer on a finger with a painful black eschar rather than systematic infection [4]. Bacteria of the genus *Exiguobacterium* distribute extensively and have been isolated from markedly diverse sources, including water, the rhizosphere of plants, and the environment of food processing plants [8]. The patient in current study was a farmer living on processing plants in humid climate of South China. Considering his early clinical symptoms, inhalation of the micro-organism might be a possible portal of entry of his pneumonia [8].

The literature review demonstrated that *Exiguobacterium* were rarely isolated as human pathogen. Furthermore, it is difficult to identify *Exiguobacterium* spp. based on traditional biochemical method. Almost all reported infective strains of this genus were misidentified when the commercial biochemical system was used, including API Coryne kit/VITEK 2 Compact system (Bio-Mérieux, France), and Becton Dickinson Diagnostic Systems [2–6]. Furthermore, Matrix-assisted laser desorption ionization–time of flight (MALDI-TOF) analysis is presently becoming a routinely used tool in many microbiology laboratories, and might be used in identifying the genus *Exiguobacterium* in future [6], however, in our study, the strain GX59 was identified as *Exiguobacterium aurantiacum* 290RLT with its score as 1.547 by using MALDI-TOF (Bruker Daltonics, MALDI Biotyper 3.1 software, 2371 species and 5989 entries included).

In current study, the pathogen could not be identified using ANC card of VITEK 2 system, and was confirmed as *Exiguobacterium* AT1b by 16s rRNA sequencing only in retrospective analysis. *Exiguobacterium* AT1b was initially isolated from a slightly alkaline, highly carbonate, and hot spring water sample from Yellowstone National Park [9], and had never documented to be isolated clinically. Therefore, the in-depth analysis of the *Exiguobacterium* sp. AT1b/GX59 isolate in present study might elucidate

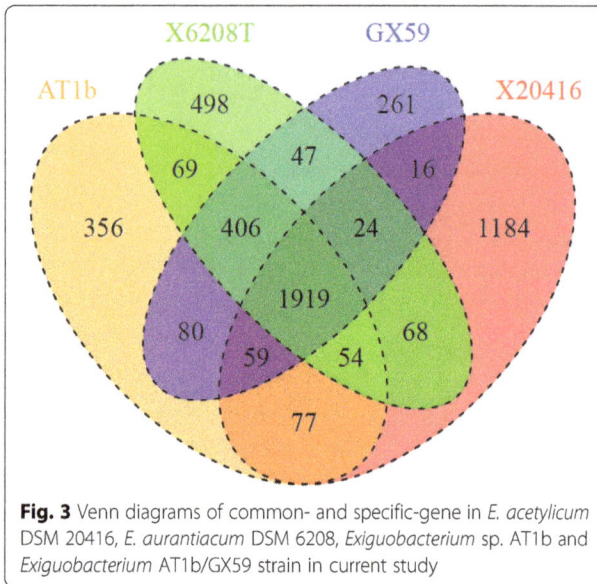

Fig. 3 Venn diagrams of common- and specific-gene in *E. acetylicum* DSM 20416, *E. aurantiacum* DSM 6208, *Exiguobacterium* sp. AT1b and *Exiguobacterium* AT1b/GX59 strain in current study

possessed 37 genes of secretion systems, encoding two translocons, including *sec* (secretion), *tat* (twin-arginine translocation), *FEA* (flagella export apparatus), *FPE* (fimbrilin-protein exporter), Type IV Pili and competence-related DNA transformation transporter (*com*).

Furthermore, 261 specific genes of *Exiguobacterium sp.* A1b/GX59 were submitted in KAAS, and 24.9% were annotated as hypothetical proteins with the BRITE functional hierarchy. In its genome, a series of unique virulence genes were identified, including *tlyC* (AT1b/GX59-P-00125 k03699) encoding hemolysin, a type of membrane-damaging toxin, *NprR* (AT1b/GX59-P-01697 k20480) encoding a quorum-sensing receptor, *mcp* (methyl accepting chemotaxis proteins) (AT1b/GX59-P-01386 k03406) and *Dam* (DNA adenine methylase) (AT1b/GX59-P-01413 k06223). Moreover, in secretion systems, *Exiguobacterium sp.* A1b/GX59 encompassed an extra gene *SecDF*, which played a role as a chaperone facilitating the translocation of *L. monocytogenes* virulence factors during infection [7].

Literature review

To better understand the characteristics of *Exiguobacterium* infections, PubMed was searched and 5 related reports were included for comparison [2–6].

Table 2 General genome features of the four *Exiguobacterium* species

Organism	Source	Size(Mb)	GC%	CDS	No. of tRNAs	No. of contigs	Genome status	GenBank No.
Exiguobacterium AT1b/GX59 strain	BALF and blood, China	2.73	47	2855	37	21	Draft	GCA_001908175.1
Exiguobacterium sp. AT1b	spring water, USA	2.99	48	3020	68	/	Complete	CP001615
E. acetylicum DSM 20416	Creamery waste, UK	3.28	47	3323	69	3	Draft	JNIR00000000
E. aurantiacum DSM 6208	Potato wash, UK	3.04	53	3067	67	2	Draft	JNIQ00000000

Table 3 Summary of reported cases of human infection due to *Exiguobacterium spp.*

Reference	2003 [2]	2006 [5]	2007 [3]	2014 [4]	2007 [6]	Our data
Cases number	1	1	1	1	6	1
Age(y)/Gender	55/M	NM/M	92/F	66/M	27/M(1), NM/M(3),neonate(1),55/M(1)	51/M
Community-acquired or hospital acquired	NM	NM	Nosocomial acquisition	Community-acquired	NM	Community-acquired
Sources	NM	NM	Catheter-related	Handled the skin of a deer and a wild boar.	NM	Respiratory tract, sugarcane farmer
Underlying disease	Alcoholic liver cirrhosis.	NM	Hypertension, hyperuricaemia and Alzheimer's disease.	Previously healthy	Intravenous drug abuse(1), multiple myeloma(2), suspected infective endocarditis(1), neonate(1), igg kappa multiple myeloma, received local radiotherapy, corticosteroids and infusion chemotherapy(1).	T2DM
Presentation	Abdominal pain and diarrhea	NM	37.4 °C; late increased to 38.6 °C.	Afebrile with no systemic symptoms. Ulcer on a finger with a painful black eschar.	NM(5), febrile at 38.2 °C and experienced rigors after the indwelling central line was flushed(1).	Fever, chills, headache, cough, expectoration, hemoptysis, and dyspnea
Diagnosis	Bacteremia	Bacteremia	Bacteremia	Cutaneous infection	Bacteremia	Bacteremia and pneumonia
Sources	Bloodstream	Bloodstream	Bloodstream	Skin infection exudate	Bloodstream	Bloodstream and BALF
Identification — Commercial identification systems	*Pantoea agglomerans* by Enterotube II (Becton Dickinson Diagnostic Systems, Sparks, MD, USA) and Phoenix Identification System PMIC/ID-30 (Becton Dickinson Diagnostic Systems)	*Oerskovia xanthincolytica* by API Coryne (biomérieux)	Not identified by API Coryne (biomérieux)	*Bacillus spp.*	*Cellulomonas/Microbacterium spp.* By API Coryne (biomérieux)	*Unidentified organism* by ANC card (biomérieux)
16 s rRNA	99% *E. profundum* (hm584043.1)	*Exiguobacterium sp.* 99% identity of 1024 nucleotides.	*E. acetylicum* (99% identity of 506 nucleotides)	*E. sibiricum* (1413 bp, and similarity was 99.6%)	*E. aurantiacum* (high sequence homology, 99.2%)	*Exiguobacteriu sp. At1b.* (1433 bp and similarity 99.7%)
AST	NM	NM	Susceptible to penicillins, cephalosporins, Aminoglycosides and quinolones	Susceptible to penicillin, imipenem, cefotaxime, cefotaxime, levofloxacin, vancomycin, clindamycin, erythromycin, gentamicin, doxycycline, linezolid, and daptomycin.	Susceptible to ampicillin, cefotaxime, chloramphenicol, ciprofloxacin, clindamycin, erythromycin, gentamicin, penicillin, rifampicin, teicoplanin, tetracycline and trimethoprim	Susceptible to penicillin, meropenem, gentamicin, ciprofloxacin, rifampin, and vancomycin, Resistant to tetracycline, erythromycin, clindamycin
Antibiotic therapy	NM	NM	Intravenous cefuroxime treatment was initiated; afterwards, cefuroxime	Ciprofloxacin for 10 days.	6th patient: intravenous ceftazidime and teicoplanin for the following 3 days, the fever persisted. Others: unknown	Imipenem, moxifloxacin and voriconazole
Outcome	Recovered	NM	Recovered	Recovered	Recovered	Died

F Female, M Male, NM Not mentioned, AST Antimicrobial Susceptibility Testing

the pathogenicity of this environmental saprophytic micro-organism. Moreover, the comparison study of the genomes of the strain GX59 and other *Exiguobacterium* spp. might then shed light on the pathogenicity of the microorganism. The publicly-available genomes of *Exiguobacterium* spp. were mostly isolated from environment. Through ortholog gene analysis, it was reasonably to speculate that several following genetic characteristics were closely related to the pathogenicity of current GX59 strain. Firstly, secretion systems identified in the strain might be involved its pathogenicity. Desvaux M [10] suggested to use the terms *sec, tat, FEA,* and *FPE* in translocation systems across the cytoplasmic membrane of both Gram-positive and -negative bacteria. The above 4 *Exiguobacterium* strains possessed 37 genes of secretion systems, encoding two translocons, including *sec, tat, FEA,* and competence-related DNA transformation transporter (*Com*). In pathogenic Gram-positive bacteria, the vast majority of proteins were exported out of cytosol by conserved general *sec* system [11] or, by *tat* system [12]. Other studies discovered *Com* proteins were required for internalization of extracellular DNA [13, 14]. Taken together, *Exiguobacterium* had the ability to export toxins to exert its full virulence and to uptake DNA to acquire a variety of virulence and resistance traits. Secondly, a series of unique virulence genes identified in the GX59 strain genome might explain its high virulence. For example, the hemolysin encoded by the gene *tlyC* was taken as a virulence factor in a variety of Gram-positive infectious bacteria. Carvalho E [15] suggested that the protein *tlyC* was not directly involved in hemolysis, but contributed to binding of Leptospira to extracellular matrix (ECM) during host infection. The non-hemolytic GX59 strain in present study contained *tlyC* genes, in consistent with Carvalho E's finding [15]. Moreover, NprR, as a major transcriptional regulator, was documented to belong to RNPP family of quorum-sensing (QS) receptors, a group of intracellular regulators activated directly by signaling oligopeptides in Gram-positive bacteria [16]. It might control sporulation and necrotrophic properties, ensuring survival and dissemination of the bacteria in clinical infections by feeding on host proteins [16]. Another pathogenetic gene uniquely detected in the GX59 strain was *mcp*, which got involved in virulence, motility, and biofilm formation of bacteria [17], possibly performing a potential function in invasive infections. Furthermore, *Dam* mediated the methylation of adenine in the 5'-GATC-3' sequence shortly after DNA replication, and was implicated as a virulence factor in bacterial pathogenesis. As documented previously, *Dam* methylation was required for efficient biofilm production in *Salmonella enterica* serovar enteritidis [18]. *Dam* was also crucial in modulating the pathogenicity of *K. pneumoniae* genotype K1 [19]. The *Dam* gene identified in the GX59 strain might participate in its invasiveness during infection. Finally, apart from the virulence factors unique in the

AT1b/GX59 strain, other common virulence factors might be involved in severe infection. For, example, the GX59 strain harboured an extra gene *SecDF*, which played a role as a chaperone that facilitates the translocation of *L. monocytogenes* virulence factors during infection [7]. Deletion of *secDF* resulted in reduced virulence and motility *Bacillus cereus* ATCC 14579 [20]. Taken together, the severe CAP and following bacteriemia in our patient was possibly explained by the high pathogenicity due to the above-identified virulence genes.

Except for high pathogenic genes, *Exiguobacterium* spp. also harboured some antimicrobial resistance genes, including tetracycline resistance genes, macrolide resistance genes, aminoglycoside resistance genes, phenicol resistance genes, cationic antimicrobial peptide, multidrug resistance efflux pumps (*abcA* and *bmrA*), and vancomycin resistance modules (*vanY, vanW*). Accordingly, although the strain remained susceptible, it would easily become resistant to many antibiotics. Generally, timely antibiotic therapy often resulted in a favorable outcome in the clinical infections due to the microorganism [2, 3, 5, 6]. However, in current study the isolate was susceptible to the antibiotics used, e.g. meropenem and ciprofloxacin, but the patient died of deteriorated infection. This might be explained by the reasons as follows. The pathogen was not identified timely, the appropriate antibiotic therapy failed to take, and furthermore, the rapidly-deteriorated severe acute type 2 respiratory failure caused his death.

Conclusions

In summary, the *Exiguobacterium* sp. AT1b/GX59 strain in current study is equipped with a variety of factors that facilitate its adaptation to a pathogenic lifestyle, such as hemolysin, secretion systems, chemotaxis proteins, and antibiotic resistance genes. The *Exiguobacterium* sp., as a potential pathogen, should attract more attention.

Abbreviations
BALF: broncho-alveolar lavage fluid; CAP: community-acquired pneumonia; T2DM: type 2 diabetes mellitus; WGS: Whole Genome Sequencing

Acknowledgements
Not applicable.

Funding
This study was partially supported by Civil Aviation General Hospital Research Funds (Grant no. 2014001) and the Science and Technology Program of Tianjin, China (No.13ZCZDSY02500).

Authors' contributions
XCC and BHL conceived and designed the experiments. LJW, JLZ, HLW, DL, and YCC collected the information about the case, contributed to the

acquisition, analysis and interpretation of data. DL, YCC and BHL conducted antibiotic sensitivity and some molecular tests, and participated in the literature review. XCC, LJW and BHL wrote and revised the manuscript. All authors read and approved the final manuscript.

Consent for publication

Written informed consent was obtained from the patient's direct relative for publication of this study. A copy of the written consent is available for review by the Editor of this journal.

Competing interests

The authors declare that they have no competing interests.

Author details

[1]Department of Laboratory Medicine, People's Hospital of Guangxi Zhuang Autonomous Region, Nanning 530021, China. [2]Department of Laboratory Medicine, Beijing Tsinghua Chang Gung Hospital, Tsinghua University, Beijing 102218, China. [3]BGI Tianjin, Tianjin 300308, China. [4]Department of Laboratory Medicine, Civil Aviation General Hospital, Peking University Civil Aviation School of Clinical Medicine, No1. Gaojing Street, Chaoyang District, Beijing 100123, China.

References

1. Collins MD, Lund BM, JAE F, Schleifer KH. Chemotaxonomic study of an alkalophilic bacterium, Exiguobacterium aurantiacum gen. Nov., sp. nov. J Gen Microbiol. 1983;129:2037–42.
2. Cheng A, Liu C-Y, Tsai H-Y, Hsu M-S, Yang C-J, Huang Y-T, Liao C-H, Hsueh P-R. Bacteremia caused by Pantoea agglomerans at a medical center in Taiwan, 2000–2010. J Microbiol Immunol Infect. 2013;46(3):187–94.
3. Keynan Y, Weber G, Sprecher H. Molecular identification of Exiguobacterium acetylicum as the aetiological agent of bacteraemia. J Med Microbiol. 2007; 56(4):563–4.
4. Tena DMN, Casanova J, García JL, Román E, Medina MJ, Sáez-Nieto JA. Possible Exiguobacterium sibiricum skin infection in human. Emerg Infect Dis. 2014;20(12):2178–9.
5. Kenny FXJ, Millar BC, McClurg RB, Moore JE. Potential misidentification of a new Exiguobacterium sp. as Oerskovia xanthineolytica isolated from blood culture. Br J Biomed Sci. 2006;63(2):86.
6. Pitt TL, Malnick H, Shah J, Chattaway MA, Keys CJ, Cooke FJ, Shah HN. Characterisation of Exiguobacterium aurantiacum isolates from blood cultures of six patients. Clin Microbiol Infect. 2007;13(9):946–8.
7. Tamar Burg-Golani YP, Rabinovich L, Sigal N, Paz RN, Herskovitsa AA. Membrane chaperone SecDF plays a role in the secretion of listeria monocytogenes major virulence factors. J Bacteriol. 2013;195(23):5262–72.
8. Vishnivetskaya TAKS, Tiedje JM. The Exiguobacterium genus: biodiversity and biogeography. Extremophiles : life under extreme conditions. 2009; 13(3):541–55.
9. Vishnivetskaya TA, Lucas S, Copeland A, Lapidus A, Glavina del Rio T, Dalin E, Tice H, Bruce DC, Goodwin LA, Pitluck S, et al. Complete genome sequence of the thermophilic bacterium Exiguobacterium sp. AT1b. J Bacteriol. 2011; 193(11):2880–1.
10. Desvaux M, Hebraud M, Talon R, Henderson IR. Secretion and subcellular localizations of bacterial proteins: a semantic awareness issue. Trends Microbiol. 2009;17(4):139–45.
11. Fagan RP, Fairweather NF. Clostridium Difficile has two parallel and essential sec secretion systems. J Biol Chem. 2011;286(31):27483–93.
12. Goosens VJ, Monteferrante CG, van Dijl JM. The tat system of gram-positive bacteria. Biochim Biophys Acta. 2014;1843(8):1698–706.
13. Inamine GS, Dubnau D. ComEA, a Bacillus Subtilis integral membrane protein required for genetic transformation, is needed for both DNA binding and transport. J Bacteriol. 1995;177(11):3045–51.
14. Muschiol S, Balaban M, Normark S, Henriques-Normark B. Uptake of extracellular DNA: competence induced pili in natural transformation of Streptococcus Pneumoniae. BioEssays. 2015;37(4):426–35.
15. Carvalho E, Barbosa AS, Gomez RM, Cianciarullo AM, Hauk P, Abreu PA, Fiorini LC, Oliveira ML, Romero EC, Goncales AP, et al. Leptospiral TlyC is an extracellular matrix-binding protein and does not present hemolysin activity. FEBS Lett. 2009;583(8):1381–5.
16. Perchat S, Talagas A, Poncet S, Lazar N, Li de la Sierra-Gallay I, Gohar M, Lereclus D, Nessler S. How quorum sensing connects sporulation to Necrotrophism in bacillus thuringiensis. PLoS Pathog. 2016;12(8):e1005779.
17. Choi Y, Kim S, Hwang H, Kim KP, Kang DH, Ryu S. Plasmid-encoded MCP is involved in virulence, motility, and biofilm formation of Cronobacter sakazakii ATCC 29544. Infect Immun. 2015;83(1):197–204.
18. Aya Castaneda Mdel R, Sarnacki SH, Noto Llana M, Lopez Guerra AG, Giacomodonato MN, Cerquetti MC. Dam methylation is required for efficient biofilm production in Salmonella enterica serovar Enteritidis. Int J Food Microbiol. 2015;193:15–22.
19. Fang CT, Yi WC, Shun CT, Tsai SF. DNA adenine methylation modulates pathogenicity of Klebsiella pneumoniae genotype K1. J Microbiol Immunol Infect. 2015. doi:10.1016/j.jmii.2015.08.022.
20. Voros A, Simm R, Slamti L, McKay MJ, Hegna IK, Nielsen-LeRoux C, Hassan KA, Paulsen IT, Lereclus D, Okstad OA, et al. SecDF as part of the sec-translocase facilitates efficient secretion of Bacillus Cereus toxins and cell wall-associated proteins. PLoS One. 2014;9(8):e103326.

15

Measuring (1,3)-β-D-glucan in tracheal aspirate, bronchoalveolar lavage fluid, and serum for detection of suspected *Candida* pneumonia in immunocompromised and critically ill patients

Kang-Cheng Su[1,2,3], Kun-Ta Chou[1,2], Yi-Han Hsiao[1,3], Ching-Min Tseng[3,4], Vincent Yi-Fong Su[1], Yu-Chin Lee[5], Diahn-Warng Perng[1,6*†] and Yu Ru Kou[3*†]

Abstract

Background: While *Candida* pneumonia is life-threatening, biomarker measurements to early detect suspected *Candida* pneumonia are lacking. This study compared the diagnostic values of measuring levels of (1, 3)-β-D-glucan in endotracheal aspirate, bronchoalveolar lavage fluid, and serum to detect suspected *Candida* pneumonia in immunocompromised and critically ill patients.

Methods: This prospective, observational study enrolled immunocompromised, critically ill, and ventilated patients with suspected fungal pneumonia in mixed intensive care units from November 2010 to October 2011. Patients with D-glucan confounding factors or other fungal infection were excluded. Endotracheal aspirate, bronchoalveolar lavage fluid and serum were collected from each patient to perform a fungal smear, culture, and D-glucan assay.

Results: After screening 166 patients, 31 patients completed the study and were categorized into non-*Candida* pneumonia/non-candidemia (*n* = 18), suspected *Candida* pneumonia (*n* = 9), and non-*Candida* pneumonia/candidemia groups (*n* = 4). D-glucan levels in endotracheal aspirate or bronchoalveolar lavage were highest in suspected *Candida* pneumonia, while the serum D-glucan level was highest in non-*Candida* pneumonia/candidemia. In all patients, the D-glucan value in endotracheal aspirate was positively correlated with that in bronchoalveolar lavage fluid. For the detection of suspected *Candida* pneumonia, the predictive performance (sensitivity/specificity/D-glucan cutoff [pg/ml]) of D-glucan in endotracheal aspirate and bronchoalveolar lavage fluid was 67%/82%/120 and 89%/86%/130, respectively, accounting for areas under the receiver operating characteristic curve of 0.833 and 0.939 (both $P < 0.05$), respectively. Measuring serum D-glucan was of no diagnostic value (area under curve $=0.510$, $P = 0.931$) for the detection of suspected *Candida* pneumonia in the absence of concurrent candidemia.

(Continued on next page)

* Correspondence: dwperng@vghtpe.gov.tw; yrkou@ym.edu.tw
†Equal contributors
[1]Department of Chest Medicine, Taipei Veterans General Hospital, No.201, Sec. 2, Shipai Rd., Beitou Dist., Taipei City 11217, Taiwan, Republic of China
[3]Institute of Physiology, School of Medicine, National Yang-Ming University, No.155, Sec.2, Linong St., Beitou Dist., Taipei City 11221, Taiwan, Republic of China

(Continued from previous page)

Conclusions: D-glucan levels in both endotracheal aspirate and bronchoalveolar lavage, but not in serum, provide good diagnostic values to detect suspected *Candida* pneumonia and to serve as potential biomarkers for early detection in this patient population.

Keywords: (1,3)-β-D-glucan, Bronchoalveolar lavage, *Candida* pneumonia, Critically ill patients, Diagnosis, Intensive care unit

Background

Candida pneumonia (CP) is life-threatening and has been associated with a high attributable mortality [1]. However, the definitive diagnosis is rarely established before overwhelming sepsis or death. Conventionally, a lung biopsy has been proposed to confirm CP [2, 3], but the procedure is too risky for patients in intensive care units (ICUs) because of the high prevalence of thrombocytopenia and coagulopathy [4]. Growth of respiratory *Candida* spp. in immunocompromised, cancer-afflicted, and critically ill patients is frequently found, but it is usually considered colonization rather than CP [5]. Indeed, growth of respiratory *Candida* spp. lacks specificity to diagnose CP [6–9], and adds little value to optimizing CP management [10, 11]. Recently, growing evidence has challenged the dogma that respiratory *Candida* spp. acts as a bystander in ICU patients [12]. The presence of respiratory *Candida* spp. has been shown to be associated with increased bacterial pneumonia development [13–16], selection of multidrug-resistant bacteria [17], and worse ICU outcomes [14, 18–20]. Accordingly, measurements of biomarkers with diagnostic value for the early detection of suspected CP are urgently needed.

Measurements of serum (1,3)-β-D-glucan (BDG), the common fungal wall antigen, can now be accomplished within hours. Measuring serum BDG has emerged as a rapid assessment to facilitate the diagnosis of invasive fungal infection, and it has proven to provide indirect mycological evidence for invasive fungal infection by a task force consensus [3]. A recent meta-analysis of 2979 patients included from 16 studies showed that using serum BDG levels to diagnose invasive fungal infection could attain a pooled sensitivity and specificity of 76.8 and 85.3%, respectively, and an area under the receiver operating characteristic curve (AUROC) of 0.89 [20]. However, none of these studies focused on respiratory *Candida* spp. infection. Additionally, it is conceivable that measuring BDG levels in respiratory specimens might be more accurate and specific for the diagnosis of pulmonary infection compared to measuring BDG levels in serum. Thus, the diagnostic value of measuring BDG levels in serum or respiratory specimens to detect suspected CP remains unclear.

In this study, we conducted a prospective, observational study aiming to compare the diagnostic value of measuring BDG levels in endotracheal aspirate (TA), bronchoalveolar lavage (BAL) fluid, and serum for the detection of suspected CP in immunocompromised and critically ill patients.

Methods

Study design

This prospective, observational study was conducted at medical and surgical ICUs in a medical center, Taipei Veterans General Hospital, in Taiwan, from November 2010 to October 2011. Eligible patients were recruited, and specimens of TA, BAL (see Additional file 1 for detail methods), and serum were collected from each individual patient on the enrollment day. BAL with or without transbronchial lung biopsy (TBLB) was a routine procedure at the discretion of the treating physicians in patients with unrecognized pulmonary lesions in our ICU. All the specimens were submitted to a bacterial culture, a fungal smear and culture, and a BDG assay. Fungal stain was applied routinely to inspect fungal structures microscopically. This study was approved by the institutional review board of Taipei Veterans General Hospital (IRB approval ID: 201011002IA) and signed informed consents were obtained from all participants.

Patients

Adult, mechanically ventilated ICU patients with suspected fungal pneumonia were recruited if they met all of the following conditions: presence of appropriate host factors defined by the task force consensus (see Additional file 1 for details about host factors) [3], non-responding or progressive pulmonary lesions despite management with broad-spectrum antibiotics for 48 to 72 h, and signature on an inform consent form. Patients were excluded if they withdrew consent, lacked respiratory specimens, had established diagnoses other than CP, or presented with factors that might confound the BDG assay (Fig. 1; see Additional file 1 for details about confounding factors) [10, 21–23]. The application of antifungal treatment depended on the treating team, which was blinded to the BDG results until ICU discharge. The final diagnosis was determined by at least 2 different ICU intensivists independently, including the primary physicians. A conference was held to determine the final diagnosis if a discrepancy existed.

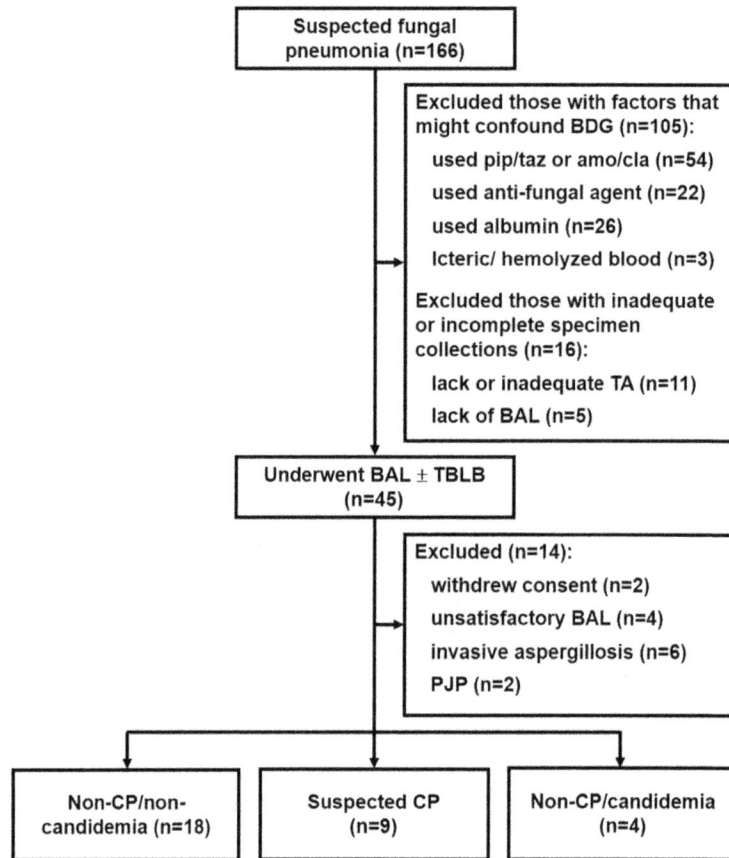

Fig. 1 Study algorithm. pip/taz = piperacillin/tazobactam; amo/cla = amoxicillin-clavulanate; TA = endotracheal aspirate; BAL = bronchoalveolar lavage fluid; TBLB = transbronchial lung biopsy; PJP = *Pneumocystis jiroveci* pneumonia

Diagnostic definitions

Suspected CP was defined if the cases met one of the 3 following conditions: 1) histopathological findings of poly-morphonuclear leukocytes infiltration in lung, while the presence of hyphae and/or pseudohyphae in the bronchial lumen with or without peribronchial tissue invasion in TBLB specimens; 2) TA and/or BAL cultural yield of *Candida* spp. with successful antifungal treatment, which was indicated by improvement in attributable symptoms and signs, radiographic resolution of chest images, and clear-ance of *Candida* spp. in repeated specimens of TA (at least 2 times per week) or BAL (at the discretion of pri-mary treating team); 3) TA and/or BAL-positive *Candida* spp. with antifungal treatment failure, which was charac-terized by persistent growth of *Candida* spp. in repeated TA or BAL specimens in conjunction with a lack of clin-ical and radiographic regression. For the later 2 condi-tions, there were no other reasonably causative factors (such as superinfection of viral or bacterial microorgan-isms) and the treatment response was modified from the guideline [24] recommended for invasive candidiasis other than CP. Non-CP indicated alternative diagnoses other than suspected CP, which included bacterial pneumonia,

viral pneumonitis, pulmonary edema or a combination of these diseases, and all of these cases were discontinued from antifungal treatment within 7 days. Candidemia was defined if the blood culture was positive for *Candida* spp. growth. Based on these definitions, the final diagnoses were categorized into 3 groups: non-CP/non-candidemia, suspected CP, and non-CP/candidemia.

Management of BDG assay

All the specimens for the BDG assay were collected and processed within 2 h of collection, followed by frozen storage at −70 °C until testing. The BDG assay was per-formed (see Additional file 1 for details about methods) using a Glucatell kit (Associates of Cape Cod, Inc., Falmouth, MA, USA) according to the manufacturer's instructions. The results of the BDG assays were not used to categorize the final diagnosis.

Statistical analysis

Data are presented as the mean ± SD, the median with inter-quartile range or a number (%), as appropriate. Continuous variables were evaluated using the Kruskal-Wallis test followed by the Mann-Whitney U test for pairwise comparisons. Categorical data were evaluated using the Chi-square or Fisher's exact test. The association between two variables was evaluated using a Pearson's correlation analysis. Analyses of ROC curves were performed to assess the predictive performance of BDG for suspected CP or candidemia in different specimens. The sensitivity, specificity, positive predictive value (PPV), and negative predictive value (NPV) of BDG levels for suspected CP were also calculated, and the best cutoff values were determined. P values <0.05 were considered significant for all tests.

Results

Patient characteristics

After enrolling 166 consecutive patients with suspected fungal pneumonia, 31 patients completed the study. The final diagnoses were categorized as non-CP/non-candidemia (n = 18, 58.1%), suspected CP (n = 9, 29.0%), or non-CP/candidemia (n = 4, 12.9%) (Fig. 1). In suspected CP group, there were 4 patients with yeast in TBLB (including one with yeast invasion in peribronchial tissue, Fig. 2) and 5 patients judged by clinical response (3 failure and 2 success). Most of the patients' characteristics were similar among the study groups (Table 1). The ICU mortality rate was 45.2% in total, but it did not significantly differ among the study group (Table 1). There were no independent factors to predict ICU mortality (please see Additional file 1: Table S1). However, all suspected CP cases demonstrated yeast evidence based on TBLB histopathology and/or BAL fungal staining, and

they also had significantly higher *Candida* culture rates in BAL (Table 1). Details about the cultural results for the *Candida* spp. are shown in Additional file 1. All the patients were treated with empirical antifungal agents initially after specimen collection due to concern about immunocompromised status and high severity scores.

BDG levels among the study groups with different diagnoses

The mean BDG level in TA (136.6 ± 37.1 pg/ml) was significant higher in patients with suspected CP than in those in non-CP/non-candidemia (85.7 ± 45.1 pg/ml, P = 0.022) and non-CP/candidemia (60.4 ± 46.6 pg/ml, P = 0.020) (Fig. 3a). The mean BDG level in BAL was also significantly higher in patients with suspected CP (217.5 ± 93.4 pg/ml) than those in the non-CP/non-candidemia (68.8 ± 46.5 pg/ml, P < 0.001) and non-CP/candidemia (77.1 ± 52.2 pg/ml, P = 0.003) groups (Fig. 3b). Conversely, the mean BDG level in serum in the non-CP/candidemia group (221.1 ± 96.0 pg/ml) was significantly higher than that in the non-CP/non-candidemia group (20.1 ± 7.5 pg/ml, P < 0.001) or the suspected CP group (22.7 ± 4.5 pg/ml, P < 0.001) (Fig. 3c).

BDG level and Candida culture results

In all the patients, the BDG level was significantly higher in specimens with growth of *Candida* spp. than in those with a negative yield in each of the 3 types of specimens (126.2 ± 34.8 vs. 73.3 ± 47.9 pg/ml, P = 0.004 in TA; 191.0 ± 92.1 vs. 56.7 ± 30.2 pg/ml, P < 0.001 in BAL;

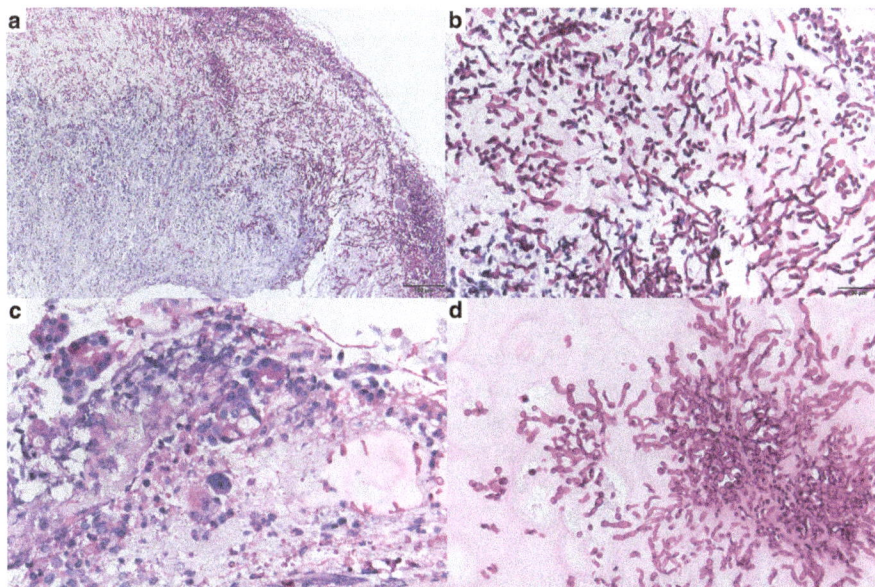

Fig. 2 Histological findings of transbronchial lung biopsy with Periodic Acid-Schiff stain. A representative section of necrotic tissue admixed with inflammatory exudate showed infiltrations of acute inflammatory cells and fungus colonies in low magnification (**a**, 100X) as well as budding yeast and hyphae/pseudohyphae appearance in high magnification (**b**, 400X). Sections of peribronchial tissue disclosed epithelial sloughing with yeast invasion in bronchial mucosa (**c**, 400X) and bronchial cartilage (**d**, 400X)

Table 1 Patients' characteristics

	All	Non-CP/non- candidemia	Suspected CP	Non-CP/ candidemia	P
Number	31	18	9	4	
Age, year	66.4 ± 16.6	65.3 ± 18.5	66.9 ± 16.5	70.3 ± 6.2	0.971[a]
Sex, male (%)	20 (64.5)	11 (61.1)	6 (66.7)	3 (75.0)	0.860[b]
APACHE II at ICU admission	22.4 ± 5.2	22.3 ± 5.2	21.1 ± 4.2	25.3 ± 6.9	0.583[a]
APACHE II on enrolled day	24.2 ± 4.8	23.2 ± 5.0	25.1 ± 3.9	27.0 ± 5.3	0.316[a]
Initial reasons for MV (%)					
Post-surgery	7 (22.6%)	3 (16.7)	2 (22.2)	2 (50.0)	0.353[b]
Pneumonia	24 (77.4%)	15 (83.3)	7 (77.8)	2 (50.0)	0.353[b]
Reasons for BAL (%)					
Non-responding pneumonia	18 (58.1)	9 (50.0)	7 (77.8)	2 (50)	0.363[b]
Newly developed infiltration	13 (41.9)	9 (50.0)	2 (22.2)	2 (50)	0.363[b]
Host factors (%)					
Recent neutropenia	10 (32.3)	5 (27.8)	2 (22.2)	3 (75.0)	0.141[b]
Prolonged steroid use	16 (51.6)	10 (55.6)	5 (55.6)	1 (25.0)	0.521[b]
Immunosuppressants	5 (16.1)	3 (16.7)	2 (22.2)	0	0.600[b]
MV days	24.2 ± 12.5	23.7 ± 14.9	22.9 ± 9.4	29.3 ± 5.7	0.129[a]
ICU stay, days	27.8 ± 11.9	28.0 ± 14.4	26.6 ± 9.2	30.0 ± 4.3	0.494[a]
ICU mortality (%)	14 (45.2)	6 (33.3)	5 (55.6)	3 (75.0)	0.241[b]
Radiographic manifestations[c] (%)					
Halo sign	1 (3.2)	0	1 (11.1)	0	0.283[b]
Single/multiple nodules	11 (35.5)	3 (16.7)	7 (77.8)	1 (25.0)	0.007[b]
Cavitary lesion	6 (19.4)	3 (16.7)	3 (33.3)	0	0.338[b]
GGO/infiltration	29 (93.5)	17 (94.4)	8 (88.9)	4 (100)	0.732[b]
Mycological evidence of yeast (%)					
TBLB[d,e]	4 (12.9)	0	4 (44.5)	0	< 0.001[b]
BAL[e]	13 (41.9)	4 (22.2)	8 (88.9)	1 (25.0)	0.003[b]
TA fungal culture	14 (45.2)	7 (38.9)	6 (66.7)	1 (25.0)	0.269[b]
BAL fungal culture	13 (41.9)	5 (27.8)	8 (88.9)	0	0.002[b]

Data are presented with means ± standard deviations

CP Candida pneumonia, APACHE acute physiology and chronic health evaluation, MV mechanical ventilation, BAL bronchoalveolar lavage, GGO ground glass opacity, TBLB transbronchial lung biopsy, TA endotracheal aspirate, BAL bronchoalveolar lavage fluid

[a]Kruskal-Wallis test

[b]Fisher's exact test

[c]Each single patient could have more than one type of radiographic manifestation

[d]A total of 19 patients underwent TBLB, including 11 in non-CP/non-candidemia, 7 in suspected CP, and 1 in non-CP/candidemia

[e]Fungal staining was applied using Grocott-Gomori methenamine silver stain in BAL and Periodic Acid-Schiff stain in TBLB

221.1 ± 96.0 vs. 21.0 ± 6.7 pg/ml, $P = 0.001$ in serum) (Fig. 4a). Additionally, the value of TA BDG was positively correlated with that of BAL BDG ($P = 0.002$, $r = 0.542$) (Fig. 4b). However, the value of neither TA BDG ($P = 0.598$; $r = 0.098$) nor BAL BDG ($P = 0.836$; $r = 0.039$) was significantly correlated with that of serum BDG.

Diagnostic value of BDG in detecting suspected CP

For the detection of suspected CP, measuring BDG levels in both TA and BAL, but not the serum BDG level, could have good diagnostic value. The results from the ROC analysis revealed that BDG levels in TA and BAL had

AUROC values of 0.833 and 0.939, respectively (Fig. 5). Given a cutoff BDG level of 120 pg/ml in TA and 130 pg/ml in BAL, the best diagnostic value could be achieved with sensitivity/specificity of 67%/82% for TA and 89%/86% for BAL (Table 2). The serum BDG level exerted excellent predictive performance for the detection of candidemia (AUROC =0.996, $P = 0.001$) but poor predictive performance for the detection of suspected CP (AUROC =0.510, $P = 0.931$, Fig. 5). In addition, measuring the BDG level in TA (AUROC =0.259, $P = 0.126$) or BAL (AUROC =0.389, $P = 0.480$) for the detection of candidemia was of no diagnostic value.

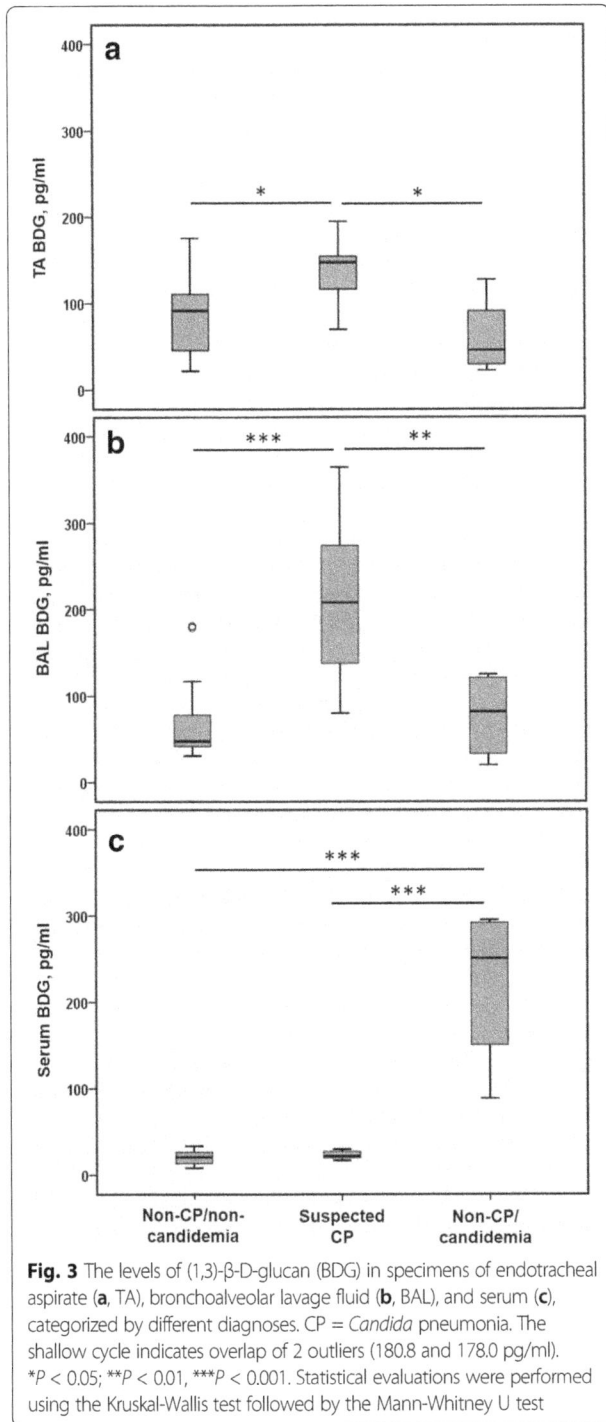

Fig. 3 The levels of (1,3)-β-D-glucan (BDG) in specimens of endotracheal aspirate (**a**, TA), bronchoalveolar lavage fluid (**b**, BAL), and serum (**c**), categorized by different diagnoses. CP = *Candida* pneumonia. The shallow cycle indicates overlap of 2 outliers (180.8 and 178.0 pg/ml). *$P < 0.05$; **$P < 0.01$, ***$P < 0.001$. Statistical evaluations were performed using the Kruskal-Wallis test followed by the Mann-Whitney U test

Discussion

To our knowledge, the present study was the first to compare the diagnostic value of measuring BDG levels in TA, BAL, and serum for the detection of suspected CP in immunocompromised and critically ill patients. The major findings were that measuring BDG levels in respiratory specimens, including both TA and BAL fluid, exerted good diagnostic value for the detection of suspected CP,

particularly in the absence of concurrent candidemia. In contrast, measuring the serum BDG level had no diagnostic value for this detection.

There are limited data regarding measuring BAL BDG levels to diagnose fungal pneumonia. The performance of BAL BDG at different cutoff value to diagnose non-*Candida* fungal pneumonia varied widely, in terms of sensitivity (53-90%) and specificity (26-88%) in different patient populations [25–28]. Among these, the largest study (268 BALs) reported by Prattes et al., who compared BAL galactomannan and BDG to diagnose proven/probable invasive pulmonary aspergillosis. They concluded that despite similar sensitivity (> 90%) and NPV (> 90%) between galactomannan and BDG, BAL BDG was less convincing due to low specificity (< 50%). This might be ascribed to frequent respiratory colonization of *Candida* spp. [28], which potentially limited the diagnostic performance of BAL BDG for non-*Candida* fungal pneumonia. In contrast, we excluded most of the possible confounding factors and focused on *Candida* pathogens. Thus, our data showed good performance (both sensitivity and specificity >85%) by means of measuring BAL BDG. Moreover, consistent with the observation reported by Reischies et al. [29], our data also showed that *Candida* culture-positive specimens had higher BDG levels (Fig. 4a), which implicates that BDG levels reflect fungal burdens indirectly. Patients with higher fungal burdens are more susceptible to fungal infection. This potentially provide the rationale to measure respiratory BDG levels as good diagnostic aid to detect suspected CP.

We further showed that the TA BDG level was positively correlated with BAL BDG (Fig. 4b). Despite with inferior value to BAL BDG, measuring TA BDG also offered good diagnostic performance for the detection of suspected CP (Fig. 5). Thus, measuring TA BDG could serve as a simple, less-invasive, alternative diagnostic for suspected CP when BAL is unavailable. Previously, most cases of CP were considered to indicate lung involvement of disseminated candidiasis rather than primary CP [1, 5]. Based on this belief, patients with CP are supposed to have as high of a serum BDG level as those with candidemia. However, our data did not correspond to this notion. Patients with suspected CP had apparently low BDG in serum (vs. those with non-CP/candidemia) and high BDG in TA and BAL (Fig. 3). These findings suggested that serum BDG might have no diagnostic value in patients with suspected CP in the absence of concurrent candidemia. Thus, we suggest clinicians should directly measure BDG in respiratory specimens in patients with suspicion of CP.

To date, there have been no universally acceptable criteria to diagnose CP, and most diagnoses have depended on lung biopsies. CP is considered uncommon based on earlier lung autopsy reports [1, 6, 8], so the clinical practice guideline does not recommend using antifungal treatment based upon the *Candida* culture alone [3, 5, 30].

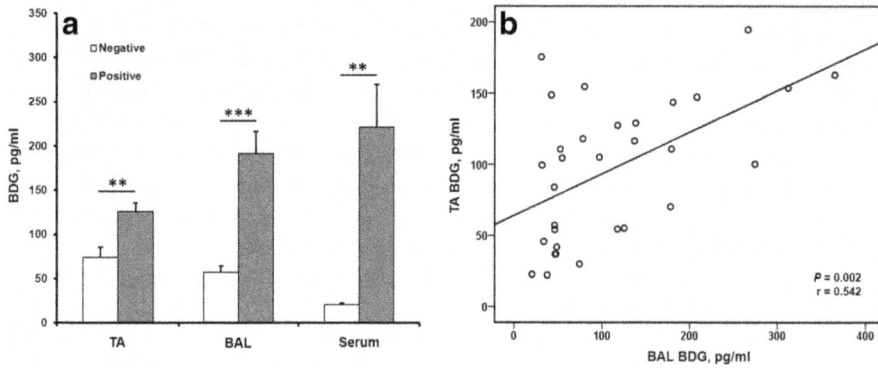

Fig. 4 a BDG levels categorized by fungal cultural results in different types of specimens. **$P < 0.01$, ***$P < 0.001$. TA = endotracheal aspirate; BAL = bronchoalveolar lavage fluid. **b** Binary correlation of values of TA BDG and BAL BDG. r = correlation coefficient. Statistical evaluations were performed using the Mann-Whitney U test in A and using Pearson's correlation coefficient in **b**

However, CP might possibly be under-diagnosed in critically ill patients because a lung biopsy is rarely performed. Indeed, even for immunocompetent ICU patients with *Candida*-positive respiratory specimens, 24.2% of physicians recommended antifungal treatment in an early questionnaire surveillance regarding CP [31] and 32.9% did so in a recent prospective study concerning ICU-acquired pneumonia [32]. These reports reflected the dissociation of managements between the guideline [3, 5, 30] and real-life ICU situations remain an unresolved issue. It is logically speculated that antifungal treatment are more frequently used for immunocompromised and critically ill ICU patients, particularly while these patients were undergoing non-responding or progressive pneumonia with the

presence of respiratory *Candida* spp. and the absence of the other causative pathogens after thorough work-ups. Thus, applying antifungal treatment response in these situations might be reasonably therapeutic diagnostics for suspected CP and could compensate the gap between the

Table 2 Predictive performance of various BDG levels for diagnosing candidemia and suspected CP in different specimens

Cutoff value	Sensitivity	Specificity	PPV	NPV
Candidemia				
Serum BDG, pg/ml				
70	100%	100%	100%	100%
80	100%	100%	100%	100%
90	75%	100%	100%	96%
Suspected CP				
TA BDG, pg/ml[a]				
90	89%	55%	44%	92%
100	89%	59%	47%	93%
110	78%	68%	50%	88%
120	67%	82%	60%	86%
130	0%	70%	0%	83%
BAL BDG, pg/ml				
110	89%	73%	57%	94%
120	89%	77%	62%	94%
130	89%	86%	73%	95%
140	89%	91%	80%	95%
150	67%	91%	75%	95%
Serum BDG, pg/ml				
20	67%	41%	32%	75%
25	33%	59%	25%	68%
30	0%	73%	0%	64%

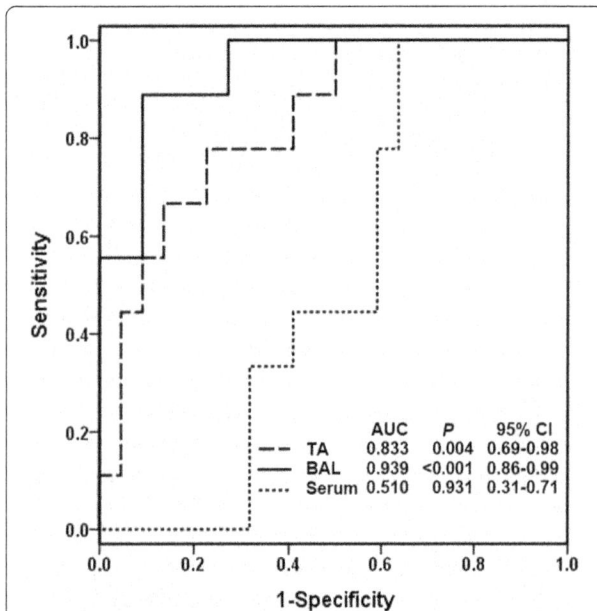

Fig. 5 The receiver operating characteristic curve of BDG levels in different types of specimens for the diagnosis of suspected *Candida* pneumonia (CP). TA = endotracheal aspirate; BAL = bronchoalveolar lavage fluid; AUC = area under the curve; CI = conference interval

PPV positive predictive value, *NPV* negative predictive value, *BDG* β-D-glucan
Refer to Table 1 for other abbreviations
[a]Adjusted to per gram of endotracheal aspirate

guideline and clinical scenario. Accordingly, more practical diagnostic criteria for detecting suspected CP are urgently needed. Our findings showed measuring respiratory BDG levels might provide valuable information to enhance these diagnostic criteria.

There were some limitations of our study. First, our data were derived from selected patients to minimize confounding factors. Particularly, we excluded many patients with concurrent use of antibiotics. The concern that if concurrent use of antibiotics possibly confounded BDG assay remains a conflicting issue [33–40]. It needs a large-scale study to validate this issue. Second, the sample size of this study was small, and future investigations with larger sample sizes will be needed to optimize the best TA or BAL BDG cutoff values. Third, our results were derived from the study of *Candida* spp.; the application of measuring BDG levels in other fungal pathogens requires further validation.

Conclusions

This study is not intended to replace lung biopsy for the diagnosis of CP, but try to use less invasive biomarker to detect suspected CP. Our results clearly showed that the BDG level in BAL or TA provided a good diagnostic value to detect suspected CP. Additionally, measuring serum BDG had no diagnostic value for detecting suspected CP in the absence of concurrent candidemia. These findings warrant a future large-scale investigation to validate the optimal cutoff value for BDG in respiratory specimens and to determine the timing to initiate antifungal treatment.

Abbreviations

AUROC: Area under the receiver operating characteristic curve; BAL: Bronchoalveolar lavage; BDG: (1,3)-β-D-glucan; CP: *Candida* pneumonia; ICU: Intensive care unit; NPV: Negative predictive value; PPV: Positive predictive value; TA: Endotracheal aspirate; TBLB: Transbronchial lung biopsy

Acknowledgements

We appreciated the great assistance of Dr. Yi-Chen, from Department of Pathology and Laboratory Medicine in Taipei Veterans General Hospital, for the preparation of histopathological findings of lung biopsy. We thank all the study participants and the Division of Experimental Surgery of the Department of Surgery for their assistance in part of laboratory work.

Funding

This study was supported by a grant V100B-032 from Taipei Veterans General Hospital, Taipei, Taiwan, and in part by grants MOST 104-2320-B-010-014-MY3, NSC 98-2628-B-320-003-MY3, and MOST 105-2314-B-075-034 from the Ministry of Science and Technology, Taiwan.

Authors' contributions

YRK and DWP had full access to all the data in the study and takes responsibility for the integrity of the data and the accuracy of the data analysis. KCS, DWP, YRK, and YCL contributed to concept generation and study design. KTC, YHH, CMT and VYS contributed to data acquisition, analysis, and the first draft. KCS contributed to grant application, data interpretation, and manuscript revision. YRK and DWP revised the manuscript critically for important intellectual content. All authors read and approved the final manuscript.

Competing interests

The authors declare that they have no competing interests.

Consent for publication

Not applicable.

Author details

[1]Department of Chest Medicine, Taipei Veterans General Hospital, No.201, Sec. 2, Shipai Rd., Beitou Dist., Taipei City 11217, Taiwan, Republic of China. [2]Center of Sleep Medicine, Taipei Veterans General Hospital, No.201, Sec. 2, Shipai Rd., Beitou Dist., Taipei City 11217, Taiwan, Republic of China. [3]Institute of Physiology, School of Medicine, National Yang-Ming University, No.155, Sec.2, Linong St., Beitou Dist., Taipei City 11221, Taiwan, Republic of China. [4]Division of Thoracic Medicine, Department of Medicine, Cheng Hsin General Hospital, No.45, Cheng Hsin St., Beitou Dist., Taipei City 11220, Taiwan, Republic of China. [5]Sijhih Cathay General Hospital, No.2, Ln. 59, Jiancheng Rd., Xizhi Dist., New Taipei City 22174, Taiwan, Republic of China. [6]School of Medicine, National Yang-Ming University, No.155, Sec.2, Linong St., Beitou Dist., Taipei City 11221, Taiwan, Republic of China.

References

1. Haron E, Vartivarian S, Anaissie E, Dekmezian R, Bodey GP. Primary Candida pneumonia. Experience at a large cancer center and review of the literature. Medicine (Baltimore). 1993;72:137–42.
2. Ascioglu S, Rex JH, de Pauw B, Bennett JE, Bille J, Crokaert F, et al. Defining opportunistic invasive fungal infections in immunocompromised patients with cancer and hematopoietic stem cell transplants: an international consensus. Clin Infect Dis. 2002;34:7–14.
3. De Pauw B, Walsh TJ, Donnelly JP, Stevens DA, Edwards JE, Calandra T, et al. Revised definitions of invasive fungal disease from the European Organization for Research and Treatment of cancer/invasive fungal infections cooperative group and the National Institute of Allergy and Infectious Diseases mycoses study group (EORTC/MSG) consensus group. Clin Infect Dis. 2008;46:1813–21.
4. Levi M, Opal SM. Coagulation abnormalities in critically ill patients. Crit Care. 2006;10:222.
5. Pappas PG, Kauffman CA, Andes D, Benjamin Jr DK, Calandra TF, Edwards Jr JE, et al. Clinical practice guidelines for the management of candidiasis: 2009 update by the Infectious Diseases Society of America. Clin Infect Dis. 2009;48:503–35.
6. Kontoyiannis DP, Reddy BT, Torres HA, Luna M, Lewis RE, Tarrand J, et al. Pulmonary candidiasis in patients with cancer: an autopsy study. Clin Infect Dis. 2002;34:400–3.
7. Rello J, Esandi ME, Diaz E, Mariscal D, Gallego M, Valles J. The role of Candida sp isolated from bronchoscopic samples in nonneutropenic patients. Chest. 1998;114:146–9.
8. el-Ebiary M, Torres A, Fabregas N, de la Bellacasa JP, Gonzalez J, Ramirez J, et al. Significance of the isolation of Candida species from respiratory samples in critically ill, non-neutropenic patients. An immediate postmortem histologic study. Am J Respir Crit Care Med. 1997;156:583–90.
9. Wood GC, Mueller EW, Croce MA, Boucher BA, Fabian TC. Candida sp. isolated from bronchoalveolar lavage: clinical significance in critically ill trauma patients. Intensive Care Med. 2006;32:599–603.
10. Ostrosky-Zeichner L. Invasive mycoses: diagnostic challenges. Am J Med. 2012;125:S14–24.
11. Albert M, Williamson D, Muscedere J, Lauzier F, Rotstein C, Kanji S, et al. Candida in the respiratory tract secretions of critically ill patients and the impact of antifungal treatment: a randomized placebo controlled pilot trial (CANTREAT study). Intensive Care Med. 2014;40:1313–22.
12. Ricard JD, Roux D. Candida colonization in ventilated ICU patients: no longer a bystander! Intensive Care Med. 2012;38:1243–5.
13. Ricard JD, Roux D. Candida pneumonia in the ICU: myth or reality? Intensive Care Med. 2009;35:1500–2.

14. Azoulay E, Timsit JF, Tafflet M, de Lassence A, Darmon M, Zahar JR, et al. Candida colonization of the respiratory tract and subsequent pseudomonas ventilator-associated pneumonia. Chest. 2006;129:110–7.

15. Nseir S, Jozefowicz E, Cavestri B, Sendid B, Di Pompeo C, Dewavrin F, et al. Impact of antifungal treatment on Candida-pseudomonas interaction: a preliminary retrospective case-control study. Intensive Care Med. 2007;33:137–42.

16. Tan X, Zhu S, Yan D, Chen W, Chen R, Zou J, et al. Candida spp. airway colonization: a potential risk factor for Acinetobacter baumannii ventilator-associated pneumonia. Med Mycol. 2016;54:557–66.

17. Hamet M, Pavon A, Dalle F, Pechinot A, Prin S, Quenot JP, et al. Candida spp. airway colonization could promote antibiotic-resistant bacteria selection in patients with suspected ventilator-associated pneumonia. Intensive Care Med. 2012;38:1272–9.

18. Delisle MS, Williamson DR, Perreault MM, Albert M, Jiang X, Heyland DK. The clinical significance of Candida colonization of respiratory tract secretions in critically ill patients. J Crit Care. 2008;23:11–7.

19. Delisle MS, Williamson DR, Albert M, Perreault MM, Jiang X, Day AG, et al. Impact of Candida species on clinical outcomes in patients with suspected ventilator-associated pneumonia. Can Respir J. 2011;18:131–6.

20. Karageorgopoulos DE, Vouloumanou EK, Ntziora F, Michalopoulos A, Rafailidis PI, Falagas ME. beta-D-glucan assay for the diagnosis of invasive fungal infections: a meta-analysis. Clin Infect Dis. 2011;52:750–70.

21. Hsu JL, Ruoss SJ, Bower ND, Lin M, Holodniy M, Stevens DA. Diagnosing invasive fungal disease in critically ill patients. Crit Rev Microbiol. 2011;37:277–312.

22. Alexander BD, Smith PB, Davis RD, Perfect JR, Reller LB. The (1,3){beta}-D-glucan test as an aid to early diagnosis of invasive fungal infections following lung transplantation. J Clin Microbiol. 2010;48:4083–8.

23. Pickering JW, Sant HW, Bowles CA, Roberts WL, Woods GL. Evaluation of a (1->3)-beta-D-glucan assay for diagnosis of invasive fungal infections. J Clin Microbiol. 2005;43:5957–62.

24. Segal BH, Herbrecht R, Stevens DA, Ostrosky-Zeichner L, Sobel J, Viscoli C, et al. Defining responses to therapy and study outcomes in clinical trials of invasive fungal diseases: Mycoses Study Group and European Organization for Research and Treatment of Cancer consensus criteria. Clin Infect Dis. 2008;47:674–83.

25. Mutschlechner W, Risslegger B, Willinger B, Hoenigl M, Bucher B, Eschertzhuber S, et al. Bronchoalveolar Lavage fluid (1,3)beta-D-Glucan for the diagnosis of invasive fungal infections in solid organ transplantation: a prospective multicenter study. Transplantation. 2015;99:e140–4.

26. Rose SR, Vallabhajosyula S, Velez MG, Fedorko DP, VanRaden MJ, Gea-Banacloche JC, et al. The utility of bronchoalveolar lavage beta-D-glucan testing for the diagnosis of invasive fungal infections. J Inf Secur. 2014;69:278–83.

27. Hoenigl M, Prattes J, Spiess B, Wagner J, Prueller F, Raggam RB, et al. Performance of galactomannan, beta-d-glucan, Aspergillus lateral-flow device, conventional culture, and PCR tests with bronchoalveolar lavage fluid for diagnosis of invasive pulmonary aspergillosis. J Clin Microbiol. 2014;52:2039–45.

28. Prattes J, Flick H, Pruller F, Koidl C, Raggam RB, Palfner M, et al. Novel tests for diagnosis of invasive aspergillosis in patients with underlying respiratory diseases. Am J Respir Crit Care Med. 2014;190:922–9.

29. Reischies FM, Prattes J, Pruller F, Eigl S, List A, Wolfler A, et al. Prognostic potential of 1,3-beta-d-glucan levels in bronchoalveolar lavage fluid samples. J Inf Secur. 2016;72:29–35.

30. Pappas PG, Kauffman CA, Andes DR, Clancy CJ, Marr KA, Ostrosky-Zeichner L, et al. Clinical practice guideline for the Management of Candidiasis: 2016 update by the Infectious Diseases Society of America. Clin Infect Dis. 2016;62:e1–e50.

31. Azoulay E, Cohen Y, Zahar JR, Garrouste-Orgeas M, Adrie C, Moine P, et al. Practices in non-neutropenic ICU patients with Candida-positive airway specimens. Intensive Care Med. 2004;30:1384–9.

32. Terraneo S, Ferrer M, Martin-Loeches I, Esperatti M, Di Pasquale M, Giunta V, et al. Impact of Candida spp. isolation in the respiratory tract in patients with intensive care unit-acquired pneumonia. Clin Microbiol Infect. 2016; 22(94):e1–8.

33. Liss B, Cornely OA, Hoffmann D, Dimitriou V, Wisplinghoff H. 1,3-beta-d-Glucan contamination of common antimicrobials. J Antimicrob Chemoth. 2016;71:913–5.

34. Liss B, Cornely OA, Hoffmann D, Dimitriou V, Wisplinghoff H. 1,3-beta-D-Glucan contamination of common antimicrobials-authors' response. J Antimicrob Chemoth. 2016; 71:2997-2999.

35. Finkelman MA. Comment on: 1,3-beta-D-Glucan contamination of common antimicrobials. J Antimicrob Chemoth. 2016;71:2996–7.

36. Hammarstrom H, Kondori N, Friman V, Wenneras C. How to interpret serum levels of beta-glucan for the diagnosis of invasive fungal infections in adult high-risk hematology patients: optimal cut-off levels and confounding factors. Eur J Clin Microbiol. 2015;34:917–25.

37. Metan G, Agkus C, Koc AN, Elmali F, Finkelman MA. Does ampicillin-sulbactam cause false positivity of (1,3)-beta-D-glucan assay? A prospective evaluation of 15 patients without invasive fungal infections. Mycoses. 2012; 55:366–71.

38. Mennink-Kersten MA, Warris A, Verweij PE. 1,3-beta-D-glucan in patients receiving intravenous amoxicillin-clavulanic acid. N Engl J Med. 2006;354: 2834–5.

39. Metan G, Agkus C, Buldu H, Koc AN. The interaction between piperacillin/ tazobactam and assays for Aspergillus galactomannan and 1,3-beta-D-glucan in patients without risk factors for invasive fungal infections. Infection. 2010;38:217–21.

40. Marty FM, Lowry CM, Lempitski SJ, Kubiak DW, Finkelman MA, Baden LR. Reactivity of (1->3)-beta-d-glucan assay with commonly used intravenous antimicrobials. Antimicrob Agents Chemother. 2006;50:3450–3.

16

The impact of virus infections on pneumonia mortality is complex in adults

Naoko Katsurada[1,2], Motoi Suzuki[3*] (ID), Masahiro Aoshima[1], Makito Yaegashi[4], Tomoko Ishifuji[3], Norichika Asoh[5], Naohisa Hamashige[6], Masahiko Abe[7], Koya Ariyoshi[3], Konosuke Morimoto[3] and on behalf of the Adult Pneumonia Study Group-Japan

Abstract

Background: Various viruses are known to be associated with pneumonia. However, the impact of viral infections on adult pneumonia mortality remains unclear. This study aimed to clarify the effect of virus infection on pneumonia mortality among adults stratified by virus type and patient comorbidities.

Methods: This multicentre prospective study enrolled pneumonia patients aged ≥15 years from September 2011 to August 2014. Sputum samples were tested by in-house multiplex polymerase chain reaction assays to identify 13 respiratory viruses. Viral infection status and its effect on in-hospital mortality were examined by age group and comorbidity status.

Results: A total of 2617 patients were enrolled in the study and 77.8% was aged ≥65 years. 574 (21.9%) did not have comorbidities, 790 (30.2%) had chronic respiratory disease, and 1253 (47.9%) had other comorbidities. Viruses were detected in 605 (23.1%) patients. Human rhinovirus (9.8%) was the most frequently identified virus, followed by influenza A (3.9%) and respiratory syncytial virus (3.9%). Respiratory syncytial virus was more frequently identified in patients with chronic respiratory disease (4.7%) than those with other comorbidities (4.2%) and without comorbidities (2.1%) ($p = 0.037$). The frequencies of other viruses were almost identical between the three groups. Virus detection overall was not associated with increased mortality (adjusted risk ratio (ARR) 0.76, 95% CI 0.53–1.09). However, influenza virus A and B were associated with three-fold higher mortality in patients with chronic respiratory disease but not with other comorbidities (ARR 3.38, 95% CI 1.54–7.42). Intriguingly, paramyxoviruses were associated with dramatically lower mortality in patients with other comorbidities (ARR 0.10, 95% CI 0.01–0.70) but not with chronic respiratory disease. These effects were not affected by age group.

Conclusions: The impact of virus infections on pneumonia mortality varies by virus type and comorbidity status in adults.

Keywords: Pneumonia mortality, Chronic respiratory disease, Respiratory syncytial virus, Respiratory virus, Influenza, Paramyxovirus

* Correspondence: mosuzuki@nagasaki-u.ac.jp
[3]Department of Clinical Medicine, Institute of Tropical Medicine, Nagasaki University, 1-12-4 Sakamoto, Nagasaki 852-8523, Japan

Background

Pneumonia is the major cause of morbidity and mortality among adults, especially in the elderly. Management of pneumonia is a critical problem in an ageing society like Japan. *Streptococcus pneumoniae* and *Haemophilus influenzae* are the leading bacterial causes of adult pneumonia, while viruses also play important roles in disease development. Recent advances in molecular diagnostic techniques have enabled us to detect multiple viruses simultaneously [1]. Studies have shown that viral infection is common in pneumonia patients [2, 3]. According to a recent systematic review and meta-analysis, viruses were detected in 24.5% of respiratory samples from community-acquired pneumonia (CAP) patients [4].

Various viruses are known to be associated with respiratory infections, including pneumonia. According to the systematic review, influenza is the most commonly detected virus in CAP, followed by human rhinovirus (HRV), respiratory syncytial virus (RSV), and human coronavirus (HCoV) [4]. In addition to these endemic respiratory viruses, emerging respiratory viruses, such as severe acute respiratory syndrome coronavirus, Middle East respiratory syndrome coronavirus, and avian influenza, are posing a particularly serious threat to global health security [5]. Studies have suggested that these emerging viral infections are associated with an increased risk of severe conditions and mortality among pneumonia patients [5, 6]. It must be noted that pneumonia mortality varies substantially according to patient characteristics, such as comorbidities, aspiration risk factors, and physical functional status [7, 8]. To establish effective control measures, high-priority viruses and patient groups must be identified. However, the prevalence of viruses in adult pneumonia and their virus-specific effects on clinical outcome remain largely unknown. To the best of our knowledge, no large-scale study has investigated the different effects of viruses on pneumonia mortality by patient characteristics.

We conducted this prospective multicentre study to determine the distribution of viruses associated with pneumonia in adults and to establish their virus-specific effects on pneumonia mortality stratified by age group and comorbidity status.

Methods

Study design, patient enrolment, and data collection

The Adult Pneumonia Study Group-Japan (APSG-J) conducted multicentre prospective hospital-based surveillance for community-onset pneumonia at four community-based hospitals in Japan. In our previous paper, the burden and aetiology of adult pneumonia were reported based on the data and clinical samples collected during the 1st phase of the study (September 2011 to January 2013) [9]. The current study included all data and samples collected during the whole study period (September 2011 to August 2014). Details of the study settings and enrolment criteria were described previously [9]. In brief, all outpatients and inpatients were screened by hospital physicians, and eligible patients were identified using a standardized case definition: patients aged ≥15 years with respiratory symptoms compatible with pneumonia and new infiltrative shadows on chest X-rays or computed tomography scans. Clinical information was collected from patients and medical charts using a standardized data collection form.

Microbiological test

Sputum, blood, and urine samples were collected at the time of diagnosis. Gram staining, sputum culture, and blood culture were performed on site. Sputum samples were further tested by in-house multiplex polymerase chain reaction (PCR) assays to identify viral and bacterial pathogens at the Institute of Tropical Medicine, Nagasaki University. Thirteen viral pathogens (influenza A virus, influenza B virus, RSV, human metapneumovirus [hMPV], human parainfluenza virus [HPIV] type 1–4, HRV, HCoV 229E/OC43, human adenovirus [HAdV], and human bocavirus [HBoV]) and six bacterial pathogens (*Streptococcus pneumoniae*, *Haemophilus influenzae*, *Moraxella Catarrhalis*, *Mycoplasma pneumoniae*, *Chlamydophila pneumoniae*, and *Legionella pneumophila*) were tested using multiplex PCR assays. Details about the primers and PCR methods used have been described previously [10, 11]. Urinary antigen testing was performed for the detection of *S. pneumoniae* and *L. pneumophila* (Binax NOW *Streptococcus Pneumoniae*, Binax NOW *Legionella*; Alere Inc., Waltham, MA, USA).

Definitions of variables

Diagnosis of viral infection was made according to PCR results. Bacterial infection was diagnosed when any of the following criteria were fulfilled: 1) culture yielded pathogenic bacteria from microscopically purulent sputum samples (i.e., Geckler's classification groups 4 and 5) or normally sterile site samples; 2) PCR assays were positive for bacterial DNA in microscopically purulent sputum samples; or 3) urinary antigen tests showed a positive result.

Patients were categorized into four age groups: 15–64 years, 65–74 years, 75–84 years, and ≥85 years. Patients' disability status was evaluated using the Eastern Cooperative Oncology Group Performance Status (PS) score [12]. Pneumonia severity was assessed using the CURB65 scoring system [13]. To estimate the effect on pneumonia mortality, viruses were categorized into four groups: 1) HRV; 2) influenza A and B viruses; 3) paramyxoviruses (RSV, hMPV, and PIV type 1–4); and 4) other viruses (HAdV, HBoV, and HCoV).

We divided patients into three groups according to comorbidity status: 1) patients without comorbidity; 2) patients with chronic respiratory disease; and 3) patients with comorbidities other than chronic respiratory disease (i.e., other comorbidities). Chronic respiratory disease included bronchial asthma, chronic obstructive pulmonary disease (COPD), interstitial pneumonia, pneumoconiosis, and bronchiectasis. Other comorbidities included diabetes mellitus, cerebrovascular disease, dementia, neuromuscular disease, cardiac failure, ischaemic heart disease, collagen disease, malignancy, renal disease, and liver disease. Patients were considered to have aspiration risk factors when they had any of the following factors: episodes of aspiration, the presence of dysphagia, consciousness disturbances, neuromuscular diseases, cerebrovascular diseases, tube feeding, and bedridden status [14].

The in-hospital death was defined as any death occurred during the hospitalization. During the first year of study, we followed up our patients after the enrolment and confirmed that no outpatient had died within 30 days of enrolment. We therefore considered the in-hospital death as a good marker of short-term mortality in pneumonia patients regardless of their hospitalization status.

Statistical analysis

Patients were categorized according to their comorbidity status (i.e., patients without comorbidity, with chronic respiratory disease, or with other comorbidities) and compared using chi-squared tests. Viral and bacterial infection status were compared by age group and comorbidity status using chi-squared tests, Fisher's exact tests, and chi-squared tests for trend. In-hospital mortality rates were calculated by viral and bacterial infection status and compared with those of the virus-negative

group. The effects of viral infection on in-hospital mortality were expressed as risk ratios with 95% confidence intervals (CI) and estimated using Poisson regression models with robust standard errors. Age, study site, comorbidity status, duration of symptoms, month of diagnosis, antibiotic use, and presence of bacteria were considered potential confounders based on prior knowledge and were included in the multiple regression models. For patients whose onset of symptoms were unknown (<5%), we coded those missing values as "unknown" and included all patients in our analysis. The data were analysed using STATA version 13 (STATA Corp., College Station, TX, USA).

Ethics

This study was approved by the institutional review boards (IRBs) of the Institute of Tropical Medicine, Nagasaki University, Ebetsu City Hospital, Kameda Medical Center, Chikamori Hospital, and Juzenkai Hospital. The requirement for obtaining written consent from all participants was waived by all IRBs because of the study's observational nature without any deviation from the current medical practice. Anonymized data were used for the analyses.

Results
Clinical characteristics

During the study period, 3816 patients were enrolled in the study. Of these, 346 were excluded because of refusal to participate in the study ($n = 48$), absence of pulmonary infiltrates ($n = 163$), and non-pneumonia diagnosis ($n = 135$). After excluding 853 (22.3%) patients whose sputum samples for PCR assays were unavailable, 2617 patients were eligible for analysis (Fig. 1).

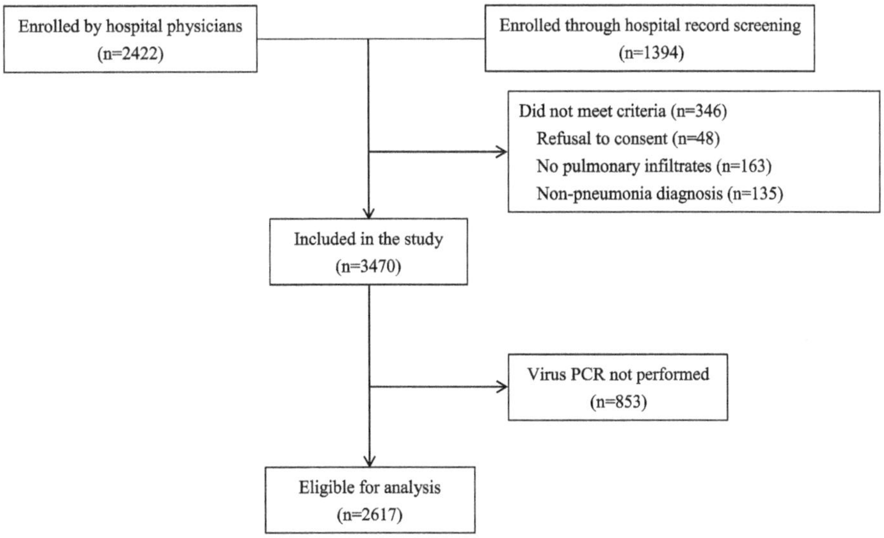

Fig. 1 Flow chart of study patients

Table 1 shows the clinical characteristics of pneumonia patients by comorbidity status. Approximately 60% of patients were male, and the median age was 73.8 years (interquartile range, 66 to 85 years). The proportions of patients aged ≥65 years and ≥85 years were 77.8 and 28.4%, respectively; 46.7% of 2545 patients had aspiration risk factors. Of all patients, 574 (21.9%) did not have comorbidities, 790 (30.2%) had chronic respiratory disease, and 1253 (47.9%) had other comorbidities. Patients with comorbidities were more likely to be male, older, more frequently required hospitalization, more frequently developed severe disease, more frequently had aspiration risk factors, had higher PS scores, and visited the hospital earlier than those without comorbidities. The proportion of patients with aspiration risk factors was particularly high (65.5%) among patients with other comorbidities. Multiple symptoms were most frequently observed in patients with chronic respiratory disease (70.1%), followed by those without comorbidities (67.9%) and those with other comorbidities (57.5%).

Detection of viral and bacterial pathogens

In total, 605 (23.1%) patients tested positive for at least one virus (Table 2). HRV was the most common virus identified ($n = 256$ [9.8%]), followed by influenza A ($n = 101$ [3.9%]) and RSV ($n = 101$ [3.9%]). Two or more viruses were detected in 31 patients (1.2%). The most frequent combinations of viruses were HRV plus influenza A ($n = 7$), followed by HRV plus RSV ($n = 4$), and HRV plus hMPV ($n = 4$). Three viruses (HRV, hMPV, and PIV type 3) were detected in one patient. Bacterial pathogens were detected in 992 (37.9%) patients, and both viral and bacterial pathogens were detected in 246 (9.4%) patients (i.e., viral-bacterial co-infection).

Viral and bacterial infection status were compared by age group (Table 2) and comorbidity status (Table 3). The proportion of overall virus-positive pneumonia did not differ by age group. RSV was more frequently identified in older age groups, while HCoV was more frequently identified in younger age groups. The proportion of influenza-

Table 1 Characteristics of enrolled pneumonia patients

	Total	No comorbidity	Chronic respiratory disease	Other comorbidities[a]	P value†
	$N = 2617$	$N = 574$	$N = 790$	$N = 1253$	
	N (%)	N (%)	N (%)	N (%)	
Male sex	1591 (60.8)	295 (51.4)	540 (68.4)	756 (60.3)	<0.001
Age group					
15–64	580 (22.2)	268 (46.7)	121 (15.3)	191 (15.2)	<0.001
65–74	447 (17.1)	91 (15.9)	141 (17.9)	215 (17.2)	
75–84	848 (32.4)	126 (22.0)	321 (40.6)	401 (32.0)	
85+	742 (28.4)	89 (15.5)	207 (26.2)	446 (35.6)	
Admission	2007 (76.7)	305 (53.1)	597 (75.6)	1105 (88.2)	<0.001
Performance status ≥3, $n = 1307$	310 (23.7)	37 (11.1)	56 (13.9)	217 (37.9)	<0.001
Severe disease (CURB65 ≥ 4), $n = 2100$	154 (7.3)	19 (4.5)	41 (6.7)	94 (8.9)	0.010
Duration of symptoms[b] > 3 days, $n = 2507$	874 (34.9)	256 (47.8)	251 (33.3)	367 (30.2)	<0.001
No. of symptoms ≥3	1664 (63.6)	390 (67.9)	554 (70.1)	720 (57.5)	<0.001
Aspiration risk, $n = 2545$	1189 (46.7)	103 (18.4)	293 (37.8)	793 (65.5)	<0.001
Period					
Spring (January to March)	645 (24.7)	129 (22.5)	195 (24.7)	321 (25.6)	0.092
Summer (April to June)	572 (21.9)	147 (25.6)	161 (20.4)	264 (21.1)	
Autumn (July to September)	641 (24.5)	151 (26.3)	189 (23.9)	301 (24.0)	
Winter (October to December)	759 (29.0)	147 (25.6)	245 (31.0)	367 (29.3)	
Study site					
Ebetsu	326 (12.4)	79 (13.8)	123 (15.6)	124 (9.9)	<0.001
Kamogawa	1379 (52.7)	348 (60.6)	416 (52.7)	615 (49.1)	
Kochi	600 (22.9)	96 (16.7)	153 (19.4)	351 (28.0)	
Nagasaki	312 (11.9)	51 (8.9)	98 (12.4)	163 (13.0)	

†Chi-square tests were performed to compare three groups
[a]Other comorbidities include diabetes mellitus, cerebrovascular disease, dementia, neuromuscular disease, cardiac failure, ischaemic heart disease, collagen disease, malignancy, renal disease, and liver disease
[b]Symptoms include cough, sputum, chest pain, fever, chill, headache, fatigue, appetite loss, myalgia, arthralgia, nausea, vomiting, diarrhoea, and dehydration

Table 2 Viral and bacterial infection status among pneumonia patients by age group

Viruses	Total N = 2617	15–64 y N = 580	65–74 y N = 447	75–84 y N = 848	85 y+ N = 742	P value*
HRV	256 (9.8)	70 (12.1)	42 (9.4)	69 (8.1)	75 (10.1)	0.185
Inf A	101 (3.9)	22 (3.8)	13 (2.9)	32 (3.8)	34 (4.6)	0.343
RSV	101 (3.9)	12 (2.1)	20 (4.5)	32 (3.8)	37 (5.0)	0.016
PIV 3	49 (1.9)	14 (2.4)	7 (1.6)	17 (2.0)	11 (1.5)	0.311
HMPV	45 (1.7)	4 (0.7)	13 (2.9)	14 (1.7)	14 (1.9)	0.286
PIV 1	26 (2.0)	5 (0.9)	3 (0.7)	10 (1.2)	8 (1.1)	0.523
Inf B	24 (0.9)	6 (1.0)	4 (0.9)	3 (0.4)	11 (1.5)	0.588
PIV 2	14 (0.5)	4 (0.7)	3 (0.7)	3 (0.4)	4 (0.5)	0.567
HCoV (229E/OC43)	13 (0.5)	6 (1.0)	3 (0.7)	2 (0.2)	2 (0.3)	0.029
HAdV	6 (0.2)	1 (0.2)	1 (0.2)	4 (0.5)	0 (0.0)	0.708
HBoV	2 (0.1)	1 (0.2)	0 (0.0)	1 (0.1)	0 (0.0)	0.394
PIV 4	0 (0.0)	0 (0.0)	0 (0.0)	0 (0.0)	0 (0.0)	NA
Any viruses	605 (23.1)	137 (23.6)	102 (22.8)	180 (21.2)	186 (25.1)	0.677
≥2 viruses	31 (1.2)	8 (1.4)	7 (1.6)	6 (0.7)	10 (1.3)	0.654
Any bacterial pathogens	992 (37.9)	265 (45.7)	194 (43.4)	288 (34.0)	245 (33.0)	<0.001
Viral-bacterial co-infection	246 (9.4)	66 (11.4)	46 (10.3)	69 (8.1)	65 (8.8)	0.056
Any viral and bacterial pathogens	1351 (51.6)	336 (57.9)	250 (55.9)	399 (47.1)	366 (49.3)	<0.001

HRV human rhinovirus, *InfA* influenza A virus, *RSV* respiratory syncytial virus, *PIV1–4* human parainfluenza virus type 1–4, *HMPV* human metapneumovirus, *InfB* influenza B virus, *HCoV* human coronavirus (229E/OC43), *HAdV* human adenovirus, *HBoV* human bocavirus
*Chi-square tests for trend were performed

Table 3 Viral and bacterial infection status among pneumonia patients by comorbidity status

Viruses	No comorbidities N = 574	Chronic respiratory disease N = 790	Other comorbidities[a] N = 1253	P value†
HRV	57 (9.9)	87 (11.0)	112 (8.9)	0.304
Inf A	21 (3.7)	29 (3.7)	51 (4.1)	0.866
RSV	12 (2.1)	37 (4.7)	52 (4.2)	0.037
PIV 3	12 (2.1)	11 (1.4)	26 (2.1)	0.492
HMPV	6 (1.1)	13 (1.7)	26 (2.1)	0.286
PIV 1	4 (0.7)	10 (1.3)	12 (1.0)	0.598
Inf B	5 (0.9)	5 (0.6)	14 (1.1)	0.596
PIV 2	3 (0.5)	4 (0.5)	7 (0.6)	1.000
HCoV (229E/OC43)	3 (0.5)	5 (0.6)	5 (0.4)	0.767
HAdV	2 (0.4)	1 (0.1)	3 (0.2)	0.764
HBoV	0 (0.0)	0 (0.0)	2 (0.2)	0.711
PIV 4	0 (0.0)	0 (0.0)	0 (0.0)	NA
Any viruses	118 (20.6)	196 (24.8)	291 (23.2)	0.183
≥2 viruses	7 (1.2)	6 (0.8)	18 (1.4)	0.386
Any bacterial pathogens	233 (40.6)	315 (39.9)	444 (35.4)	0.043
Viral-bacterial co-infection	54 (9.4)	88 (11.1)	104 (8.3)	0.101
Any viral and bacterial pathogens	297 (51.7)	423 (53.5)	631 (50.4)	0.373

HRV human rhinovirus, *InfA* influenza A virus, *RSV* respiratory syncytial virus, *PIV1–4* human parainfluenza virus type 1–4, *HMPV* human metapneumovirus, *InfB* influenza B virus, *HCoV* human coronavirus (229E/OC43), *HAdV* human adenovirus, *HBoV* human bocavirus
† Chi-square tests or Fisher's exact tests were performed to compare the three groups
[a]Other comorbidities include diabetes mellitus, cerebrovascular disease, dementia, neuromuscular disease, cardiac failure, ischaemic heart disease, collagen disease, malignancy, renal disease, and liver disease

positive pneumonia was similar across all age groups. Bacterial pathogens were more frequently identified in younger patients. For patients' comorbidity status, RSV was most frequently identified in patients with chronic respiratory disease (4.7%), followed by those with other comorbidities (4.2%) and without comorbidities (2.1%) (p = 0.037); the frequencies of other viruses were almost identical between the three groups (Table 3). Bacterial pathogens were more frequently identified in patients without comorbidities than in those with comorbidities.

We explored symptoms of patients with each respiratory virus groups (Additional file 1: Table S1). The proportion of patients with multiple symptoms (i.e., the number of symptoms ≥3) was higher in patients with paramyxovirus infection than those without viral infection (75.0% vs 61.3%, p < 0.001). In the group of patients with aspiration risk factors, those with paramyxovirus were more likely to have a cough than patients without virus (71.1% vs 46.2%, p < 0.001).

In-hospital mortality of pneumonia and virus detection

Among 2617 patients, 193 patients died before discharge, with an overall in-hospital mortality of 7.4%. The mortalities among virus-positive and -negative groups were 5.8 and 7.9%, respectively, and the overall effect (adjusted risk ratio [ARR]) of viruses on mortality was 0.76 (95% CI 0.53–1.09, p = 0.140). Intriguingly, when the effect of specific virus type was analysed, paramyxoviruses, including RSV, hMPV, and PIV type 1–4, were associated with a dramatically lower mortality (ARR 0.29, 95% CI 0.12–0.71, p = 0.007). Among 212 paramyxovirus-positive pneumonia, five died: three were RSV-positive, one was HMPV-positive, and one was HMPV-positive at the enrolment. RSV alone was also associated with a lower mortality (ARR 0.48, 95% CI 0.18–1.29, p = 0.146), but the association did not reach a statistically significant level. None of the other virus types were associated with mortality.

The virus type-specific effects were further investigated after patients were stratified by age group and comorbidity status (Tables 4 and 5). Similar effects of viruses were seen across all age groups. However, influenza virus A and B were strongly associated with higher mortality in patients with chronic respiratory disease (ARR 3.38, 95% CI 1.54–7.42, p = 0.002), while no influenza-related death was observed in those without comorbidity. Intriguingly, paramyxoviruses were associated with markedly lower mortality in patients with other comorbidities (ARR 0.10, 95% CI 0.01–0.70, p = 0.020), but this association was not observed in other groups. HRV was not associated with mortality in the three groups. Virus only, bacteria only, and both virus- and bacteria-positive pneumonia demonstrated higher mortality than virus- and bacteria-negative pneumonia in patients with chronic respiratory disease, but these associations did not reach statistically significant levels.

We explored the association between viruses and in-hospital mortality in patients with aspiration risk factors (Additional file 1: Table S2). Paramyxovirus was the only virus type significantly associated with reduced mortality in this category of patients (ARR 0.28, 95% CI 0.09–0.85, p = 0.024). Influenza A and B were not associated with mortality (ARR 1.78, 95% CI 0.92–3.47, p = 0.089). The mortality was higher among patients with cough than those without cough (11.7% vs 4.9%, p < 0.001).

Discussion

In this multicentre prospective study, 23.1% of adult pneumonias were associated with viruses. HRV was the leading virus identified, followed by influenza A and RSV. This pattern was almost identical across all age groups. Influenza was strongly associated with higher mortality in patients with chronic respiratory disease but not in other groups. Paramyxoviruses, including RSV, hMPV, and PIV type 1–4, were associated with improved survival in patients with other comorbidities, especially in those with aspiration risk factors. To the best of our knowledge, this study is the first to systematically investigate virus-specific effects on pneumonia mortality by age group and comorbidity status among adults.

Viruses are frequently observed in pneumonia patients. According to previous studies, viruses were positive in 23, 34, 30 and 28% of CAP patents in the US [2], Norway [3], UK [15], and China [16], respectively, and HRV, influenza A, and RSV were the leading viruses identified; these findings were confirmed in our study. However, the role of viruses in pneumonia development and progression has not been fully established. A systematic review showed that the risk of death was higher in patients with viral infection, although the association did not reach a statistically significant level (odds ratio 1.3, 95% CI 0.8–2.2) [4]. The major limitation of previous studies is that all viruses and patient groups were pooled, which may have overlooked their intergroup differences. In fact, in the current study, viruses overall were not associated with increased mortality among all pneumonia patients (ARR 0.76, 95% CI 0.53–1.09), but the effects were different by viruses and patient characteristics.

Influenza increased pneumonia mortality by 3.4-fold (95% CI 1.54–7.42) in our patients with chronic respiratory disease but did not change the mortality in other patients. Although influenza is known to be an important cause of pneumonia and death, only a few studies have formally compared the mortality of influenza pneumonia with that of non-influenza pneumonia, and the findings have been inconsistent [17, 18]. On the other hand, previous studies have demonstrated that chronic respiratory disease increases the risk of severe outcome among influenza patients [19, 20]. Bronchial epithelial cells of COPD are susceptible to replication of influenza virus because of their

Table 4 Viral and bacterial infection status and in-hospital mortality among pneumonia patients by age group

	Total, n = 2617		15–64 y, n = 580		65–74 y, n = 447		75–84 y, n = 848		85 y+, n = 742	
	No. death/no. cases (% mortality)	ARR[a] (95% CI)	No. death/no. cases (% mortality)	ARR[a] (95% CI)	No. death/no. cases (% mortality)	ARR[a] (95% CI)	No. death/no. cases (% mortality)	ARR[a] (95% CI)	No. death/no. cases (% mortality)	ARR[a] (95% CI)
HRV	14/234 (6.0)	0.86 (0.51–1.45)	2/63 (3.2)	1.60 (0.38–6.65)	3/37 (8.1)	1.16 (0.38–3.59)	3/66 (4.6)	0.55 (0.17–1.74)	6/68 (8.8)	0.87 (0.40–1.93)
Inf A/B	10/110 (9.1)	1.13 (0.60–2.13)	1/25 (4.0)	1.74 (0.17–17.74)	1/15 (6.7)	1.03 (0.12–8.86)	3/31 (9.7)	0.93 (0.29–2.99)	5/39 (12.8)	1.44 (0.58–3.61)
Paramyxovirus (RSV/hMPV/PIV1–4)	5/212 (2.4)	0.29 (0.12–0.71)	0/35 (0.0)	0.00 (0.00–0.00)	1/40 (2.5)	0.41 (0.06–3.01)	3/70 (4.3)	0.44 (0.14–1.39)	1/67 (1.5)	0.15 (0.02–1.05)
Other viruses (H-AdV/HBoV/HCoV)	2/18 (11.1)	1.62 (0.42–6.18)	1/6 (16.7)	4.30 (0.63–29.53)	0/3 (0.0)	0.00 (0.00–0.00)	1/7 (14.3)	1.66 (0.26–10.64)	0/2 (0.0)	0.00 (0.00–0.00)
Multiple viruses	4/31 (12.9)	1.69 (0.67–4.27)	0/8 (0.0)	0.00 (0.00–0.00)	1/7 (14.3)	2.63 (0.37–18.75)	0/6 (0.0)	0.00 (0.00–0.00)	3/10 (30.0)	2.72 (0.88–8.46)
No virus	158/2012 (7.9)	Reference ARR[b](95% CI)	15/443 (3.4)	Reference ARR[b](95% CI)	25/345 (7.3)	Reference ARR[b](95% CI)	62/668 (9.3)	Reference ARR[b](95% CI)	56/556 (10.1)	Reference ARR[b](95% CI)
Only viruses	19/359 (5.3)	0.66 (0.41–1.07)	2/71 (2.8)	0.96 (0.18–5.02)	1/56 (1.8)	0.27 (0.03–2.20)	7/111 (6.3)	0.70 (0.32–1.56)	9/121 (7.4)	0.68 (0.34–1.39)
Only bacterial pathogens	51/746 (6.8)	0.90 (0.65–1.25)	5/199 (2.5)	0.82 (0.28–2.42)	10/148 (6.8)	1.02 (0.48–2.17)	21/219 (9.6)	1.05 (0.64–1.74)	15/180 (8.3)	0.76 (0.43–1.35)
Viral-bacterial co-infection	16/246 (6.5)	0.85 (0.51–1.41)	2/66 (3.0)	1.31 (0.25–6.80)	5/46 (10.9)	1.75 (0.67–4.60)	3/69 (4.4)	0.46 (0.14–1.49)	6/65 (9.2)	0.85 (0.37–1.94)
No viral or bacterial pathogens	107/1266 (8.5)	Reference	10/244 (4.1)	Reference	15/197 (7.6)	Reference	41/449 (9.1)	Reference	41/376 (10.9)	Reference

ARR adjusted risk ratio, CI confidence interval, HRV human rhinovirus, InfA influenza A virus, RSV respiratory syncytial virus, PIV1–4 human parainfluenza virus type 1–4, HMPV human metapneumovirus, InfB influenza B virus, HCoV human coronavirus (229E/OC43), HAdV human adenovirus, HBoV human bocavirus

[a]Adjusted for age, study site, comorbidity status, duration of symptoms, month of diagnosis, antibiotic use, and presence of bacteria

[b]Adjusted for age, study site, comorbidity status, duration of symptoms, month of diagnosis, and antibiotic use

Table 5 Viral and bacterial infection status and in-hospital mortality among pneumonia patients by comorbidity status

	Without comorbidities, n = 574		With chronic respiratory disease, n = 790		With other comorbidities[a], n = 1253	
	No. death/no. cases (% mortality)	ARR[b] (95% CI)	No. death/no. cases (% mortality)	ARR[b] (95% CI)	No. death/no. cases (% mortality)	ARR[b] (95% CI)
HRV	2/53 (3.8)	0.73 (0.18–2.96)	4/83 (4.8)	0.78 (0.28–2.14)	8/98 (8.2)	0.97 (0.48–1.96)
Inf A/B	0/22 (0.0)	0.00 (0.00–0.00)	6/31 (19.4)	3.38 (1.54–7.42)	4/57 (7.0)	0.73 (0.26–2.02)
Paramyxovirus (RSV/hMPV/PIV1–4)	1/32 (3.1)	0.47 (0.07–3.26)	3/71 (4.2)	0.66 (0.20–2.13)	1/109 (0.9)	0.10 (0.01–0.70)
Other viruses (HAdV/HBoV/HCoV)	0/4 (0.0)	0.00 (0.00–0.00)	1/5 (20.0)	4.55 (0.58–35.5)	1/9 (11.1)	1.33 (0.21–8.66)
Multiple viruses	0/7 (0.0)	0.00 (0.00–0.00)	1/6 (16.7)	3.98 (0.68–23.24)	3/18 (16.7)	1.68 (0.56–5.03)
No virus	26/456 (5.7)	Reference	44/594 (7.4)	Reference	88/962 (9.2)	Reference
		ARR[c] (95% CI)		ARR[c] (95% CI)		ARR[c] (95% CI)
Only viruses	1/64 (1.6)	0.24 (0.03–1.78)	9/108 (8.3)	1.28 (0.59–2.81)	9/187 (4.8)	0.51 (0.26–1.01)
Only bacterial pathogens	8/179 (4.5)	0.83 (0.36–1.93)	16/227 (7.1)	1.13 (0.61–2.09)	27/340 (7.9)	0.84 (0.54–1.31)
Viral-bacterial co-infection	2/54 (3.7)	0.58 (0.14–2.38)	6/88 (6.8)	1.29 (0.55–3.06)	8/104 (7.7)	0.77 (0.38–1.59)
No viral or bacterial pathogens	18/277 (6.5)	Reference	28/367 (7.6)	Reference	61/622 (9.8)	Reference
		ARR[b] (95% CI)		ARR[b] (95% CI)		ARR[b] (95% CI)
Multiple viruses	0/7 (0.0)	0.00 (0.00–0.00)	1/6 (16.7)	3.22 (0.52–19.81)	3/18 (16.7)	2.98 (0.91–9.78)
Single virus	3/111 (2.7)	Reference	14/190 (7.4)	Reference	14/273 (5.1)	Reference

ARR adjusted risk ratio, CI confidence interval, HRV human rhinovirus, InfA influenza A virus, RSV respiratory syncytial virus, PIV1–4 human parainfluenza virus type 1–4, HMPV human metapneumovirus, InfB influenza B virus, HCoV human coronavirus (229E/OC43), HAdV human adenovirus, HBoV human bocavirus

[a] Other comorbidities include diabetes mellitus, cerebrovascular disease, dementia, neuromuscular disease, cardiac failure, ischaemic heart disease, collagen disease, malignancy, renal disease, and liver disease

[b] Adjusted for age, study site, duration of symptoms, month of diagnosis, antibiotic use and presence of bacteria

[c] Adjusted for age, study site, duration of symptoms, month of diagnosis, and antibiotic use

impaired antiviral immunity [21]; thus, the effect of influenza on disease progression may be stronger in patients with this condition. According to the Cochrane review, influenza vaccination reduces exacerbations in patients with COPD [22]. Seasonal influenza vaccination campaigns must therefore pay special attention to this patient group.

Interestingly, paramyxoviruses including RSV were associated with improved survival in our patients with other comorbidities. Inconsistent findings have been reported about the effect of paramyxoviruses on pneumonia severity. A multinational study showed that older patients who had been infected with RSV were more likely to be hospitalized than those with other respiratory viruses [23], while a study conducted in the US demonstrated that patients with RSV infection were less frequently hospitalized than those with influenza infection [24]. A retrospective cohort study conducted in Hong Kong showed that the 30-day and 60-day mortality rates were similar between adult patients hospitalized with RSV and those with seasonal influenza [25]. These inconsistent findings suggest that the effects of paramyxovirus infection substantially vary by patients' conditions. In fact, in the current study, compared with virus-negative pneumonia, the mortality of paramyxovirus-associated pneumonia was substantially lower among patients with other comorbidities but this finding was not observed among patients without comorbidities and patients with chronic respiratory disease. The low mortality of paramyxovirus-associated pneumonia in this groups may be associated with its high prevalence of multiple symptoms. In our study, the proportion of patients with multiple symptoms (i.e., the number of symptoms ≥ 3) was higher in patients with paramyxovirus infection than those without viral infection. Patients with paramyxovirus-associated pneumonia are more likely to develop symptoms and are probably more likely to visit hospitals, and this benefit may be observed in patients with comorbidities. In the group of patients with aspiration risk factors, those with paramyxovirus-associated pneumonia were more likely to have a cough than patients without virus (71.1% vs 46.2%, $p < 0.001$), and the mortality was higher among patients with cough than those without cough (11.7% vs 4.9%, $p < 0.001$). The low mortality of paramyxovirus-associated pneumonia in patients with aspiration risk factors also suggests that these viruses may stimulate the cough reflex and improve patients' survival; however, our study does not provide conclusive evidence. Further studies are needed to unveil the mechanisms of potential benefits of paramyxovirus infection on pneumonia mortality.

In our study, multiple viruses were identified in 5.1% of virus-associated pneumonia and were associated with higher mortality than single viral infection in patients with chronic respiratory disease and other comorbidities.

The association between multiple viral infections and pneumonia mortality remains uncertain [26]. Systematic reviews have shown that multiple viral infections in patients with respiratory disease are not associated with disease severity [27, 28]; however, the majority of previous studies included young children but not adults. The effect of multiple viruses on disease progression may be different in children and adults. Consistent with previous studies [3, 29, 30], half of the viral pneumonia patients were co-infected with bacterial pathogens. A systematic review showed that viral-bacterial co-infection increased mortality [4]; however, this association was not observed in our study. Viral infections of the lower respiratory tract may increase the risk of secondary bacterial infection, which may increase the risk of pneumonia and mortality [26]. However, sputum samples were collected once in our study; thus, we were unable to determine the time course of viral and bacterial infections. A cohort study with sequential respiratory sampling may be a preferable design to establish a causal association between viral-bacterial co-infection and pneumonia mortality.

Advances in molecular diagnostic techniques have enabled virus detection in clinical settings. Our findings raise the question of whether all pneumonia patients should be tested for viruses. The increased mortality of influenza-associated pneumonia in patients with chronic respiratory disease suggests the importance of early diagnosis of influenza and initiation of antivirals for this patient group. On the other hand, no substantial increase of mortality was found for other viruses. Screening for viruses in all pneumonia patients may be unnecessary in clinical settings.

Our study has limitations. First, sputum samples were not available for 25% of the enrolled patients. However, the clinical characteristics of patients without sputum samples did not differ from those of patients with sputum samples. Exclusion of this group did not affect our findings. Second, we used PCR to detect viruses. The detection of viral RNA and DNA in respiratory samples does not always indicate the presence of a causal pathogen; particularly, the detection of viruses in nasopharyngeal swabs may not be reflecting lower respiratory infections in pneumonia patients. We, therefore, used sputum samples from pneumonia patients, and the presence of viruses in the lower respiratory tract must be very likely causative [31]. Third, due to the nature of an observational study design, unmeasured confounding factors may have remained in our risk factor analyses for pneumonia mortality.

Conclusions

Viral infections are common in adult pneumonia, and their impact on pneumonia mortality varies by viruses and comorbidities. Variable impacts of viruses by population characteristics must be considered in the development of antiviral drugs and vaccines.

Abbreviations

ARR: Adjusted risk ratio; CAP: Community-acquired pneumonia; CI: Confidence intervals; COPD: Chronic obstructive pulmonary disease; HAdV: Human adenovirus; HBoV: Human bocavirus; HCoV: Human coronavirus; hMPV: Human metapneumovirus; HPIV: Human parainfluenza virus; HRV: Human rhinovirus; PCR: Polymerase chain reaction; PS: Performance Status; RSV: Respiratory syncytial virus

Acknowledgements

We are grateful to all the laboratory staff at the participating hospitals. We would like to thank Rina Shiramizu (Institute of Tropical Medicine, Nagasaki University, Nagasaki, Japan) and Kyoko Uchibori (Institute of Tropical Medicine, Nagasaki University, Nagasaki, Japan) for performing PCR and Yumi Araki (Institute of Tropical Medicine, Nagasaki University, Nagasaki, Japan) for administrative work. Adult Pneumonia Study Group—Japan (APSG-J) are: Takao Wakabayashi[1], Naoto Hosokawa[2], Norihiro Kaneko[3], Kei Nakashima[3], Yoshihito Otsuka[4], Eiichiro Sando[5], Kaori Shibui[5], Daisuke Suzuki[2], Kenzo Tanaka[6], Kentaro Tochitani[2], Masayuki Chikamori[7], Masayuki Ishida[7], Hiroshi Nakaoka[7], Hiroyuki Ito[8], Kei Matsuki[8], Yoshiko Tsuchihashi[8], Bhim G Dhoubhadel[9], Akitsugu Furumoto[9], Sugihiro Hamaguchi[1,9], Shungo Katoh[1,9], Satoshi Kakiuchi[9], Emi Kitashoji[9], Takaharu Shimazaki[9], Masahiro Takaki[9], Kiwao Watanabe[9], Lay-Myint Yoshida[10].
1. Department of General Internal Medicine, Ebetsu City Hospital, Hokkaido, Japan.
2. Department of Infectious Diseases, Kameda Medical Center, Chiba, Japan.
3. Department of Pulmonology, Kameda Medical Center, Chiba, Japan.
4. Department of Laboratory Medicine, Kameda Medical Center, Chiba, Japan.
5. Department of General Internal Medicine, Kameda Medical Center, Chiba, Japan.
6. Emergency and Trauma Center, Kameda Medical Center, Chiba, Japan.
7. Department of Internal Medicine, Chikamori Hospital, Kochi, Japan.
8. Department of Internal Medicine, Juzenkai Hospital, Nagasaki, Japan.
9. Department of Clinical Medicine, Institute of Tropical Medicine, Nagasaki University, Nagasaki, Japan.
10. Department of Pediatric Infectious Diseases, Institute of Tropical Medicine, Nagasaki University, Nagasaki, Japan.

Funding

This study was supported by Nagasaki University and Pfizer Japan Inc. The authors were independent from the sponsors.

Authors' contributions

This study was conceived by NK, MS, MAO, KM, and KA. MAB, MY, TI, NA, NH, and MAO collected data. NK, MS, and KM performed data analysis and wrote the manuscript. All authors approved the final manuscript.

Consent for publication

Not applicable

Competing interests

The authors declare that they have no competing interests.

Author details

[1]Department of Pulmonology, Kameda Medical Center, 929 Higashi-cho, Kamogawa, Chiba, Japan. [2]Division of Respiratory Medicine, Department of Internal Medicine, Kobe University Graduate School of Medicine, 7-5-1 Kusunoki-cho, Chuo-ku, Kobe, Japan. [3]Department of Clinical Medicine, Institute of Tropical Medicine, Nagasaki University, 1-12-4 Sakamoto, Nagasaki 852-8523, Japan. [4]Department of General Internal Medicine, Kameda Medical Center, 929 Higashi-cho, Kamogawa, Chiba, Japan. [5]Department of Internal Medicine, Juzenkai Hospital, 7-18 Kagomachi, Nagasaki, Japan. [6]Department of Internal Medicine, Chikamori Hospital, 1-1-16 Okawasuji, Kochi, Japan. [7]Department of General Internal Medicine, Ebetsu City Hospital, 6 Wakakusacho, Ebetsu, Hokkaido, Japan.

References

1. Johansson N, Kalin M, Tiveljung-Lindell A, Giske CG, Hedlund J. Etiology of community-acquired pneumonia: increased microbiological yield with new diagnostic methods. Clin Infect Dis. 2010;50:202–9.
2. Jain S, Self WH, Wunderink RG, Fakhran S, Balk R, Bramley AM, et al. Community-acquired pneumonia requiring hospitalization among U.S. adults. N Engl J Med. 2015;373:415–27.
3. Holter JC, Muller F, Bjorang O, Samdal HH, Marthinsen JB, Jenum PA, et al. Etiology of community-acquired pneumonia and diagnostic yields of microbiological methods: a 3-year prospective study in Norway. BMC Infect Dis. 2015;15:64.
4. Burk M, El-Kersh K, Saad M, Wiemken T, Ramirez J, Cavallazzi R. Viral infection in community-acquired pneumonia: a systematic review and meta-analysis. Eur Respir Rev. 2016;25:178–88.
5. Berry M, Gamieldien J, Fielding BC. Identification of new respiratory viruses in the new millennium. Viruses. 2015;7:996–1019.
6. Zumla A, Hui DS, Perlman S. Middle East respiratory syndrome. Lancet. 2015;386:995–1007.
7. Ma HM, Tang WH, Woo J. Predictors of in-hospital mortality of older patients admitted for community-acquired pneumonia. Age Ageing. 2011;40:736–41.
8. Komiya K, Rubin BK, Kadota JI, Mukae H, Akaba T, Moro H, et al. Prognostic implications of aspiration pneumonia in patients with community acquired pneumonia: a systematic review with meta-analysis. Sci Rep. 2016;6:38097.
9. Morimoto K, Suzuki M, Ishifuji T, Yaegashi M, Asoh N, Hamashige N, et al. The burden and etiology of community-onset pneumonia in the aging Japanese population: a multicenter prospective study. PLoS One. 2015;10:e0122247.
10. Yoshida LM, Suzuki M, Yamamoto T, Nguyen HA, Nguyen CD, Nguyen AT, et al. Viral pathogens associated with acute respiratory infections in central vietnamese children. Pediatr Infect Dis J. 2010;29:75–7.
11. Vu HT, Yoshida LM, Suzuki M, Nguyen HA, Nguyen CD, Nguyen AT, et al. Association between nasopharyngeal load of Streptococcus Pneumoniae, viral coinfection, and radiologically confirmed pneumonia in Vietnamese children. Pediatr Infect Dis J. 2011;30:11–8.
12. Oken MM, Creech RH, Tormey DC, Horton J, Davis TE, McFadden ET, et al. Toxicity and response criteria of the eastern cooperative oncology group. Am J Clin Oncol. 1982;5:649–55.
13. Lim WS, van der Eerden MM, Laing R, Boersma WG, Karalus N, Town GI, et al. Defining community acquired pneumonia severity on presentation to hospital: an international derivation and validation study. Thorax. 2003;58:377–82.
14. Reza Shariatzadeh M, Huang JQ, Marrie TJ. Differences in the features of aspiration pneumonia according to site of acquisition: community or continuing care facility. J Am Geriatr Soc. 2006;54:296–302.
15. Gadsby NJ, Russell CD, McHugh MP, Mark H, Conway Morris A, Laurenson IF, et al. Comprehensive molecular testing for respiratory pathogens in community-acquired pneumonia. Clin Infect Dis. 2016;62:817–23.
16. JX Q, Gu L, ZH P, XM Y, Liu YM, Li R, et al. Viral etiology of community-acquired pneumonia among adolescents and adults with mild or moderate severity and its relation to age and severity. BMC Infect Dis. 2015;15:89.
17. Bewick T, Myles P, Greenwood S. Nguyen-van-tam JS, Brett SJ, Semple MG, et al. clinical and laboratory features distinguishing pandemic H1N1 influenza-related pneumonia from interpandemic community-acquired pneumonia in adults. Thorax. 2011;66:247–52.
18. Sohn CH, Ryoo SM, Yoon JY, Seo DW, Lim KS, Kim SH, et al. Comparison of clinical features and outcomes of hospitalized adult patients with novel influenza a (H1N1) pneumonia and other pneumonia. Acad Emerg Med. 2013;20:46–53.
19. Loubet P, Samih-Lenzi N, Galtier F, Vanhems P, Loulergue P, Duval X, et al. Factors associated with poor outcomes among adults hospitalized for influenza in France: a three-year prospective multicenter study. J Clin Virol. 2016;79:68–73.
20. Garg S, Jain S, Dawood FS, Jhung M, Perez A, D'Mello T, et al. Pneumonia among adults hospitalized with laboratory-confirmed seasonal influenza virus infection-United States, 2005-2008. BMC Infect Dis. 2015;15:369.
21. Hsu AC, Starkey MR, Hanish I, Parsons K, Haw TJ, Howland LJ, et al. Targeting PI3K-p110alpha suppresses influenza virus infection in chronic obstructive pulmonary disease. Am J Respir Crit Care Med. 2015;191:1012–23.

22. Poole PJ, Chacko E, Wood-Baker RW, Cates CJ. Influenza vaccine for patients with chronic obstructive pulmonary disease. Cochrane Database Syst Rev. 2006;(1):CD002733.
23. Falsey AR, McElhaney JE, Beran J, van Essen GA, Duval X, Esen M, et al. Respiratory syncytial virus and other respiratory viral infections in older adults with moderate to severe influenza-like illness. J Infect Dis. 2014; 209:1873–81.
24. Sundaram ME, Meece JK, Sifakis F, Gasser RA Jr, Belongia EA. Medically attended respiratory syncytial virus infections in adults aged >/= 50 years: clinical characteristics and outcomes. Clin Infect Dis. 2014;58:342–9.
25. Lee N, Lui GC, Wong KT, Li TC, Tse EC, Chan JY, et al. High morbidity and mortality in adults hospitalized for respiratory syncytial virus infections. Clin Infect Dis. 2013;57:1069–77.
26. Ruuskanen O, Lahti E, Jennings LC, Murdoch DR. Viral pneumonia. Lancet. 2011;377:1264–75.
27. Goka EA, Vallely PJ, Mutton KJ, Klapper PE. Single and multiple respiratory virus infections and severity of respiratory disease: a systematic review. Paediatr Respir Rev. 2014;15:363–70.
28. Asner SA, Science ME, Tran D, Smieja M, Merglen A, Mertz D. Clinical disease severity of respiratory viral co-infection versus single viral infection: a systematic review and meta-analysis. PLoS One. 2014;9:e99392.
29. Jennings LC, Anderson TP, Beynon KA, Chua A, Laing RT, Werno AM, et al. Incidence and characteristics of viral community-acquired pneumonia in adults. Thorax. 2008;63:42–8.
30. Takaki M, Nakama T, Ishida M, Morimoto H, Nagasaki Y, Shiramizu R, et al. High incidence of community-acquired pneumonia among rapidly aging population in Japan: a prospective hospital-based surveillance. Jpn J Infect Dis. 2014;67:269–75.
31. Falsey AR, Formica MA, Walsh EE. Yield of sputum for viral detection by reverse transcriptase PCR in adults hospitalized with respiratory illness. J Clin Microbiol. 2012;50:21–4.

17

Atypical pathogens in hospitalized patients with community-acquired pneumonia

Andrea Gramegna[1], Giovanni Sotgiu[2], Marta Di Pasquale[1], Dejan Radovanovic[3], Silvia Terraneo[4], Luis F. Reyes[5], Ester Vendrell[6], Joao Neves[7], Francesco Menzella[8], Francesco Blasi[1], Stefano Aliberti[1*], Marcos I. Restrepo[5] and on behalf of the GLIMP Study Group

Abstract

Background: Empirical antibiotic coverage for atypical pathogens in community-acquired pneumonia (CAP) has long been debated, mainly because of a lack of epidemiological data. We aimed to assess both testing for atypical pathogens and their prevalence in hospitalized patients with CAP worldwide, especially in relation with disease severity.

Methods: A secondary analysis of the GLIMP database, an international, multicentre, point-prevalence study of adult patients admitted for CAP in 222 hospitals across 6 continents in 2015, was performed. The study evaluated frequency of testing for atypical pathogens, including *L. pneumophila*, *M. pneumoniae*, *C. pneumoniae*, and their prevalence. Risk factors for testing and prevalence for atypical pathogens were assessed through univariate analysis.

Results: Among 3702 CAP patients 1250 (33.8%) underwent at least one test for atypical pathogens. Testing varies greatly among countries and its frequency was higher in Europe than elsewhere (46.0% vs. 12.7%, respectively, $p < 0.0001$). Detection of *L. pneumophila* urinary antigen was the most common test performed worldwide (32.0%). Patients with severe CAP were less likely to be tested for both atypical pathogens considered together (30.5% vs. 35.0%, $p = 0.009$) and specifically for legionellosis (28.3% vs. 33.5%, $p = 0.003$) than the rest of the population. Similarly, *L. pneumophila* testing was lower in ICU patients. At least one atypical pathogen was isolated in 62 patients (4.7%), including *M. pneumoniae* (26/251 patients, 10.3%), *L. pneumophila* (30/1186 patients, 2.5%), and *C. pneumoniae* (8/228 patients, 3.5%). Patients with CAP due to atypical pathogens were significantly younger, showed less cardiovascular, renal, and metabolic comorbidities in comparison to adult patients hospitalized due to non-atypical pathogen CAP.

Conclusions: Testing for atypical pathogens in patients admitted for CAP in poorly standardized in real life and does not mirror atypical prevalence in different settings. Further evidence on the impact of atypical pathogens, expecially in the low-income countries, is needed to guidelines implementation.

Keywords: CAP, Atypical pathogens, Epidemiology

* Correspondence: stefano.aliberti@unimi.it
[1]Department of Pathophysiology and Transplantation, University of Milan, Internal Medicine Department, Respiratory unit and Adult Cystic Fibrosis Center, Fondazione IRCCS Ca' Granda Ospedale Maggiore Policlinico, Via Francesco Sforza 35, 20122 Milan, Italy

Background

Community-acquired pneumonia (CAP) is a leading cause of hospitalization and death worldwide [1]. The annual estimated CAP burden in the Unites States of America (USA) accounts for more than 1.5 million adult hospitalizations and one third of hospitalized patients die within 1 year [2]. The assessment of the epidemiology of CAP-related pathogens is crucial to target appropriate empiric therapy in order to improve patients' outcomes. The empirical coverage for atypical pathogens, including *Mycoplasma pneumoniae*, *Chlamydia pneumoniae*, and *Legionella pneumophila*, is still a matter of debate [3].

Several Authors reported on an increased trend of atypical pathogens over the last 15 years, with prevalences ranging from 6 to 40% in both Europe and USA [4]. One study performed in China showed atypical pathogens as the most frequent cause of CAP with incidence rates far exceeding *Streptococcus pneumoniae* [5]. Other studies described similar prevalences of atypical pathogens [6].

Epidemiological data are mainly based on retrospective studies or secondary analyses of local or national datasets with key design limitations, such as: 1) cultures for atypicals are rarely performed and a standardized diagnostic approach has not been adopted; 2) serology for atypical pathogens could be prescribed for epidemiological studies according to international guidelines and an all-encompassing microbiological work-up should be carried out only for hospitalized patients with severe CAP [1, 7]; 3) information on testing frequency of atypical pathogens and which population subgroups are more likely to be investigated are missing. Finally, the only published description on atypical pathogens in CAP is a secondary analysis of a retrospective database [6].

The aim of this study was to provide a real-life description of both testing frequency and prevalence of atypical pathogens in hospitalized patients with CAP worldwide, along with the evaluation of predisposing conditions for testing and risk factors for CAP caused by atypical pathogens.

Methods

Study design and population

The present study is based on a secondary analysis of the Global Initiative for MRSA Pneumonia (GLIMP) international database [8]. This project was not funded and relied upon voluntary site and investigator participation. The GLIMP methodology has been already published elsewhere [8]. The coordinating center (University of Texas Health at San Antonio –UT Health-, Texas, USA) received project approval by the Institutional Review Board (IRB# HSC20150184E). All participating centers followed their local law and regulations. Study participants were enrolled on a single day in the months of March, April, May, and June in 2015.

All adults (> 18 years old) hospitalized with CAP were screened for study selection. CAP was defined by the evidence of new radiological pulmonary infiltrates during the first 48 h of hospitalization and by ≥1 of the following criteria: 1) new or increased cough with/without sputum production and/or purulent respiratory secretions; 2) fever (documented rectal or oral temperature ≥ 37.8 °C) or hypothermia (documented rectal or oral temperature < 36 °C); 3) systemic inflammation (e.g., white blood cell count > 10,000/cm^3 or < 4000/cm^3, C-reactive protein or procalcitonin values above the local upper limit of normality). Patients hospitalized with a diagnosis of hospital-acquired and/or ventilator-associated pneumonia were excluded. Patients without any bacterial tests for atypical pathogens collected within 24 h after hospital admission were also excluded.

Data collection and microbiology for atypical pathogens

Data were collected using REDCap™ (Research Electronic Data Capture), an electronic data capture tool hosted on the UT Health server. After study enrolment, participating centers were allowed 7 days to complete electronic data entry and confirm microbiological results.

Physicians taking care of CAP patients decided the microbiological work-up according to local standard operating procedures. Serology for atypical pathogens and urinary antigen test for *L. pneumophila* were performed by local hospital laboratories according to standard techniques. Atypical pathogens were considered: *M. pneumoniae*, *C. pneumoniae*, and *L. pneumophila*.

Study groups

Definition of CAP caused by atypical pathogens was based on species-specific serology or urinary antigen positivity. Patients tested for atypical pathogens were defined as having at least one of the following tests: urinary antigen test for *L. pneumophila*, serology for *L. Pneumophila*, *C. pneumoniae*, and *M. pneumoniae*.

Study definitions

CAP was deemed severe when patients were prescribed one of the following interventions: intensive care unit (ICU) admission, invasive or non-invasive mechanical ventilation, or vasopressor/inotrope administration during the first 24 h after hospital admission.

Definition of immunodepression was based on the diagnosis of ≥1of the following medical conditions in the six-month period before hospital admission: hematological malignancy, asplenia, aplastic anemia, neutropenia, long-term exposure to biological drugs or steroids or chemotherapy or immunosuppressive therapy for hematological/solid organ transplantation other than lung transplant, HIV/AIDS, and congenital or genetic immunodepression. All site investigators were provided with a protocol including the above-mentioned clinical definitions.

Statistical analysis

Testing frequency of atypical pathogens was calculated on all CAP patients in the dataset. Prevalence of an atypical pathogen was computed based on positive results of serology and/or urinary antigen test for *L. pneumophila* performed during the first 24 h of hospital stay. Categorical variables, expressed as absolute frequencies and percentages, were compared between groups using the Chi-squared test. Regressions analyses were performed to compare prevalence and compute odds ratios (OR) with their 95% confidence interval (CI); furthermore, theywere performed to assess the relationship between atypical pathogen-related pneumonia and demographic, epidemiological, and clinical variables. Circular relation analysis using the Chi-squared test was performed to compare the prevalence between countries and continents. Statistical significance when P was < 0.05. All statistical analyses were performed with IBM SPSS, Statistics for Mac, version 22.0, and STATA 13. Prevalence maps were created using Stat Planet software.

Results

Testing for atypical pathogens

A total of 3702 hospitalized CAP patients were recruited in 54 countries across 6 continents. Among them, 1250 (33.8%) patients were tested for atypical pathogens: 1186 (32.0%) for *L. pneumophila* (either urinary antigen or serology), 251 (6.8%) for *M. pneumoniae* (serology), and 228 (6.1%) for *C. pneumoniae* (serology). Distribution of testing frequencies across countries is showed in Fig. 1a.

The frequency of patients tested for atypicals was significantly higher in Europe in comparison with the rest of the world (46.0% VS. 12.7%, $P < 0.0001$). The lowest testing frequency was recorded in Africa and South America (5.8 and 5.0%, respectively). The highest frequencies of patients tested for atypicals in countries enrolling > 100 CAP patients were detected in Spain (70.8%), Italy (63.8%), Portugal (43.3%), Germany (23.1%), and USA (21.4%) (Table 1). Data on testing for *L. pneumophila*, *M. pneumoniae*, and *C. pneumoniae* are reported in the additional files (Additional file 1: Table A). Detection of *L. pneumophila* urinary antigen was the most prevalent test performed worldwide (32.0%).

The frequencies of patients tested for atypical pathogens were lower among those with severe CAP in comparison with those with non-severe CAP (30.5% VS. 35.0% for atypical pathogens other than *L. pneumophila*, $P = 0.009$; 28.3% VS. 33.5% for *L. pneumophila*, $P = 0.003$). *L. pneumophila* testing was lower in ICU patients. Univariate analysis comparing characteristics of tested and non-tested patients is reported in Table 3, column A.

Prevalence of atypical pathogens

At least one atypical pathogen was isolated in 63 (4.7%) patients out of those tested for atypicals. *L. pneumophila* was detected in 30 (2.5%), *M. pneumoniae* in 26 (10.3%), and *C. pneumoniae* in 8 (3.5%) patients. The prevalence of atypical pathogens ranged from 0.0 to 36.4% and from 0.0 to 66.7% across different continents and countries, see Fig. 1b. Italy showed the highest prevalence of atypical pathogens in comparison with the rest of the world (7.5% VS. 4.2%, $P = 0.022$), whereas Spain showed the lowest prevalence (2.2% VS. 6.5%, $P = 0.001$) (Table 2).

Patients with CAP caused by atypical pathogens were significantly younger, showed less cardiovascular, renal, and metabolic comorbidities in comparison with patients with CAP caused by other pathogens CAP (Table 3, column B and Table 4).

Discussion

This secondary analysis of the GLIMP database found that only a third of patients hospitalized for CAP were tested for atypical pathogens worldwide, with a large variability among continents and countries. Patients with severe CAP were less likely to be tested for all atypical pathogens. Furthermore, *L. pneumophila* testing frequency was lower in ICU patients. Among those tested for, the prevalence of CAP caused by atypical pathogens was low. Younger age, female gender, and having a less comorbidities (cardiovascular disease, chronic renal failure) were factors associated with CAP due to atypicals.

The most frequent test for atypical pathogens performed in hospitalized patients with CAP was the *Legionella* urinary antigen (32.0%), followed by *Legionella* serology, whereas frequency of serological testing for any atypical pathogens was very low (6.8 and 6.1% for *M. pneumoniae* and *C. pneumoniae*, respectively).

However, information on molecular biology was not retrieved in the GLIMP dataset based on missing recommendations by international guidelines [1, 7]. Although molecular techniques was found helpful in the diagnosis of CAP caused by *L. pneumophila*, findings from different studies showed that single available tests were not reliable for the detection of *M. pneumoniae* and *C. pneumoniae* in CAP patients [9–11]. In addition, molecular studies carried out in large population groups found financial limitations and lack of standardization [6, 12, 13]. Finally, these results are intended to be a real-life snapshot of what it is really done in different countries worldwide; we deem that it is unrealistic a worldwide shift to PCR techniques considering that data presented here suggest that even the most common and affordable test, the urinary antigen for *Legionella*, is not routinely prescribed.

One of the major implications of a poor standardized approach for atypical pathogen testing is the wide heterogeneity across continents and countries. In Europe,

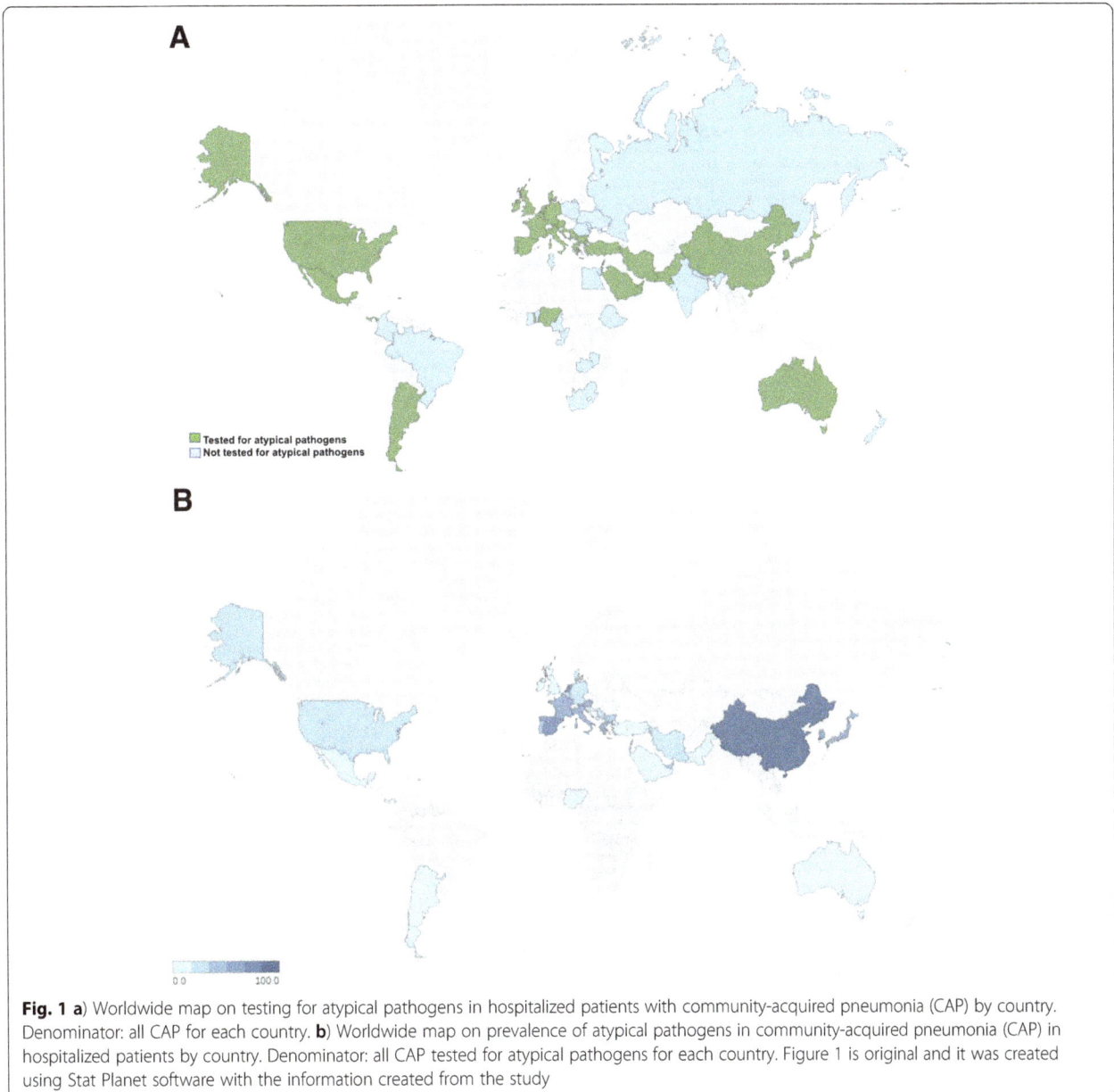

Fig. 1 a) Worldwide map on testing for atypical pathogens in hospitalized patients with community-acquired pneumonia (CAP) by country. Denominator: all CAP for each country. **b**) Worldwide map on prevalence of atypical pathogens in community-acquired pneumonia (CAP) in hospitalized patients by country. Denominator: all CAP tested for atypical pathogens for each country. Figure 1 is original and it was created using Stat Planet software with the information created from the study

almost half of the patients in the GLIMP database was investigated for atypical pathogens, thus resulting in the highest testing frequency. However, among European countries a significant variability was found. For example, the testing frequency was higher in the Mediterranean countries than in Northern Europe, ranging from 10.7% in United Kingdom to 70.8% in Spain. This significant difference may be caused by several factors, including the importance given to atypical pathogens in relation with national epidemiological reports and the lack of interest for this microbiological work-up in countries where extensive empirical therapy is routinely offered to patients. Interestingly, although large differences in frequencies of testing were found, prevalence of atypical pathogens seems to be quite similar in Europe, ranging from 1.6 to 6.5%, with the only exception of Italy and Spain.

Furthermore, our data did not suggest significant clinical differences between patients who underwent testing for atypical pathogens and those who did not. The recent guidelines for the management of CAP published by the European Respiratory Society suggest a comprehensive microbiological work-up in severe patients [1]. However, we found that severe CAP was not a relevant driver for testing. Same results were obtained for other severity indicators, such as ICU admission, invasive/non-invasive mechanical ventilation, and administration of vasopressors. The low frequency testing may be explained by the

Table 1 Testing frequency for atypical pathogens (all) in hospitalized patients with community-acquired pneumonia across different continents and countries

Continent/Country	Tested/Total (%)	Rest of the world Tested/Total (%)	P
Europe	1078/2344 (46%)	172/1358 (12.7%)	< 0.0001
North America	105/529 (19.8%)	1145/3173 (36.1%)	< 0.0001
Asia	44/415 (10.6%)	1206/3287 (36.7%)	< 0.0001
Oceania	3/40 (7.5%)	1247/3662 (34.1%)	< 0.0001
Africa	9/156 (5.8%)	1241/3546 (35%)	< 0.0001
South America	11/218 (5%)	1239/3484 (35.6%)	< 0.0001
Spain	455/643 (70.8%)	795/3059 (26%)	< 0.0001
Italy	293/459 (63.8%)	957/3243 (29.5%)	< 0.0001
Greece	54/87 (62.1%)	1196/3615 (33.1%)	< 0.0001
France	40/66 (60.6%)	1210/3636 (33.3%)	< 0.0001
Portugal	58/134 (43.3%)	1192/3568 (33.4%)	0.018
Bulgaria	21/51 (41.2%)	1229/3651 (33.7%)	0.260
Denmark	26/89 (29.2%)	1224/3613 (33.9%)	0.358
Germany	40/173 (23.1%)	1210/3529 (34.3%)	0.002
US	102/477 (21.4%)	1148/3225 (35.6%)	< 0.0001
Serbia	10/56 (17.9%)	1240/3646 (34%)	0.011
Croatia	16/103 (15.5%)	1234/3599 (34.3%)	< 0.0001
UK	20/186 (10.8%)	1230/3516 (35%)	< 0.0001
Argentina	11/190 (5.8%)	1239/3512 (35.3%)	< 0.0001
Pakistan	6/109 (5.5%)	1244/3593 (34.6%)	< 0.0001

recommendation of several guidelines on broad empirical coverage in severe patients [1, 14–16]. Notably, despite cost-effectiveness and ease of use of urinary antigen test, *L. pneumophila* testing frequency was also lower in ICU patients. These data are consistent with those showed by Singanayagam who demonstrated that pneumonia severity scores, such as PSI and CURB-65, are poor predictors of microbial etiology and that atypical pathogens are more prevalent in patients with less disease severity at their presentation [17].

The present study showed that the estimated prevalence of atypical pathogens in hospitalized CAP patients is low during a non-epidemic season (i.e., from March to June).

Table 2 Prevalence of atypical pathogens in hospitalized patients with community-acquired pneumonia across different continents

Continent	Tested/Total (%)	Rest of the world Tested/Total (%)	P
Africa	2/9 (22.2%)	60/1241 (4.8%)	0.070
Asia	2/44 (4.5%)	60/1206 (5%)	1
Europe	50/1078 (4.6%)	12/172 (7%)	0.091
North America	6/105 (5.7%)	56/1145 (4.9%)	0.922
Oceania	0/3 (0%)	62/1247 (5%)	1
South America	5/11 (45%)	57/1239 (4.6%)	0.001

The proportional distribution was heterogeneous and the majority of the reported cases were from Europe. Intercontinent differences suggest that prevalence is lower in Africa and South America. *L. pneumophila* and *M. pneumoniae* seem to be the most frequent pathogens worldwide. The prevalence of *M. pneumoniae* is highest in South America, whereas *L. pneumophila* did show a homogeneous geographical distribution. *L. pneumophila* prevalence was similar to that recorded by Viasus (5.4% among 3934 immunocompetent hospitalized CAP patients after a 15-year study) [18]. Conversely, our data might underestimate the high incidence of legionellosis (12%) in the US population as previously reported by Vergis [19].

The CAPO database reported on a prevalence for atypical pathogens ranging from 20 to 28% across 21 countries over a five-year period (epidemic seasons included) [6]. The Authors performed a very comprehensive microbiological work-up including PCR for atypicals for the majority of CAP patients, but it is unclear the proportion of cases diagnosed by serological or molecular techniques. National and regional epidemiological reports showed a prevalence ranging from 9 to 50% [20–24]. Singanayagam and Coworkers recently published a secondary analysis of four independent prospective CAP datasets with atypical pathogens accounting for a global frequency of 14% in patients with identified microbiological positivity [17]. Interestingly, most of these

Table 3 Clinical characteristics of tested and non-tested patients for both all atypical pathogens and L. pneumophila (column A) and of patients with community-acquired pneumonia caused and not caused by atypical pathogen (column B)

Variables	Column A			Column B		
	Tested patients (N = 1250)	Non-tested patients (N = 2452)	P	Atypical pathogen CAP (N = 63)	Non-atypical pathogen CAP (N = 1187)	P
Demographic characteristics						
Age, years	68 (46–75)	70 (51–81)	0.43	62 (43–72)	71 (56–81)	0.015
Male, n (%)	714 (57)	1459 (59)	0.83	27 (43)	687 (58)	0.027
Underweight, n (%)	56 (4.5)	110 (4.5)	0.36	3 (4.8)	53 (4.5)	1
Obesity, n (%)	208 (16.6)	369 (15)	0.21	11 (17.4)	197 (16.6)	0.811
Respiratory past medical history						
Active lung cancer, s (%)	27 (2.2)	82 (3.3)	0.50	0 (0)	27 (2.3)	0.64
Asthma, n (%)	85 (6.8)	176 (7.2)	0.73	3 (4.8)	82 (6.9)	0.79
Bronchiectasis, n (%)	61 (4.9)	117 (4.6)	0.87	1 (1.6)	60 (5)	0.36
Chronic aspiration, n (%)	71 (5.7)	186 (7.6)	0.03	0 (0)	71 (6)	0.45
COPD, n (%)	327 (26.2)	609 (24.8)	0.38	14 (22.2)	313 (26.3)	0.51
FEV1 ≤ 30%, n (%)	27 (2.2)	73 (3)	0.16	0 (0)	27 (2.2)	0.64
Current/former smoker, n (%)	427 (34.2)	818 (33.4)	0.63	18 (28.5)	409 (34.4)	0.382
Interstitial lung disease, n (%)	34 (2.7)	61 (2.5)	0.66	1 (1.6)	33 (2.8)	1
Obstructive sleep apnea, n (%)	51 (4.1)	79 (3.2)	0.19	0 (0)	51 (4.3)	0.17
Oxygen therapy at home, n (%)	83 (6.6)	141 (5.7)	0.30	4 (6.4)	79 (6.6)	1
Lung transplantation, n (%)	1 (0.8)	6 (0.2)	0.44	0 (0)	1 (0.8)	1
Tracheostomy, n (%)	15 (1)	38 (1.5)	0.45	0 (0)	15 (1.3)	1
Cardiovascular past medical history						
Arrhythmia, n (%)	218 (17.4)	309 (12.6)	< 0.001	11 (17.7)	207 (17.4)	0.947
Coronary artery disease, n (%)	178 (14.2)	345 (14.1)	0.88	3 (4.8)	175 (14.7)	0.030
Heart failure, n (%)	88 (7)	210 (8.2)	0.26	2 (3.2)	86 (7.2)	0.312
Hypertension, n (%)	183 (14.6)	323 (13)	0.14	4 (6.5)	179 (14.4)	0.790
Chronic medications						
Inhaled corticosteroids use, n (%)	207 (16.6)	383 (15.6)	0.47	4 (6.5)	203 (17.1)	0.028
Proton Pump Inhibitor use, n (%)	401 (32)	627 (25.6)	< 0.001	17 (27.4)	384 (32.3)	0.423
Statins use, n (%)	285 (22.8)	470 (19.2)	0.011	9 (14.5)	276 (23.2)	0.111
Steroids use, n (%)	86 (6.8)	208 (8.5)	0.09	4 (6.5)	82 (6.9)	1
Chronic interventions						
Enteric tube feeding, n (%)	11 (0.88)	41 (1.7)	0.05	0 (0)	11 (1)	1
Haemodialysis, n (%)	12 (1)	40 (1.6)	0.11	0 (0)	12 (1)	1
Indwelling catheter, n (%)	18 (1.4)	61 (2.5)	0.04	2 (3.2)	16 (1.4)	0.22
Immunosuppressive conditions						
Active solid tumour, n (%)	88 (7)	199 (8.1)	0.27	1 (1.6)	87 (7.3)	0.12
HIV infection, n (%)	28 (2.24)	95 (3.9)	0.009	2 (3.2)	26 (2.2)	0.64
AIDS, n (%)	15 (1.2)	50 (2)	0.08	2 (3.2)	13 (1.1)	0.16
Aplastic anaemia, n (%)	6 (0.3)	8 (0.3)	0.57	0 (0)	6 (0.5)	1
Asplenia, n (%)	6 (0.3)	6 (0.2)	0.24	0 (0)	6 (0.5)	1
Biological drug use, n (%)	14 (1.1)	23 (0.9)	0.60	0 (0)	14 (1.2)	1
Chemotherapy in the last 3 months, n (%)	48 (3.8)	97 (3.8)	0.92	1 (1.6)	47 (4)	0.51
Haematological malignancy, n (%)	73 (5.8)	89 (3.6)	=0.003	2 (3.2)	71 (6)	0.57
Immunocompromised patients, n (%)	230 (18.4)	435 (17.7)	0.62	12 (19.4)	218 (18.4)	0.84

Table 3 Clinical characteristics of tested and non-tested patients for both all atypical pathogens and L. pneumophila (column A) and of patients with community-acquired pneumonia caused and not caused by atypical pathogen (column B) *(Continued)*

Variables	Column A			Column B		
	Tested patients (N = 1250)	Non-tested patients (N = 2452)	P	Atypical pathogen CAP (N = 63)	Non-atypical pathogen CAP (N = 1187)	P
Neutropenia, n (%)	13 (1.8)	35 (1.4)	0.36	0 (0)	13 (1.1)	1
Other chronic medical conditions						
Chronic renal failure, n (%)	144 (11.5)	256 (10.4)	0.31	2 (3.2)	142 (12)	0.036
Dementia, n (%)	136 (18.9)	272 (11.1)	0.87	5 (8.1)	131 (11)	0.46
Diabetes mellitus, n (%)	266 (21.3)	516 (21)	0.86	7 (11.3)	259 (21.8)	0.049
Liver disease, n (%)	59 (4.72)	81 (3.03)	0.36	4 (6.5)	55 (4.6)	0.53
Malnutrition, n (%)	95 (7.6)	0 (0)	0.08	4 (6.5)	91 (7.7)	1
Mental illness, n (%)	83 (6.6)	0 (0)	0.73	4 (6.5)	79 (6.6)	1
Prosthetic material, n (%)	41 (3.3)	75 (3)	0.76	1 (1.6)	40 (3.4)	0.71
Recurrent skin infections, n (%)	14 (1.1)	44 (1.8)	0.13	1 (1.6)	13 (1.1)	0.51
Other non-medical conditions						
Bedridden, n (%)	110 (8.8)	305 (12.4)	0.001	3 (4.8)	86 (7.2)	0.61
Contact sport, n (%)	1 (0.1)	5	0.67	0 (0)	1 (1)	1.0
Healthcare worker, n (%)	20 (1.6)	27 (1.1)	0.21	5 (7.9)	15 (1.3)	0.002
Homeless, n (%)	12 (1.8)	23 (0.9)	1.0	0 (0)	12 (1)	1
Living in crowded conditions, n (%)	236 (18.9)	485 (19.8)	0.54	0 (0)	9 (0.8)	1
Nursing home resident, n (%)	86 (6.88)	216 (8.8)	0.042	11 (17.7)	225 (18.9)	0.81
Chronic aspiration, n (%)	71 (5.7)	186 (7.6)	0.034	0 (0)	62 (5.3)	0.047
Previous infections/colonization						
Prior mycobacterial diseases, n (%)	31 (2.5)	65 (2.6)	0.82	3 (4.8)	28 (2.4)	0.19
Prior MRSA infection/colonisation, n (%)	30 (2.4)	56 (2.3)	0.82	0 (0)	30 (2.5)	0.39
Prior ESBL-producing bacterial infection, n (%)	21 (1.7)	34 (1.4)	0.48	1 (1.6)	20 (1.7)	1
Prior Pseudomonas spp. infection, n (%)	30 (2.4)	71 (2.9)	0.45	1 (1.6)	29 (2.4)	1
Current pneumonia episode						
Severe CAP, n (%)	314 (25.1)	716 (29.2)	0.009	21 (33)	293 (24.7)	0.103
ICU or HDU admission, n (%)	277 (22.2)	619 (25.2)	=0.039	18 (28)	259 (22)	0.181
Either invasive or non-invasive ventilation, n (%)	206 (16.5)	456 (17.9)	0.11	12 (19)	194 (16.3)	0.531
Invasive ventilation, n (%)	114 (9.1)	240 (9.4)	0.55	3 (4.8)	111 (9.3)	0.230
Non-invasive ventilation, n (%)	118 (9.4)	231 (9)	1	9 (14.3)	109 (9.1)	0.161

CAP; Community-acquired pneumonia, MRSA; Methicillin resistant Staphylococcus aureus, COPD; Chronic obstructive pulmonary disease, FEV$_1$; Forced expiratory volume during the first second, CAD; Coronary artery disease, ESBL; extended-spectrum beta-lactamases, LRTI; lower respiratory tract infections

studies suggested that atypical pathogens are more relevant in the outpatient population [17, 20–24].

The prevalence estimates on atypical microorganisms might be limited. Even if the combination of serology and molecular techniques was suggested to increase sensitivity, diagnostic tools only accounted on serology for atypical pathogens and urinary antigen for *Legionella* [1, 25]. Then, prevalence estimation can depend on frequency and comprehensiveness of the microbiological work-up.

Second, since patients have been enrolled on a single day in the months of March, April and May, most of data come from non-epidemic season in northern hemisphere, thus biasing a plausible estimation of atypical pathogen epidemiology.

However, the low testing frequency underscores the poor emphasis given by physicians or local health authorities to the role of atypicals. Therefore, the controversy on empiric coverage for atypical pathogens should be addressed after a more adequate description of the epidemiological burden and a sensitization of attending physicians.

Potential risk factors for atypical pathogens were also investigated. In this analysis cardiovascular disease as well as chronic renal failure act as protective factors for atypical etiology. Our understanding is that these results

Table 4 Protective factors for atypical pathogens in hospitalized patients with community-acquired pneumonia

	OR (95% CI)	P
Age	0.583 (0.350–0.973)	0.039
Cardiovascular disease	> 0.0001	< 0.0001
Diabetes mellitus	0.464 (0.207–1.043)	0.063
Chronic renal failure	0.203 (0.480–0.865)	0.031
Severe CAP	1.769 (0.516–3.073)	0.364
Mechanical ventilation	0.288 (0.810–1.031)	0.056
ICU admission	1.156 (0.311–4.294)	0.826

ICU: intensive care unit; OR: Odds ratio; CI: confidence interval

might be a function of age, being patients with atypical pneumonia younger than others.

Conclusions

In conclusion, this real-life study demonstrates that testing for atypical pathogens in hospitalized patients with CAP is not routinely performed worldwide.

Testing for atypical pathogens is poorly standardized and a wide inter-country heterogeneity was found. Testing rates could not appropriately describe prevalence of atypicals in different settings. Further studies are needed to better assess the epidemiological burden and the utility of the current microbiological and clinical recommendations.

Abbreviations
CAP: Community-acquired pneumonia; GLIMP: Global Initiative for MRSA Pneumonia; ICU: Intensive care unit

Acknowledgments
GLIMP investigators
Argentina—Patricia Karina Aruj (Department of Internal Medicine, University Hospital Alfredo Lanari, Buenos Aires, Argentina); Silvia Attorri (Hospital Luis Lagomaggiore, Mendoza, Argentina); Enrique Barimboim (Hospital Central de Mendoza, Argentina); Juan Pablo Caeiro, María I Garzón (Hospital Privado Universitario, Córdoba, Argentina); Victor Hugo Cambursano (V H Dr Cazaux A Servicio de Neumologia, Hospital Rawson, Córdoba, Argentina); Adrian Ceccato (Hospital Nacional Prof Alejandro Posadas, Argentina); Julio Chertcoff , Florencia Lascar, Fernando Di Tulio (Critical Care Unit and Respiratory Medicine, Buenos Aires British Hospital, Buenos Aires, Argentina); Ariel Cordon Díaz (Hospital General Alvear, Ciudad, Mendoza, Argentina); Lautaro de Vedia (Respiratory Intensive Care Unit, Hospital Muñiz, Buenos Aires, Argentina); Maria Cristina Ganaha (Infectious Diseases Ward, Hospital Interzonal General de Agudos, Vicente Lopez y Planes from General Rodriguez, Buenos Aires, Argentina); Sandra Lambert (Hospital El Cruce - Alta Complejidad en Red, Argentina); Gustavo Lopardo, Hospital Bernardo Houssay, Vicente López, Argentina); Carlos M Luna (Pulmonary Medicine Division, Department of Medicine, Hospital de Clínicas, Universidad de Buenos Aires, Argentina); Alessio Gerardo Malberti (Hospital Nuestra Señora del Carmen, Argentina); Nora Morcillo and Silvina Tartara (Hospital Zonal Especializado de Agudos y Crónicos Dr Antonio A Cetrangolo, Argentina); Claudia Pensotti (Infectious Diseases and Infection Control Department, Buenos Aires, Clinica Privada Monte Grande, Argentina); Betiana Pereyra (Hospital San Roque, Córdoba, Argentina); Pablo Gustavo Scapellato (Infectious Diseases Department, Hospital D F Santojanni, Argentina); Juan Pablo Stagnaro (HZGA Mi Pueblo, Florencio Varela, Argentina). Australia—Sonali Shah (Department of General Medicine, Austin Hospital, Heidelberg, Australia).

Austria–Felix Lötsch, Florian Thalhammer (Division of Infectious Diseases and Tropical Medicine, Department of Medicine I, Medical University of Vienna, Austria). Belgium—Jean Louis Vincent (Department of Intensive Care, Erasme University Hospital, Université Libre de Bruxelles, Brussels, Belgium); Kurt Anseeuw (ZNA Campus Stuivenberg, Antwerp, Belgium); Camille A Francois (Anesthesia and critical care department, Erasme university hospital, Brussels, Belgium); Eva Van Braeckel (Department of Respiratory Medicine, Ghent University Hospital, Ghent, Belgium). Benin—Marcel Zannou Djimon, Jules Bashi, Dodo Roger (Centre Hospitalier Universitaire HKM of Cotonou, Benin). Brazil—Simone Aranha Nouér (Federal University of Rio de Janeiro, Rio de Janeiro, Brazil). Bulgaria—Peter Chipev, Milena Encheva (Clinic of Pulmonary Diseases, Military Medical Academy, Sofi a, Bulgaria); Darina Miteva (UMHAT "St. Marina", Varna, Bulgaria); Diana Petkova (University Hospital Varna, Bulgaria. Cameroon—Balkissou Adamou Dodo (Yaounde Jamot Hospital, Yaounde, Cameroon); Mbatchou Ngahane Bertrand Hugo (Douala General Hospital, Douala, Cameroon). China—Ning Shen (Respiratory Medicine, Peking University Third Hospital, Beijing, China); Jin-fu Xu, (Department of Respiratory Medicine, Shanghai Pulmonary Hospital, Tongji University, China). Colombia— Carlos Andres Bustamante Rico, Ricardo Buitrago (Clinica Shaio, Bogota, Colombia); Fernando Jose Pereira Paternina (Las Americas Clinic, Medellin, Colombia). Congo—Kayembe Ntumba Jean-Marie (Cliniques Universitaires de Kinshasa, DR Congo). Croatia—Vesna Vladic Carevic (Interne Medicine, Dubrovnik, Croatia); Marko Jakopovic (Medical School, University of Zagreb, Department for Respiratory Diseases Jordanovac, University Hospital Centre Zagreb, Zagreb, Croatia); Mateja Jankovic (University Hospital Center Zagreb, Department for Respiratory Diseases, Zagreb, Croatia); Zinka Matkovic (University Hospital Dubrava, Zagreb, Croatia); Ivan Mitrecic (Karlovac general hospital, Karlovac, Croatia). Denmark—Marie-Laure Bouchy Jacobsson (Emergency Department in North Zealand Hospital – Hillerød, Denmark); Anette Bro Christensen (Department of Anaethesiology, Viborg Region Hospital, Denmark); Uff e Christian HeitmannBødtger (Department of Pulmonology, Naestved Hospital, Denmark); Christian Niels Meyer (Department of Internal Medicine, Roskilde Hospital, Copenhagen University Hospital, Roskilde, Denmark); Andreas Vestergaard Jensen, Gertrud Baunbæk-knudsen, Pelle Trier Petersen and Stine Andersen (Department of Lung and Infectious Diseases, Nordsjællands Hospital-Hillerød, Denmark). Egypt—Ibrahim El-Said Abd El-Wahhab (Thoracic Medicine, Faculty of Medicine, Mansoura University, Egypt); Nesreen Elsayed Morsy (Pulmonary, Critical Care and Sleep Medicine, Faculty of Medicine, Mansoura University, Mansoura, Egypt); Hanaa Shafi ek (Chest diseases department, Faculty of Medicine, Alexandria University, Egypt); Eman Sobh (Chest Diseases Department, Al-Azhar University, Cairo, Egypt). France— Fabrice Bertrand (Critical care Unit, Robert Ballanger Hospital, Aulnay sous Bois, France); Christian Brun- Buisson (Univ Hospital Henri Mondor, 94000 Créteil, France); Etienne de Montmollin (Intensive care unit, Hôpital Delafontaine, Centre hospitalier de Saint-Denis, Saint-Denis, France); Muriel Fartoukh (Unité de réanimation médico-chirurgicale, Pôle Thorax Voies aériennes, Hôpital Tenon, Groupe Hospitalier Est Parisien, France); Jonathan Messika (Publique-Hôpital de Paris, Service de Réanimation Médicochirurgicale, Hôpital Louis Mourier, Colombes, France, and Université Paris Diderot, IAME, UMR 1137, Sorbonne Paris Cité, Paris, France); Pierre Tattevin (Infectious Diseases & ICU, Pontchaillou University Hospital, Rennes, France). Germany—Michael Dreher (Department of Cardiology, Pneumology, Vascular Medicine and Intensive Care Medicine, University Hospital Aachen, Aachen, Germany); Martin Kolditz (Division of Pulmonology, Medical Department I, University Hospital Carl Gustav Carus, Technische Universität Dresden, Germany); Matthias Meisinger (Klinikum Niederlausitz GmbH, Klinik für Innere Medizin und Intensivmedizin, Senftenberg, Germany); Mathias W Pletz and Stefan Hagel (Center for Infectious Diseases and Infection Control, Jena University Hospital, Germany); Jan Rupp (Department of Molecular and Infectious Diseases, University of Lübeck, Lübeck, Germany); Tom Schaberg (Zentrum für Pneumologie, Agaplesion Diakonieklinikum Rotenburg, Germany); Marc Spielmanns (Internal Medicine Department, Pulmonary rehabilitation and Department of Health, School of Medicine, University Witten- Herdecke, St Remigius-Hospital, Leverkusen, Germany). Ghana—Beatrice Siaw-Lartey (Komfo-Anokye Teaching Hospital, Kumasi, Ghana). Greece—Katerina Dimakou (5th Rerpiratory Medicine Dpt, "SOTIRIA" Chest Hospital, Athens, Greece); Dimosthenis Papapetrou

(Medical Group of Athens, Paleo Faliro Clinic, Athens, Greece); Evdoxia Tsigou and Dimitrios Ampazis, Agioi Anargiroi Hospital, Kifi ssia, Athens, Greece). India—Mohit Bhatia (S S Hospital IMS BHU Varanasi, India); Raja Dhar (Fortis Hospitals, Kolkata, India); George D'Souza (Department of Pulmonary Medicine, St John's Medical College Hospital, Bangalore, India); Rajiv Garg (Department of Respiratory Medicine, King George's Medical University UP, Lucknow, India); Parvaiz A Koul (Department of Internal & Pulmonary Medicine, SheriKashmir Institute of Medical Sciences, Srinagar, India); P A Mahesh and B S Jayaraj (Department of Pulmonary Medicine, JSS Medical College, JSS University, Mysore, India); Kiran Vishnu Narayan (Pulmonary Medicine, Government Medical College Kozhikode, Kerala, India); Hirennappa B Udnur and Shashi Bhaskara Krishnamurthy (Columbia Asia Hospital, Hebbal, Bengaluru, Karnataka, India). Iran—Keihan Golshani (Isfahan University of Medical Sciences, Iran). Ireland—Vera M Keatings (Letterkenny General Hospital, Co. Donegal, Ireland); Ignacio Martin-Loeches (Multidisciplinary Intensive Care Research Organization (MICRO), St James's University Hospital, Trinity Centre for Health Sciences Dublin, Ireland). Israel—Yasmin Maor (Infectious Disease Unit, Affi liated to Tel Aviv University, Wolfson Medical Center, Holon, Israel); Jacob Strahilevitz (Department of Clinical Microbiology & Infectious Diseases, Hadassah-Hebrew University, Jerusalem, Israel). Italy—Salvatore Battaglia (University of Palermo, Pneumologia DiBiMIS, Palermo, Italy); Maria Carrabba (Internal Medicine Department, Fondazione IRCCS Ca' Granda Ospedale Maggiore Policlinico, Milano, Italy); Piero Ceriana (Pulmonary rehabilitation, IRCCS Fondazione Maugeri, Pavia Italy); Marco Confalonieri (Department of Pulmunology, University Hospital, Trieste, Italy); Antonella d'Arminio Monforte (Department of Health Sciences, Clinic of Infectious Disease, San Paolo Hospital, University of Milan, Italy); Bruno Del Prato (Interventional Pneumology, Hospital Antonio Cardarelli, Naples, Italy); Marino De Rosa (UOC Pneumologia San Filippo Neri ASL RM E, Rome, Italy); Riccardo Fantini (Respiratory Diseases Clinic, Policlinico di Modena, Modena, Italy); Giuseppe Fiorentino (UOC Fisiopatologia e Riabilitazione Respiratoria AO Ospedali dei Colli PO, Monaldi, Italy); Maria Antonia Gammino (Pulmonary Medicine Unit, San Martino Hospital, ASL 5 Oristano, Sardegna, Italy); Francesco Menzella (Department of Cardiac-Thoracic-Vascular and Intensive Care Medicine, Pneumology Unit, IRCCS-Arcispedale Santa Maria Nuova, Reggio Emilia, Italy); Giuseppe Milani (Azienda Ospedaliera Sant Anna di Como, Presidio Ospedale S Anna Nuovo, Unità Operativa di Pneumologia, Como, Italy); Stefano Nava (Alma Mater University of Bologna, DIMES, Respiratory and Critical Care Unit Sant'Orsola Malpighi Hospital, Italy); Gerardo Palmiero (Respiratory Unity, Versilia Hospital, Azienda USL 12 Viareggio, Lido di Camaiore, Lucca, Italy); Roberta Petrino and Barbra Gabrielli (Emergency Medicine Unit, S. Andrea Hospital, Vercelli, Italy); Paolo Rossi (Internal Medicine Department, Azienda Ospedaliero-Universitaria S. Maria della Misericordia, Udine, Italy); Claudio Sorino (Pulmonology Unit, AO Sant'Anna di Como, Italy); Gundi Steinhilber (Spedali Civili Brescia, UO Pneumologia e Fisiopatologia Respiratoria, Brescia, Italy); Alessandro Zanforlin (ULSS 18 Rovigo, Ospedale San Luca, Trecenta, Italy). Japan—Kiyoyasu Kurahashi (Yokohama City University Medical Center, Japan). Lebanon—Zeina Aoun Bacha (Medicine school, St Joseph University, Beyrouth, Lebanon). Mexico—Daniel Barajas Ugalde (National Institute of Respiratory Diseases, Mexico); Omar Ceballos Zuñiga (Hospital General de Mexicali, Mexicali, Baja California, Mexico); José F Villegas (Hospital Universitario Monterrey, México). Montenegro—Milic Medenica, Hospital for Lung Diseases—Brezovik, Niksic, Montenegro). Netherlands—E M W van de Garde (Dept. Clinical Pharmacy, St Antonius Hospital, Utrecht/Nieuwegein, Netherlands). Nepal—Deebya Raj Mihsra (Internal Medicine, BP Koirala Institute of Health Sciences, Nepal); Poojan Shrestha, Oxford University Clinical Research Unit, Patan Hospital, Nepal). New Zealand—Elliott Ridgeon (Medical Research Institute of New Zealand). Nigeria—Babatunde Ishola Awokola (Department of Family Medicine & Primary Care, Lily Hospitals Limited, Warri, Nigeria); Ogonna N O Nwankwo (University of Calabar Teaching Hospital, Calabar, Nigeria); Adefuye Bolanle Olufunlola (Olabisi Onabanjo University teaching hospital, Sagamu, Ogun State, Nigeria); Segaolu Olumide (Department of Medicine, Pulmonary Unit, University College Hospital, Ibadan, Nigeria); Kingsley N Ukwaja (Department of Medicine, Federal Teaching Hospital

Abakaliki, Ebonyi State, Nigeria). Pakistan—Muhammad Irfan (Section of Pulmonary and Critical Care Medicine, Department of Medicine, Aga Khan University, Karachi, Pakistan). Poland—Lukasz Minarowski (Department of Lung Diseaes and Tuberculosis, Medical University of Bialystok, Poland); Skoczyński Szymon (Department of Pneumology, School of Medicine in Katowice, Medical University of Silesia, Katowice, Institute of Occupational Medicine and Environmental Health, Sosnowiec, Poland). Portugal—Felipe Froes (Hospital Pulido Valente - CHLN, Lisboa, Portugal); Pedro Leuschner (Centro Hospitalar do Porto, Porto, Portugal); Mariana Meireles, Cláudia Ferrão, Pedro Leuschner and João Neves (Serviço de Medicina, Centro Hospitalar do Porto, Largo, Abel Salazar, Porto, Portugal); Sofi a B Ravara (Faculty of Health Sciences, University of Beira Interior; Cova da Beira Hospital Center, Covilhã, Portugal). Moldova—Victoria Brocovschii (Department of Pneumology & Allergology, State University of Medicine and Pharmacy "Nicolae Testemitanu", Moldova); Chesov Ion (Clinic of Anesthesia and Intensive Care "Valeriu Ghrerg", Institute of Emergency Medicine, State University of Medicine and Pharmacy "Nicolae Testemitanu", Chisinau, Moldova); Doina Rusu (SMFU "N Testemitanu", Chisinau, Moldova); Cristina Toma (Department of Pneumology & Allergology, State University of Medicine and Pharmacy "Nicolae Testemitanu", Chisinau, Moldova). Romania—Daniela Chirita (Hospital Sfantul Stefan, Bucharest, Romania). Russia—Alexei Birkun (Department of Anesthesiology, Critical Care and Emergency Medicine, Medical Academy named after S I Georgievsky, Russia); Anna Kaluzhenina (Volgograd State Medical University, Russia). Saudi Arabia—Abdullah Almotairi (King Fahad medical City (KFMC), Riyadh, Saudi Arabia); Zakeya Abdulbaqi Ali Bukhary (College of Medicine, Taibah University, Medina, Saudi Arabia); Jameela Edathodu (Al Faisal University, King Faisal Specialist Hospital, Riyadh, Saudi Arabia); Amal Fathy (Pulmonary and respiratory critical care Medicine, Mansoura University Egypt, Affi liate at Taibah University, Saudi Arabia); Abdullah Mushira Abdulaziz Enani and Nazik Eltayeb Mohamed (Infectious Diseases Section, Medical Specialties Department, King Fahad Medical City, Riyadh, Saudi Arabia); Jawed Ulhadi Memon (Pulmonology Division, Department of Internal Medicine, King Fahad Hospital, Hofuf, Al Ahasa, 31982, Saudi Arabia). Serbia—Nada Bogdanović (Pulmonary department of KHC Dr Dragiša Mišović, Belgrade, Serbia); Branislava Milenkovic (Clinic for Pulmonary Diseases, Clinical Centre of Serbia, Faculty of Medicine, University of Belgrade, Belgrade, Serbia); Dragica Pesut (University of Belgrade School of Medicine, Teaching Hospital of Pulmonology, Clinical Centre of Serbia, Belgrade, Serbia). Spain—Luis Borderìas, Respiratoy and Sleep Unit, Hospital San Jorge, Huesca, Spain); Noel Manuel Bordon Garcia (Barcelona Policlínic and Moises Broggi Hospital at sant Joan Despí, Spain); Hugo Cabello Alarcón, Sant Hospital Seu de Urgell, Catalonia, Spain); Catia Cilloniz and Antoni Torres (Department of Pneumology, Institut Clinic del Tórax, Hospital Clinic of Barcelona - Institut d'Investigacions Biomèdiques August Pi i Sunyer (IDIBAPS), University of Barcelona, Ciber de Enfermedades Respiratorias (CIBERES), Spain); Vicens Diaz-Brito and Xavier Casas (Infectious diseases Unit and Pneumology Service, Parc Sanitari Sant Joan de Deu, Sant Boi, Barcelona, Spain); Alicia Encabo González (Hospital Complex of Pontevedra, Spain); Maria Luisa FernándezAlmira (Medicina Interna, Hospital Universitario Central de Asturias, Spain); Miguel Gallego (Department of Respiratory Medicine, Hospital de Sabadell, Institut Universitari Parc Taulí-UAB, Sabadell, Spain. CIBER de Enfermedades Respiratorias, CIBERES, Bunyola, Spain); Inmaculada Gaspar-García (Department of Respiratory Medicine, Hospital Costa del Sol, Marbella, Málaga, Spain); Juan González del Castillo (Emergency Department, Hospital Universitario Clínico San Carlos, Madrid, Spain); Patricia Javaloyes Victoria (Hospital General Universitario de Alicante, Alicante, Spain); Elena Laserna Martínez (Hospital Mollet, Barcelona, Spain); Rosa Malo de Molina (University Hospital Puerta de Hierro Majadahonda, Madrid); Pedro J Marcos (Servicio de Neumología, Complejo Hospitalario Universitario de A Coruña CHUAC, INIBIC, Sergas, Universidade de A Coruña, Spain); Rosario Menéndez (Pneumology Service, Universitary and Polytechnic Hospital La Fe, Valencia, Spain); Ana Pando-Sandoval (Hospital Universitario Central de Asturias. Area de Gestion Clinica de Pulmon. Servicio de Neumologia, Oviedo, Spain); Cristina Prat Aymerich, Alicia Lacoma del la Torre, and Ignasi García-Olivé

(Microbiology Department and Pneumology Department, Hospital Universitari Germans Trias i Pujol, Institut d'Investigació Germans Trias i Pujol, Badalona, Spain; Universitat Autònoma de Barcelona; CIBER Enfermedades Respiratorias, Instituto de Salud Carlos III, Spain); Jordi Rello and Silvia Moyano (Critical Care Department, Hospital Vall d'Hebron, Barcelona, Spain); Francisco Sanz (Servicio de Neumología, Consorci Hospital General Universitari de Valencia, Valencia, Spain); Oriol Sibila and Ana Rodrigo-Troyano (Servei de Pneumologia, Hospital de la Santa Creu i Sant Pau, IIB-Sant Pau, Barcelona, Spain); Jordi Solé-Violán (Hospital Universitario de Gran Canaria Dr Negrín, Las Palmas de Gran Canaria, Spain); Ane Uranga (Pulmology Department, Hospital of Galdakao-Usansolo, Spain); Job FM van Boven (Hospital Universitari Son Espases, Palma de Mallorca, Spain); Ester Vendrell Torra and Jordi Almirall Pujol (Intensive Care Medicine, Hospital de Mataró, Spain). South Africa—Charles Feldman (Division of Pulmonology, Department of Internal Medicine, Charlotte Maxeke Johannesburg Academic Hospital, Faculty of Health Sciences, University of the Witwatersrand, Johannesburg, South Africa). South Korea—Ho Kee Yum (Inje Univ. Seoul Paik Hospital, South Korea). Togo—Arnauld Attannon Fiogbe (Pulmonology and Infectious Diseases Service/University hospital of Sylvanus Olympio, Lomé, Togo). Tunisia—Ferdaous Yangui (Department of Pneumology, Hospital of Internal Forces Security (I.F.S), Marsa, Tunis, Tunisia). Turkey—Semra Bilaceroglu (Izmir Dr Suat Seren Training and Research Hospital for Thoracic Medicine and Surgery, Izmir, Turkey); Levent Dalar (Pulmonary Medicine, Istanbul Bilim University, Istanbul, Turkey); Ufuk Yilmaz (Suat Seren Chest Disease and Surgery Training and Research Hospital, İzmir, Turkey). Ukraine—Artemii Bogomolov (Vinnitsa National Pirogov Memorial Medical University, Vinnitsa regional antituberculosis hospital, Vinnitsa, Ukraine). United Arab Emirates—Naheed Elahi (Dubai Hospital, UAE.); UK—Devesh J Dhasmana (Victoria Hospital, Kirkcaldy, NHS Fife, UK); Rhiannon Ions, Julie Skeemer, and Gerrit Woltmann (University Hospitals of Leicester NHS Trust and University of Leicester, Leicester, UK); Carole Hancock (Royal Respiratory Research Team, Royal Liverpool University Hospital, Liverpool, UK); Adam T Hill (Royal Infirmary and University of Edinburgh, UK); Banu Rudran (The Royal London Hospital, Barts Health Trust, London, UK); Silvia Ruiz-Buitrago and Marion Campbell (Hairmyres Hospital, Eaglesham Road, East Kilbride, UK); Paul Whitaker (Department of Respiratory Medicine, St James's Hospital, Leeds, UK). USA—Karen S Allen (University of Oklahoma Health Sciences Center, OK, USA); Veronica Brito (Texas A&M Health Science Center, Division of Pulmonary, Critical Care and Sleep Medicine Baylor Scott & White Health, TX, USA); Jessica Dietz (Fargo VA Health Care System, Fargo, ND, USA); Claire E Dysart and Susan M Kellie (Clement J Zablocki VA Medical Center, Milwaukee, WI, USA, Division of Infectious Diseases, University of New Mexico School of Medicine, Raymond G Murphy VA Medical Center, Albuquerque, NM, USA); Ricardo A Franco-Sadud and Garnet Meier (Division of Hospital Medicine, Cook County Hospital, Chicago, MI, USA); Mina Gaga (7th Resp Med Dept and Asthma Center, Athens Chest Hospital, USA); Thomas L Holland and Stephen P Bergin (Department of Medicine, Duke University Medical Center and School of Medicine, Duke Clinical Research Institute, NC, USA); Fayez Kheir (Department Pulmonary Diseases, Critical Care & Environmental Medicine, Tulane University Health Sciences Center, New Orleans, LA, USA); Mark Landmeier (Division of Pulmonary and Critical Care Medicine, Northwestern Memorial Hospital, Chicago, IL, USA); Manuel Lois (John Peter Smith Hospital, Fort Worth, TX, USA); Girish B Nair (Interstitial Lung Disease Program and Pulmonary Rehabilitation, SUNY Stony Brook Winthrop University Hospital, Mineola, NY, USA); Hemali Patel (Department of Medicine, Division of General Internal Medicine, Hospital Medicine Group, University of Colorado, USA); Katherine Reyes (Henry Ford Hospital, Detroit, IL, USA); William Rodriguez-Cintron (Pulmonary/Critical Care Medicine VA Caribbean Healthcare System, USA); Shigeki Saito (Tulane University, New Orleans, USA); Nilam J Soni, Julio Noda, Cecilia I Hinojosa, Stephanie M Levine, Luis F Angel, and Antonio Anzueto (Divisions of Hospital Medicine & Pulmonary/Critical Care Medicine, South Texas Veterans Health Care System, University of Texas Health Science Center San Antonio, San Antonio, TX, USA); K Scott Whitlow, John Hipskind, and Kunal Sukhija (Kaweah Delta Health Care District, Department of Emergency Medicine,

Visalia, CA, USA); Richard G. Wunderink and Ray D Shah (Northwestern University Feinberg School of Medicine, Chicago, IL, USA). Zambia—Kondwelani John Mateyo (Department of Internal Medicine, University Teaching Hospital, Lusaka, Zambia).

Funding
The authors did not receive any funding for this study.

Authors' contributions
AG, SA and GS analyzed the dataset. AG, SA, GS, MDP, DR and ST interpreted the patient data. LFR took charge of Figs. EV, JN, FM, FB and MIR along with all the auothors read and approved the final manuscript.

Consent for publication
Not applicable.

Competing interests
The authors declare that they have no competing interests for this study.

Author details
[1]Department of Pathophysiology and Transplantation, University of Milan, Internal Medicine Department, Respiratory unit and Adult Cystic Fibrosis Center, Fondazione IRCCS Ca' Granda Ospedale Maggiore Policlinico, Via Francesco Sforza 35, 20122 Milan, Italy. [2]Clinical Epidemiology and Medical Statistics Unit, Department of Clinical and Experimental Medicine, University of Sassari, Sassari, Italy. [3]Department of Biomedical and Clinical Sciences (DIBIC), University of Milan, Section of Respiratory Diseases, Ospedale L. Sacco, ASST Fatebenefratelli-Sacco, Milan, Italy. [4]Respiratory Unit, San Paolo Hospital, Department of Medical Sciences, University of Milan, Milan, Italy. [5]Division of Pulmonary Diseases and Critical Care Medicine, The University of Texas Health Science Center at San Antonio, San Antonio, TX, USA. [6]Intensive Care Unit, Hospital de Mataró, Consorci Sanitari del Maresme, Carretera de Cirera s/n, 08304 Mataró, Barcelona, Spain. [7]Internal Medicine Department, Centro Hospitalar do Porto, Porto, Portugal. [8]Department of Medical Specialties, Pneumology Unit, IRCCS Arcispedale Santa Maria Nuova, Azienda USL Reggio Emilia, Italy.

References
1. Mandell LA, Wunderink RG, Anzueto A, et al. Infectious Diseases Society of America; American Thoracic Society. Infectious Diseases Society of America/American Thoracic Society consensus guidelines on the management of community-acquired pneumonia in adults. Clin Infect Dis. 2007;44(suppl 2):S27–72.
2. Ramirez JA, Wiemken TL, Peyrani P, Arnold FW, Kelley R, Mattingly WA, Nakamatsu R, Pena S, Guinn BE, Furmanek SP, Persaud AK, Raghuram A, Fernandez F, Beavin L, Bosson R, Fernandez-Botran R, Cavallazzi R, Bordon J, Valdivieso C, Schulte J, Carrico RM. University of Louisville Pneumonia Study Group. Adults hospitalized with pneumonia in the United States: incidence, epidemiology, and mortality. Clin Infect Dis. 2017 Nov 13;65(11):1806–12.
3. Eliakim-Raz N, Robenshtok E, Shefet D, Gafter-Gvili A, Vidal L, Paul M, Leibovici L. Empiric antibiotic coverage of atypical pathogens for community-acquired pneumonia in hospitalized adults. Cochrane Database of Systematic Reviews 2012, Issue 9. Art. No.: CD004418.
4. Arnold FW, Summersgill JT, Ramirez JA. Role of atypical pathogens in the etiology of community-acquired pneumonia. Semin Respir Crit Care Med. 2016 Dec;37(6):819–28 Epub 2016 Dec 13.
5. Tao LL, Hu BJ, He LX, Wei L, Xie HM, Wang BQ, Li HY, Chen XH, Zhou CM, Deng WW. Etiology and antimicrobial resistance of community-acquired pneumonia in adult patients in China. Chin Med J. 2012 Sep;125(17):2967–72.
6. Arnold FW, Summersgill JT, Lajoie AS, Peyrani P, Marrie TJ, Rossi P, Blasi F, Fernandez P, File TM Jr, Rello J, Menendez R, Marzoratti L, Luna CM, Ramirez JA. Community-acquired pneumonia organization (CAPO) investigators. A worldwide perspective of atypical pathogens in community-acquired pneumonia. Am J Respir Crit Care Med. 2007 May 15;175(10):1086–93.

7. Woodhead M, Blasi F, Ewig S, Garau J, Huchon G, Ieven M, Ortqvist A, Schaberg T, Torres A, van der Heijden G, Read R, Verheij TJ. Joint taskforce of the European Respiratory Society and European Society for Clinical Microbiology and Infectious Diseases. Guidelines for the management of adult lower respiratory tract infections--full version. Clin Microbiol Infect. 2011 Nov; 17(Suppl 6):E1–59. https://doi.org/10.1111/j.1469-0691.2011.03672.x.

8. Aliberti S, Reyes LF, Faverio P, Sotgiu G, Dore S, Rodriguez AH, Soni NJ, Restrepo MI, investigators GLIMP. Global initiative for meticillin-resistant Staphylococcus aureus pneumonia (GLIMP): an international, observational cohort study. Lancet Infect Dis. 2016 Dec;16(12):1364–76. https://doi.org/10.1016/S1473-3099(16)30267-5.

9. Martinez MA, Ruiz M, Zunino E, Luchsinger V, Avendano LF. Detection of mycoplasma pneumoniae in adult community-acquired pneumonia by PCR and serology. J Med Microbiol. 2008;57(Pt 12):1491–5.

10. von BH, Welte T, Marre R, Suttorp N, Luck C, Ewig S. Mycoplasma pneumoniae pneumonia revisited within the German competence network for community-acquired pneumonia (CAPNETZ). BMC Infect Dis. 2009;9:62.

11. Thurman KA, Walter ND, Schwartz SB, et al. Comparison of laboratory diagnostic procedures for detection of mycoplasma pneumoniae in community outbreaks. Clin Infect Dis. 2009;48:1244–9.

12. Welte T, Suttorp N, Marre R. CAPNETZ: community-acquired pneumonia competence network. Infection. 2004;32:234–8.

13. Raeven VM, Spoorenberg SM, Boersma WG, van de Garde EM, Cannegieter SC, Voorn GP, Bos WJ, van Steenbergen JE, Alkmaar study group, Ovidius study group. Atypical aetiology in patients hospitalised with community-acquired pneumonia is associated with age, gender and season; a data-analysis on four Dutch cohorts. BMC Infect Dis. 2016 Jun 17;16:299. https://doi.org/10.1186/s12879-016-1641-9.

14. Lim WS, Baudouin SV, George RC, et al. BTS guidelines for the management of community acquired pneumonia in adults: update 2009. Thorax 2009; 64: Suppl. 3, iii1–ii55.

15. Yanagihara K, Kohno S, Matsusima T. Japanese guidelines for the management of community-acquired pneumonia. Int J Antimicrob Agents. 2001;18(Suppl. 1): S45–8.

16. Working Group of the South African Thoracic Society. Management of community-acquired pneumonia in adults. S Afr Med J. 2007;97:1296–306.

17. Singanayagam A, Aliberti S, Cillóniz C, et al. Evaluation of severity score-guided macrolide use in community-acquired pneumonia. Eur Respir J. 2017;50:1602306.

18. Viasus D, Di Yacovo S, Garcia-Vidal C, Verdaguer R, Manresa F, Dorca J, Gudiol F, Carratalà J. Community- acquired legionella pneumophila pneumonia:a single- center experience with 214 hospitalized sporadic cases over 15 years. Medicine. 2012;92:51–60.

19. Vergis EN, Indorf A, File TM Jr, Phillips J, Bates J, Tan J, Sarosi GA, Grayston JT, Summersgill J, Yu VL. Azithromycin vs cefuroxime plus erythromycin for empirical treatment of community-acquired pneumonia in hospitalized patients: a prospective, randomized, multicenter trial. Arch Intern Med. 2000 May 8;160(9):1294–300.

20. Luchsinger V, Ruiz M, Zunino E, Martínez MA, Machado C, Piedra PA, Fasce R, Ulloa MT, Fink MC, Lara P, Gebauer M, Chávez F, Avendaño LF. Community- acquired pneumonia in Chile: the clinical relevance in the detection of viruses and atypical bacteria. Thorax. 2013;68:1000–6.

21. Spoorenberg SM, Bos WJ, Heijligenberg R, Voorn PG, Grutters JC, Rijkers GT, van de Garde EM. Microbial aetiology, outcomes, and costs of hospitalisation for community-acquired pneumonia; an observational analysis. BMC Infect Dis. 2014;14:335–43.

22. Shibli F, Chazan B, Nitzan O, Flatau E, Edelstein H, Blondheim O, Raz R, Colodner R. Etiology of community-acquired pneumonia in hospitalized patients in northern Israel. Isr Med Assoc J. 2010;12:477–82.

23. Chen K, Jia R, Li L, Yang C, Shi Y. The aetiology of community associated pneumonia in children in Nanjing, China and aetiological patternsassociated with age and season. BMC Public Health. 2015;15:113–8.

24. Arancibia F, Cortes CP, Valdés M, Cerda J, Hernández A, Soto L, Torres A. Importance of legionella pneumophila in the etiology of severe community-acquired pneumonia in Santiago. Chile Chest. 2014;145:290–6.

25. Templeton KE, Scheltinga SA, van den Eeden WC, Graffelman AW, van den Broek PJ, Claas EC. Improved diagnosis of the etiology of community-acquired pneumonia with real-time polymerase chain reaction. Clin Infect Dis. 2005;41:345–51.

18

Etiologic spectrum and occurrence of coinfections in children hospitalized with community-acquired pneumonia

Wujun Jiang[1†], Min Wu[1†], Jing Zhou[1], Yuqing Wang[1*], Chuangli Hao[1], Wei Ji[1], Xinxing Zhang[1], Wenjing Gu[1] and Xuejun Shao[2]

Abstract

Background: Co-infections are common in childhood community acquired pneumonia (CAP). However, their etiological pattern and clinical impact remains inconclusive.

Methods: Eight hundred forty-six consecutive children with CAP were evaluated prospectively for the presence of viral and bacterial pathogens. Nasopharyngeal aspirates were examined by direct immunofluorescence assay or polymerase chain reaction (PCR) for viruses. PCR of nasopharyngeal aspirates and enzyme-linked immunosorbent assays were performed to detect M. pneumoniae. Bacteria was detected in blood, bronchoalveolar lavage specimen, or pleural fluid by culture.

Results: Causative pathogen was identified in 70.1% (593 of 846) of the patients. The most commonly detected pathogens were respiratory syncytial virus (RSV) (22.9%), human rhinovirus (HRV) (22.1%), M. pneumoniae (15.8%). Coinfection was identified in 34.6% (293 of 846) of the patients. The majority of these (209 [71.3%] of 293) were mixed viral-bacterial infections. Age < 6 months (odds ratio: 2.1; 95% confidence interval: 1.2–3.3) and admission of PICU (odds ratio: 12.5; 95% confidence interval: 1.6–97.4) were associated with mix infection. Patients with mix infection had a higher rate of PICU admission.

Conclusions: The high mix infection burden in childhood CAP underscores a need for the enhancement of sensitive, inexpensive, and rapid diagnostics to accurately identify pneumonia pathogens.

Keywords: Community-acquired pneumonia, Children, Coinfection

Background

Childhood community-acquired pneumonia (CAP) is the leading cause of mortality in children aged less than 5 years. Pneumonia causes almost 1 in 5 under-five deaths worldwide: more than 2 million children each year [1–3]. Despite this large disease burden, critical gaps in our knowledge about pediatric pneumonia remain [4], especially establishing the cause of pneumonia, because distinguishing possible prolonged shedding or colonization from active infection can be difficult.

In China, incidence of CAP ranged from 0.06-0.27 episodes per person-year and mortality ranged from 184 to 1223 deaths per 100,000 population for children <5 years [5]. The most common pathogens of CAP are viruses, followed by bacteria and atypical bacteria [6]. Co-infections are common in childhood CAP, especially in younger children [6, 7]. Previous studies from western countries revealed that the coinfection rate ranged from 23% to 35% [6, 8–11]. These studies showed appreciable differences in the frequencies of causative agents, which seemed to be related to seasonal, geographical, and racial factors. A study conducted in eight eastern cities in China revealed the mix infection rate was 14.4% [12]. However, in their study, they included a combination of traditional Chinese medicine and western medicine hospitals. Mix infection rate was significantly lower in

* Correspondence: wang_yu_qing@126.com
†Equal contributors
[1]Department of Respiratory Medicine, Children's Hospital of Soochow University, Suzhou, China

traditional Chinese medicine hospitals compared with western medicine hospitals (1% vs 28.5%). As a matter of fact, there has been few well-defined prospective studies on the etiology and occurrence of coinfections of childhood CAP in China.

The objective of this study was to investigate the etiologic spectrum and occurrence of coinfections in children with CAP. Furthermore, the study provides data that will facilitate age-appropriate antibiotic selection and candidate vaccines for CAP.

Methods
Subjects
Eight hundred forty-six consecutive children with CAP admitted to Children's Hospital of Soochow University were evaluated prospectively from January 2015 through Dec 2015. Children's Hospital of Soochow University is a 1000 bed tertiary referral teaching hospital located in southeastern Jiangsu Province of East China. It has over 50,000 patients admitted to hospital each year. Children were included in this study if they were 1 month to 14 years old, had preceding fever (defined as body temperature ≥ 38 °C), and had clinical (chest retractions, tachypnea, nasal flaring, hypoxia, or abnormal auscultatory findings) and radiologic evidence of CAP. Children were excluded if they had preterm birth ≤34 weeks' gestation, recent hospitalization (4 weeks before admission), immunodeficiency, history of a diagnosis of chronic lung disease, or congenital heart disease.

This study was approved by the Medical Ethics Committee of Children's Hospital of Soochow University. The parents of the children enrolled in this study gave written informed consent before enrollment.

Specimen collection
Nasopharyngeal aspirates were obtained from all the patients enrolled within 24 h after admission. A suction catheter was used to passed through the nose into the lower part of the pharynx. The depth of penetration was set at 7-9 cm. A total of 2 ml nasopharyngeal aspirates was obtained and sent for analysis within 30 min. It is centrifuged at 500×g for 10 min and resuspended in 2 ml saline and divided into 2 aliquots for pathogen detection using direct immunofluorescence assay (DFA) and PCR.

Blood, Pleural fluid (if indicated), and bronchoalveolar (BAL) (if indicated) specimens obtained for clinical care were also collected.

Viral detection
DFA was used to detect syncytial virus infection (RSV), influenza virus A (IVA), influenza virus B (IVB), parainfluenza virus (PIV) I, PIV II, PIV III, and adenovirus (ADV). All assay kits were purchased from Chemicon

(USA) and all staining procedures were performed according to the manufacturer's instructions. Immunostained preparations were viewed with a fluorescence microscope (Leica 020-518.500, Germany).

RNA was extracted from nasopharyngeal specimens using Trizol (Invitrogen, USA). cDNA was synthesized by reverse transcription. The cyclic temperature settings were 94 °C, 30 s; 55 °C, 30 s; 68 °C, 30 s; amplified by 45 cycles with the last at 68 °C for 7 min. Human metapneumovirus (hMPV) and rhinoviruses (HRV) was assayed by fluorescent real-time PCR (BIO-RAD iCycler). For hMPV detection, primers were designed to specifically amplify the N gene (213 bps). The forward and reverse primers were hMPV-F: 5′-AACCGTGTAC TAAGTGATGCACTC-3′ and hMPV-R: 5′-CATTGT TTGACCGGCCCCATAA-3′, respectively. For HRV detection, the primers and probe sequences were HRV-F: 5′-TGGACAGGGTGTGAAGAGC -3′; HRV-R:5′-CAAA GTAGTCGGTCCCATCC-3′; HRV-probe: FAM-TCCT CCGGCCCCTGA ATG-TAMRA. The cyclic temperature settings were 94 °C, 30 s; 56 °C, 30 s; 72 °C, 30 s; amplified, 40 cycles.

Nasopharyngeal specimen DNA was extracted as described above, and human bocavirus (hBoV)-DNA was detected by real-time fluorescent PCR. For HBoV VP1 gene detection, the primers and probe sequences were HBoV-F: 5′-TGACATTCAACTACCAACAACCTG-3′;HBoV-R:5′-CAGATCCTTTTCCTCCTCCAATAC-3′;HBoV-probe: FAM-AGCACCACAAAACACCTCAGGGG-TAMRA. The cyclic temperature settings were 94 °C, 30 s; 56 °C, 30 s; 72 °C, 30 s; amplified by 40 cycles.

Bacterial detection
A bacterial pathogen was defined as detection of H. influenza, M.catarrhalis and other Gram-negative bacteria, S. aureus, S. anginosus/mitis, S. pneumoniae, or S. pyogenes in blood, BAL specimen, or pleural fluid by culture, or a significant rise in M. pneumoniae IgG, or the presence of IgM antibodies together with M. pneumoniae DNA. Other bacteria were considered contaminants according to the previous study [6].

A ELISA kit (Serion ELISA classic M. pneumoniae IgG/IgM, Würzburg, Germany) was used to detect M. pneumoniae IgM and IgG antibodies in paired serum samples of patients on admission and one week after admission, respectively. The cut-off value of the test was 0.5 × mean optical density (OD) of the kit control serum. A significant rise in M. pneumoniae IgG titre was defined as a doubling of the OD value above the cut-off.

A quantitative diagnostic kit (DaAn Gene Co., Ltd. Guangzhou, China) for M. pneumoniae DNA was performed to identify the 16S rRNA gene of MP extracted from nasopharyngeal specimens. The primers and probe sequences were MP-F: 5'-GCAAGGGTTCGTTATTTG-3' and MP-R: 5'-CGCCTGCGCTTGCTTTAC-3', and MP-probe: FAM-AGGTAATGGCTAGAGTTTGACTG-TAMRA.

Radiographic confirmation

A senior radiologist (G.W.L.), blinded to demographic and clinical information, reviewed all chest radiographs. The radiologist assigned standardized and mutually exclusive diagnoses that included unequivocal focal or segmental consolidation with or without pleural effusion, atelectasis, consolidation indistinguishable from atelectasis, or interstitial pneumonia.

Statistical analysis

Statistical analyses were performed using the Statistical Package for the Social Sciences (version 17.0). Data were expressed as number with percentage, mean and standard deviation (SD) or, median and interquartile range as appropriate. Normally distributed continuous variables were compared using the Student t test and non-normally distributed variables were analyzed using Mann-Whitney U test. Categorical data were analyzed using the chi-squared (χ2) test or Fisher's exact test. Posthoc multiple comparisons were performed to determine the origins of significant differences, and the results were adjusted by using the Bonferroni method. Backward stepwise logistic-regression analyses were performed to determine the best predictors of mix infections (viral and bacterial, viral and viral, bacterial and bacterial infections). Covariates included in the regression model were age (<6 month /≥6 months), gender, fever, wheeze, dyspnea, pleural effusion, WBC count, percentage of neutrophils, CRP, need of oxygen and pediatric intensive care unit (PICU) admission. Only variables from the univariate analyses that were significant at the .05 level were entered into the multivariate logistic-regression analyses. Goodness of fit of the regression model was tested with the Hosmer–Lemeshow test, with $P > 0.05$ considered to indicate lack of deviation between the model and observed event rate. The area under ROC curves (AUROC) of predictors for predicting mix infections were calculated. P value < .05 was considered statistically significant.

Results

Patients

Eight hundred forty-six children with CAP met the inclusion criteria for enrollment. Of these patients, 489 (57.8%) were male. Ages ranged from 1 month to 14 years (median: 11 months). Two hundred ninety-four (34.8%) children were <6 months old, 161(19%) were 6 months to <1 years old, 208 (24.6%) were 1 to <3 years

old, 117 (13.8%) were 3 to <5 years old, and 66(7.8%) were ≥5 years old.

Etiology

At least 1 respiratory pathogen was identified in 70.1% (593 of 846) of the patients. Pathogens were documented in 70.7% of patients <6 months old, 76.1% of patients 6 months to <1 years old, 70.2% of patients 1 to <3 years old, 74.0% of patients 3 to <5 years old, and 78.0% of patients ≥5 years old. The most commonly detected pathogens were RSV (22.9%), HRV (22.1%), M. pneumoniae (15.8%), hBoV (6.0%), PIV (4.0%) and S. pneumoniae (3.0%) (Fig. 1). RSV (24.6% vs. 3%, $P < 0.01$) was more commonly detected in children <5 years old compared with older children; M. pneumoniae (42.4% vs. 13.6%, $P < 0.01$) was more commonly detected in children ≥5 years old compared with younger children. Monthly distributions of commonly detected pathogens were shown in Fig. 2.

Mixed infections

Coinfection was identified in 34.6% (293 of 846) of the patients. Of the 293 patients with coinfection, two pathogens were identified in 220 (75.1%) patients, three were identified in 60 (20.5%) patients and four in 13(4.4%) patients. The majority of these (209 [71.3%] of 293) were mixed viral-bacterial infections. Mixed viral-viral infections were identified in 56 (19.1%) patients and mixed bacterial -bacterial in 28 (9.6%) patients.

Coinfections were documented in 59.9% of patients <6 months old, 65.8% of patients 6 months to <1 years old, 60.6% of patients 1 to <3 years old, 52.1% of patients

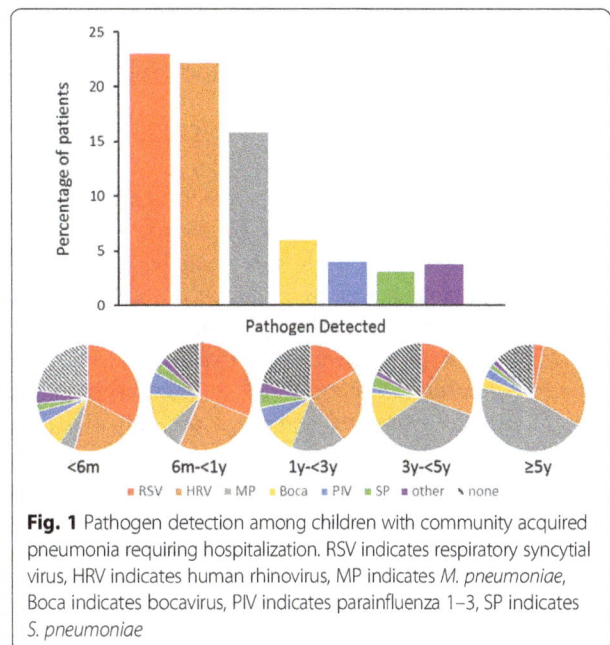

Fig. 1 Pathogen detection among children with community acquired pneumonia requiring hospitalization. RSV indicates respiratory syncytial virus, HRV indicates human rhinovirus, MP indicates *M. pneumoniae*, Boca indicates bocavirus, PIV indicates parainfluenza 1–3, SP indicates *S. pneumoniae*

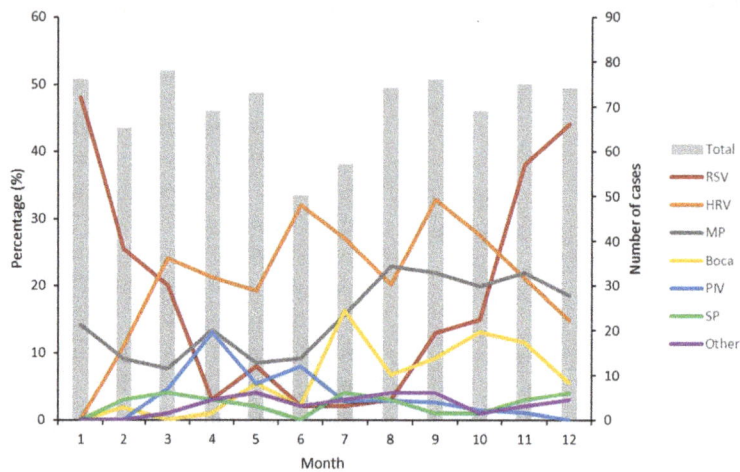

Fig. 2 Monthly distributions of commonly detected pathogens were shown in Fig. 2. RSV indicates respiratory syncytial virus, HRV indicates human rhinovirus, MP indicates *M. pneumoniae*, Boca indicates bocavirus, PIV indicates parainfluenza 1–3, SP indicates *S. pneumoniae*

3 to <5 years old, and 34.8% of patients ≥5 years old. Mixed viral-bacterial infections were the major coinfections in each age group. Mixed viral-viral infections were more commonly detected in children <3 years old compared with older children (9.2% vs 1.5%, $P < 0.01$) For children <3 years, RSV/HRV was the most common combination (48.6%) of viral-viral infections, followed by RSV/hBoV (22.9%) and HRV/hBoV (14.3%). HRV/ M. pneumoniae (34.9%) was the most common combination of viral-bacterial infections, followed by M. pneumoniae /hBoV (24.4%) and RSV/ M. pneumoniae (18.6%) (Fig. 3).

The coinfection status of varied pathogens is shown in Table 1. Co-infection was found significantly more frequently among patients with hBoV (64.7%), M. pneumoniae (51.5%) and HRV (47.6%) than those with RSV (30.9%) and PIV (23.5%) ($P < 0.01$, respectively).

Comparisons of clinical characteristics of the patients with single and mix infections

The demographic and clinical characteristics of the patients with single/mix infections are shown in Table 2. Their median age of children with single bacterial infections (35 months), as well as those with mixed bacterial pathogens (30 months) was significantly greater than that of children infected with single viruses (12 months) or mixed viruses (12 months) ($P < 0.01$, respectively). The duration of symptoms and usage of antibiotics preceding admission was similar among all groups of patients. The proportion of children presenting with wheezing was lowest among children with single bacterial infection, while the proportion of children presenting with fever, as well as percentage of neutrophils was lowest among children with single virus infection (all $P < 0.01$). Children with single virus infection had a

higher proportion of oxygen therapy compared with single bacterial infection (11.4% vs 2.7%, $P < 0.01$), while the PICU admission rate did not differ between the two groups. The type of infection was not associated with length of hospital of stay.

We further performed multivariate logistic-regression analyses to determine the best predictors of mix infections. Multivariate logistic-regression analyses revealed that only 2 variables were associated with mix infections: age < 6 months (odds ratio: 2.1; 95% confidence interval: 1.2–3.3) and admission of PICU (odds ratio: 12.5; 95% confidence interval: 1.6–97.4). Hosmer–Lemeshow statistic was 0.51, which indicated a lack of deviation between the model and observed event rate. The AUROC for age was 0.71 (95% CI, 0.58-0.92), and for admission of PICU was 0.67 (95% CI, 0.54-0.88).

Discussion

Eight hundred forty-six children immunocompetent children hospitalized were studied prospectively to elucidate the etiologic spectrum and occurrence of coinfections. A comprehensive investigation combining microbiologic, serologic, and molecular tests was undertaken to maximize the diagnostic yield. Overall, a pathogen was identified in 76.5% of children. Coinfection was identified in 34.6% of the patients.

The most commonly detected pathogens in our study were RSV (22.9%) and HRV (22.1%). In a recent population-based surveillance in USA, RSV was detected among 28% of children and HRV was 27% detected among <15 years old hospitalized with pneumonia similar to our results [6]. In another 6-year prospective study conducted in children <14 years, the most frequently detected virus was RSV with 41.6% of positive patients

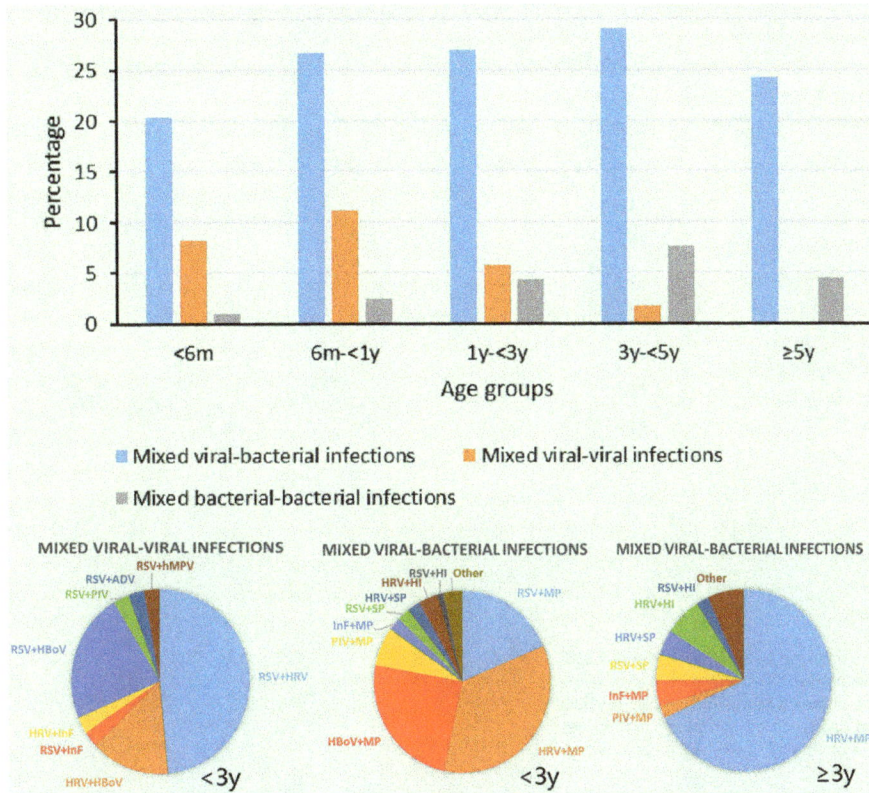

Fig. 3 Distribution of pathogen coinfections associated with community acquired pneumonia, stratified by age. RSV indicates respiratory syncytial virus, HRV indicates human rhinovirus, MP indicates M. pneumoniae, HBoV indicates bocavirus, PIV indicates parainfluenza 1–3, SP indicates S, pneumoniae, ADV indicates adenovirus, InF indicates influenza virus A and B, hMPV indicates human metapneumovirus, HI indicates H. influenza

Table 1 Pathogens Identified in Hospitalized Children with Community-Acquired Pneumonia

Pathogen	No. of Episodes			Total No. of Episodes
	Coinfection	Coinfection With Viruses[a]	Coinfection With Bacteria[a]	
Viruses[b]				
RSV	60 (30.9)	31 (16.0)	35 (18.0)	194
Rhinovirus	89 (47.6)	23 (12.3)	73 (39.0)	187
Bocavirus	33 (64.7)	13 (25.5)	21 (41.2)	51
Parainfluenza 1–3	8 (23.5)	1 (2.9)	8 (23.5)	34
Influenza A or B[c]	4	2	3	8
Metapneumovirus[c]	2	1	1	3
Adenovirus[c]	1	1	0	4
Bacteria[b]				
M. pneumoniae	69 (51.5)	63 (47.0)	14 (10.4)	134
S. pneumoniae	13 (52.0)	5 (20.0)	8 (32.0)	25
H. influenzae	7 (63.6)	4 (36.4)	3 (27.3)	11
M.catarrhalis[c]	6	3	3	8
S. aureus[c]	1	1	0	2

[a]The categories of coinfection with bacteria and with viruses are not mutually exclusive
[b]Data are n (%)
[c]The percentages are not listed because the total episodes is too small

Table 2 The Demographic and Clinical Characteristics of 593 Patients with Community-acquired Pneumonia Associated with Single/mix infections

Characteristics	Single virus	Single bacteria	Mixed viruses	Mixed bacteria/viruses	Mixed bacteria	P value
No. of patients	118	182	28	209	56	–
Age, months[a]	12[cd]	35[cef]	12[eg]	20 [f]	30[dg]	<0.01
Gender, % male	62.8	54.0	67.9	56.9	66.1	0.10
Duration of symptoms before admission, days[b]	7.0	6.5	6	5.8	7.2	0.43
Antibiotic therapy during preceding 2 weeks, %	76.3	70.2	73.2	66.6	70.5	0.21
Fever, %	35.6[cdef]	67.5[cg]	51.8[dg]	53.7[e]	57.3[f]	<0.01
Wheeze, %	50.8[c]	32.4[cdef]	51.9[d]	47.8[e]	44.1[f]	<0.01
Dyspnea, %	9.0	7.9	7.7	8.5	8.1	0.41
WBC count, ×10⁹/L[b]	11.3	10.2	11.9	11.3	11.8	0.25
Percentage of neutrophils[b]	34.9[cde]	47.9[c]	40.1	45.2[d]	49.4[e]	<0.01
CRP, mg/L[b]	10.6	13.6	22.5	14.3	15.6	0.07
Pleural effusion, %	1.5	3.2	3.7	2.5	1.5	0.64
Need of oxygen, %	11.4[c]	2.7[cd]	11.1	9.5[d]	8.1	0.02
PICU admission, %	0[c]	0.6	7.4[c]	3.5	2.2	0.01

[a]The median value was used
[b]The mean value was used
[c]Significant differences were observed between each pair of values
[d]Significant differences were observed between each pair of values
[e]Significant differences were observed between each pair of values
[f]Significant differences were observed between each pair of values
[g]Significant differences were observed between each pair of values

followed by RV (26.2%), which was also in line with our study [13].

S. pneumoniae was detected in 3% of the study population, which is similar with a recent study in USA (4%) [6], but lower than an earlier US pediatric pneumonia etiology study. The 7-valent pneumococcal conjugate vaccine was introduced to China in 2008, it has been covered in around 15% of the children in the last seven years [14]. While our data, as well as the recent study in USA [6], partly reflect the substantial reduction of pneumococcal disease due to conjugate vaccines, bacterial culture-based diagnostics have limited sensitivity and bacteremia is detected in a minority of pneumococcal pneumonias [6].

In our study, the proportion of mix infection was 34.6%, the majority (71.3%) of which were mixed viral-bacterial infections. Our study is similar to a previous study which had a mix infection rate of 35%, they also found that most of the coinfections were mixed viral-bacterial infections [11]. Michelow et al. conducted a prospective diagnostic study and found that mix infection rate was 34%, they also found that the majority of which were mixed viral-bacterial infections [10]. It has been speculated that viruses may induce pneumonia, either directly or by rendering the host more susceptible to bacterial infection. The high prevalence of mixed viral-bacterial infection found in our study, as well as the previous studies raise the important question of

whether sequential or concurrent viral and bacterial infections have a synergistic impact on the evolution of disease in children [15]. However, in Jain et al. study, they found that the proportion of pathogen co-detection was 26%, the majority of which were mixed viral-viral infections [6]. The difference of coinfection rate and pattern of coinfection may be related to seasonal, geographical, and racial factors.

In our study, children with proven single/mix viral infections tended to be younger than children with single/mix bacterial infections. This is also approved in Michelow's study [10]. In their study, they also found that the proportion of children presenting with wheezing was lowest among children with bacterial infection, while the proportion of children presenting with fever, as well as percentage of neutrophils, was lowest among children with virus infection. However, in their study, they neither compared the clinical characteristics between single and mix virus infection, nor compared between single and mix bacterial infection. Interestingly, in our study, children with mix viral infections presented with a higher proportion of fever compared with those with single viral infection, which suggested that a combination of virus infections had more degree of inflammation than single virus infection. Besides, we also found that children with mix bacterial infections presented with a higher proportion of wheeze compared with those with single bacterial infection. The higher proportion of wheeze in children with mix bacterial infections may be attributed to the protracted bacterial bronchitis (PBB). PBB is disease characterized by protracted wet cough >4 weeks and bacterial culture-positive BALF. A high proportion of wheezing episodes was reported in children with PBB [16, 17]. Our previous study found that wheezing was presented in 90% of the children with PBB [18]. Actually, in our study, 11 patients were diagnosed as PPB. Nine of the 11 patients had the mix bacterial infection.

To date, the relationship between the clinical severity and infection status with single vs. multiple respiratory pathogens remains inconclusive. Asner et al. Reported that equivalent clinical severity was observed between children with single virus infection and virus coinfection [19]. In adult, previous works also pointed that CAP patients requiring ICU admission did not point out any relationship between viral-bacterial coinfection and severity [20, 21]. However, other studies found that coinfection was associated with higher rate of intensive care unit admission and receipt of mechanical ventilation as well as longer hospital stay in children and adult [22–26]. In our study, we found that patients with mix infection had a higher rate of PICU admission, while the type of infection was not associated with length of hospital of stay. Further studies with larger populations may explore this point, with comparing the severity and prognosis of CAP patients according to the type of virus as well as the different type of virus/bacteria combinations.

In our study, 73 patients (8.6%) infected with three or four pathogens. Interestingly, compared with 220 (75.1%) patients with pathogens, children with three or four pathogens had a longer duration of hospital stay, after adjusted by age ($P < 0.01$), while oxygen therapy or the PICU admission rate did not differ between the two groups (data not shown). This interesting phenomenon may reflect the fact that patients with multiple pathogen infection has a more effective mechanism for evading the innate immune response, resulting in slower pathogenic clearance and greater lung injury.

Our study has some limitations. As previous study documented [27–29], detection of pathogens in the upper respiratory tract may not represent causation of pneumonia. Although thoracocentesis may provide more solid evidence of pathogens, invasive procedures were not commonly performed due to feasibility considerations. Second, prevalence of each pathogens varied yearly, their association with CAP may also variable. Third, the tests used for virus detection were heterogeneous, as some were detected by immune-fluorescence and some other by PCR. Fourth, our virus tests did not cover all the common viruses, such as coronaviruses, which had positive rate of around 3% in patients with acute respiratory infections in a recent Chinese study [30]. Finally, although our study investigated large populations with standardized procedures, our findings in a single center may not be representative of the entire Chinese pediatric population.

Conclusion

In conclusion, virus accounted for the majority of identifiable infections in children hospitalized with CAP in this series. Effective anti-viral vaccines or treatments, particularly for RSV and HRV could have an impact on pediatric pneumonia. Mixed infections were identified in 34.6% of the patients with CAP. The majority of these were mixed viral-bacterial infections. The high mix infection burden in childhood CAP underscores a need for the enhancement of sensitive, inexpensive, and rapid diagnostics to accurately identify pneumonia pathogens.

Abbreviations
ADV: Adenovirus; BAL: Bronchoalveolar; CAP: Community acquired pneumonia; DFA: Direct immunofluorescence assay; hMPV: Human metapneumovirus; HRV: Human rhinoviruses; IVA: Influenza virus A; IVB: Influenza virus B; OD: Optical density; PBB: Protracted bacterial bronchitis; PCR: Polymerase chain reaction; PICU: Pediatric intensive care unit; PIV: Parainfluenza virus; RSV: Syncytial virus infection; SD: Standard deviation

Acknowledgements
The authors thank all nursing staff working in our department for keeping extremely detailed patient records, which contributed greatly to the completion of this research.

Funding
This work was supported by a grant from the National Natural Science Foundation of China (Grant No.81573167). The funding body had no role in the design of the study and collection, analysis, and interpretation of data and in writing the manuscript.

Authors' contributions
WJJ and MW wrote the main manuscript text. CLH and YQW conceptualized and designed the study, drafted the initial manuscript, and approved the final manuscript. JZ and WJ carried out the initial analyses, reviewed and revised the manuscript, and approved the final manuscript. XXZ, WJG and XJS did the microbiological detection. All authors read and approved the final manuscript.

Consent for publication
Not applicable.

Competing interests
The authors declare that they have no competing interests.

Author details
[1]Department of Respiratory Medicine, Children's Hospital of Soochow University, Suzhou, China. [2]Department of Clinical Laboratory, Children's Hospital of Soochow University, Suzhou, China.

References

1. Rudan I, Boschi-Pinto C, Biloglav Z, Mulholland K, Campbell H. Epidemiology and etiology of childhood pneumonia. Bull World Health Organ. 2008;86: 408–16.
2. Rudan I, Tomaskovic L, Boschi-Pinto C, Campbell H, Group WHOCHER. Global estimate of the incidence of clinical pneumonia among children under five years of age. Bull World Health Organ. 2004;82:895–903.
3. Nair H, Simoes EA, Rudan I, Gessner BD, Azziz-Baumgartner E, Zhang JS, et al. Global and regional burden of hospital admissions for severe acute lower respiratory infections in young children in 2010: a systematic analysis. Lancet. 2013;381:1380–90.
4. Bradley JS, Byington CL, Shah SS, Alverson B, Carter ER, Harrison C, et al. Executive summary: the management of community-acquired pneumonia in infants and children older than 3 months of age: clinical practice guidelines by the Pediatric Infectious Diseases Society and the Infectious Diseases Society of America. Clin Infect Dis. 2011;53:617–30.
5. Guan X, Silk BJ, Li W, Fleischauer AT, Xing X, Jiang X, et al. Pneumonia incidence and mortality in mainland China: systematic review of Chinese and English literature, 1985-2008. PLoS One. 2010;5:e11721.
6. Jain S, Williams DJ, Arnold SR, Ampofo K, Bramley AM, Reed C, et al. Community-acquired pneumonia requiring hospitalization among U.S. children. N Engl J Med. 2015;372:835–45.
7. Miller EK, Gebretsadik T, Carroll KN, Dupont WD, Mohamed YA, Morin LL, et al. Viral etiologies of infant bronchiolitis, croup and upper respiratory illness during 4 consecutive years. Pediatr Infect Dis J. 2013;32:950–5.
8. Cilla G, Onate E, Perez-Yarza EG, Montes M, Vicente D, Perez-Trallero E. Viruses in community-acquired pneumonia in children aged less than 3 years old: high rate of viral coinfection. J Med Virol. 2008;80:1843–9.
9. Honkinen M, Lahti E, Osterback R, Ruuskanen O, Waris M. Viruses and bacteria in sputum samples of children with community-acquired pneumonia. Clin Microbiol Infect. 2012;18:300–7.
10. Michelow IC, Olsen K, Lozano J, Rollins NK, Duffy LB, Ziegler T, et al. Epidemiology and clinical characteristics of community-acquired pneumonia in hospitalized children. Pediatrics. 2004;113:701–7.
11. Tsolia MN, Psarras S, Bossios A, Audi H, Paldanius M, Gourgiotis D, et al. Etiology of community-acquired pneumonia in hospitalized school-age children: evidence for high prevalence of viral infections. Clin Infect Dis. 2004;39:681–6.
12. Wang XF, Liu JP, Shen KL, Ma R, Cui ZZ, Deng L, et al. A cross-sectional study of the clinical characteristics of hospitalized children with community-acquired pneumonia in eight eastern cities in China. BMC Complement Altern Med. 2013;13:367.
13. Garcia-Garcia ML, Calvo C, Pozo F, Villadangos PA, Perez-Brena P, Casas I. Spectrum of respiratory viruses in children with community-acquired pneumonia. Pediatr Infect Dis J. 2012;31:808–13.
14. Boulton ML, Ravi NS, Sun X, Huang Z, Wagner AL. Trends in childhood pneumococcal vaccine coverage in shanghai, China, 2005-2011: a retrospective cohort study. BMC Public Health. 2016;16:109.
15. O'Brien KL, Walters MI, Sellman J, Quinlisk P, Regnery H, Schwartz B, et al. Severe pneumococcal pneumonia in previously healthy children: the role of preceding influenza infection. Clin Infect Dis. 2000;30:784–9.
16. De Schutter I, Dreesman A, Soetens O, De Waele M, Crokaert F, Verhaegen J, et al. In young children, persistent wheezing is associated with bronchial bacterial infection: a retrospective analysis. BMC Pediatr. 2012;12:83.
17. Le Bourgeois M, Goncalves M, Le Clainche L, Benoist MR, Fournet JC, Scheinmann P, et al. Bronchoalveolar cells in children < 3 years old with severe recurrent wheezing. Chest. 2002;122:791–7.
18. Wang Y, Hao C, Chi F, Yu X, Sun H, Huang L, et al. Clinical characteristics of protracted bacterial bronchitis in Chinese infants. Sci Rep. 2015;5:13731.
19. Asner SA, Rose W, Petrich A, Richardson S, Tran DJ. Is virus coinfection a predictor of severity in children with viral respiratory infections? Clin Microbiol Infect. 2015;21:264. e1-6
20. Choi SH, Hong SB, Ko GB, Lee Y, Park HJ, Park SY, et al. Viral infection in patients with severe pneumonia requiring intensive care unit admission. Am J Respir Crit Care Med. 2012;186:325–32.
21. Karhu J, Ala-Kokko TI, Vuorinen T, Ohtonen P, Syrjala H. Lower respiratory tract virus findings in mechanically ventilated patients with severe community-acquired pneumonia. Clin Infect Dis. 2014;59:62–70.
22. Reed C, Kallen AJ, Patton M, Arnold KE, Farley MM, Hageman J, et al. Infection with community-onset Staphylococcus Aureus and influenza virus in hospitalized children. Pediatr Infect Dis J. 2009;28:572–6.
23. Finelli L, Fiore A, Dhara R, Brammer L, Shay DK, Kamimoto L, et al. Influenza-associated pediatric mortality in the United States: increase of Staphylococcus Aureus coinfection. Pediatrics. 2008;122:805–11.
24. Techasaensiri B, Techasaensiri C, Mejias A, McCracken GH Jr, Ramilo O. Viral coinfections in children with invasive pneumococcal disease. Pediatr Infect Dis J. 2010;29:519–23.
25. Voiriot G, Visseaux B, Cohen J, Nguyen LB, Neuville M, Morbieu C, et al. Viral-bacterial coinfection affects the presentation and alters the prognosis of severe community-acquired pneumonia. Crit Care. 2016;20:375.
26. Johansson N, Kalin M, Hedlund J. Clinical impact of combined viral and bacterial infection in patients with community-acquired pneumonia. Scand J Infect Dis. 2011;43:609–15.
27. Turner RB, Lande AE, Chase P, Hilton N, Weinberg D. Pneumonia in pediatric outpatients: cause and clinical manifestations. J Pediatr. 1987;111:194–200.
28. Ruuskanen O, Nohynek H, Ziegler T, Capeding R, Rikalainen H, Huovinen P, et al. Pneumonia in childhood: etiology and response to antimicrobial therapy. Eur J Clin Microbiol Infect Dis. 1992;11:217–23.
29. Claesson BA, Trollfors B, Brolin I, Granstrom M, Henrichsen J, Jodal U, et al. Etiology of community-acquired pneumonia in children based on antibody responses to bacterial and viral antigens. Pediatr Infect Dis J. 1989;8:856–62.
30. Zhang D, He Z, Xu L, Zhu X, Wu J, Wen W, et al. Epidemiology characteristics of respiratory viruses found in children and adults with respiratory tract infections in southern China. Int J Infect Dis. 2014;25:159–64.

19

Effects of a clinical pathway on antibiotic use in patients with community-acquired pneumonia

Liping Zhu[1], Jie Bai[1], Yongcong Chen[2] and Di Xue[1*]

Abstract

Background: Community-acquired pneumonia (CAP) is a common condition with high mortality, morbidity and healthcare costs. This study aimed to determine whether clinical pathway (CP) implementation in different hospitals in China increased antibiotic compliance with the national CP in inpatients with CAP.

Methods: Chart reviews of CAP cases were conducted in 18 public hospitals from 3 different regions of China in 2015. Chi-square tests and the t-test were used to compare differences between hospitals that implemented CP (CP group) and those that did not (non-CP group). Multivariate logistic analysis was adopted to test whether CP implementation for CAP in hospitals affected their overall antibiotic use compliance rates with the national CP for CAP.

Results: The overall compliance rate with the national CP for inpatients with CAP was 43.69%. The compliance rates for timely initial antibiotic use, recommended antibiotic use and use of the recommended combination of antibiotics and the overall compliance rate were substantially higher in the CP group than in the non-CP group. A multivariate logistic model for overall compliance in inpatients with CAP showed that the hospitals in the CP group had greater overall compliance than those in the non-CP group (odds ratio [OR] = 1.76; 95% confidence interval [CI] = 1.16–2.71) after controlling for hospital and inpatient characteristics.

Conclusion: In China, the overall compliance rate with the national CP for inpatients with CAP was low, but inpatients with CAP in the hospitals in the CP group received antibiotics more concordantly with the national CP. Since adherence to evidence-based care has been shown to improve clinical outcomes, internal and external support from hospitals is required to facilitate CP implementation for inpatients with CAP. Additionally, governmental commitment, hospital input and population involvement are required to improve antibiotic utilization.

Keywords: Clinical pathway, Antibiotic, Implementation, Community-acquired pneumonia

Background

Community-acquired pneumonia (CAP) is a common condition with high mortality, morbidity and costs [1] and is also the most common infectious cause of death worldwide [2]. Empiric antibiotic therapy is the cornerstone of CAP treatment. According to the guideline for inpatients with CAP outside of the intensive care unit (ICU), the preferred antibiotics are β-lactams* plus macrolides in the United States, amoxicillin plus macrolides in Britain and aminopenicillin with or without macrolides in Europe.

Respiratory fluoroquinolones are alternative antibiotics in the CAP guidelines in all of these countries or regions [3–5]. Similar to many other countries, the national CAP guideline for inpatients with CAP outside of the ICU in China recommends the use of a β-lactam/β-lactamase inhibitor and a 2nd-generation cephalosporin, cefotaxime or ceftriaxone with or without macrolides; the alternative recommendation is application of a respiratory quinolone [6, 7].

However, inappropriate antibiotic use for CAP treatment has been well documented [8]. The World Health Organization (WHO) has reported that antibiotic resistance causes 2.50 thousand deaths annually in the European Union and 204.94 thousand illnesses and 2.30

* Correspondence: xuedi@shmu.edu.cn
[1]NHC Key Laboratory of Health Technology Assessment (Fudan University), Department of Hospital Management, School of Public Health, Fudan University, Shanghai, People's Republic of China

thousand deaths annually in the United States [9]. Antibiotic resistance also has a significant economic impact due to the need for more drugs and longer hospital stays [10]. A large-scale study reported that antibiotic use was several-times higher in China than in other developing countries [11]. In 2010, 49.63% of patients in tertiary hospitals in China were prescribed antibiotics, and 32% of inpatients received antibiotic combination therapy [12]. Because of inappropriate antibiotic use, China has experienced the most rapid growth of antibiotic resistance worldwide [13]. *Clostridium difficile* infection (CDI) is another incidental complication related to antibiotic use [14] and has become a major public health problem associated with significant morbidity, mortality and hospital costs [15, 16].

With the increase in antibiotic resistance, the decline in antibiotic development and the frequent occurrence of adverse events, antibiotics should be used wisely for greater effectiveness and lower risks [17]. One strategy to address the antibiotic crisis is adoption of clinical guidelines (CGs) and clinical pathways (CPs) [18, 19]. Although both CGs and CPs have been embraced as strategies to decrease clinical practice variation, CPs, which are operational structures usually based on pre-existing CGs, are more explicit concerning the participants, sequence, timing and provision of interventions for patients with specific medical conditions [20–22]. In China, national CPs are issued by the National Health Commission (NHC) in accordance with national CGs. A total of 1010 CPs had been issued in China by the end of 2016 [23]. Hospitals in China can modify national CPs slightly to make them more practical for local use, and some hospitals require physicians to provide medical care that adheres to CPs (including recommended antibiotic use).

In 1988, the Infectious Diseases Society of America (IDSA) initially published CPs to improve antibiotic use in inpatients and to minimize or eliminate the increased morbidity, mortality and health care costs attributed to antibiotics [24]. Recently, a positive correlation between the implementation of CPs and improvement in antibiotic use was found in some studies in China [25, 26]. However, many previous studies on the effects of CPs on antibiotic use in China are limited to one hospital or by a small sample size. Therefore, testing the effects of CP implementation on general antibiotic use is difficult.

This study aimed to determine whether CP implementation in different hospitals from three representative regions of China increased antibiotic compliance with the national CP for inpatients with CAP.

Methods

Survey sample

This retrospective study was conducted in Shanghai, Hubei Province and Gansu Province, which represented high, middle and low socioeconomic status levels and

the eastern, central and western regions of China in 2015, respectively. In the Hubei and Gansu provinces, 3 areas (cities or autonomous prefectures) were selected to represent high, middle and low socioeconomic status levels in each province. In each surveyed area of the Hubei and Gansu provinces, 1 tertiary and 1 secondary public hospital were selected as the surveyed hospitals. Because the tertiary public general hospitals in Shanghai were not evenly distributed among districts, 3 tertiary public general hospitals were selected in Shanghai to represent tertiary hospitals owned by a university, the Shanghai government and the district government. In Shanghai, 3 secondary public general hospitals were also selected from 3 districts to represent hospitals in urban, suburban and rural areas.

Data sources

Chart reviews were conducted to collect information on antibiotic use from inpatients with CAP who were admitted to any of the 18 surveyed hospitals in 2014. We identified all inpatients with CAP admitted to each hospital in 2014 based on the International Statistical Classification of Diseases and Related Health Problems, 10th Revision (ICD-10) codes. Inpatients admitted to the ICU during their hospitalization were excluded from this study. For most hospitals, hospital electronic information systems were used to identify cases and to collect information from the first pages of medical records (including information regarding patient characteristics and diagnoses). However, for hospitals in rural areas without electronic health information systems, cases were identified, and information on the first pages of medical records was collected manually.

To ensure that the sample was evenly distributed throughout the year, 2–3 cases were selected each month; thus, 30 cases were sampled from each hospital. For the hospitals with electronic medical information systems, we selected 2–3 medical records per month with a random sampling method using the randomizing formula in Excel. For the hospitals without electronic medical information systems, we used the convenient sampling method to select 2–3 medical records per month. If a hospital admitted fewer than 30 inpatients with CAP in 2014, then all medical records from 2014 and some records from late 2013 or even all of 2013 were extracted so that 30 records could be extracted for each condition in each hospital.

We developed an audit chart according to the elements in the CP for CAP (issued by the NHC) related to antibiotic use [27]. Then, the auditors extracted information from the medical records corresponding to each item in the audit chart for each inpatient. To ensure the quality and consistency of the chart audit, we trained 5 auditors (master's or PhD students with specialties in social medicine and health service management) on the meaning of each item on the checklist and how to judge adherence to antibiotic use according to the national CP for CAP. In addition, two experts were invited to review medical records from two hospitals that were reviewed by the auditors to analyse the consistency of the review between the experts and the auditors. The consistency rate between the auditors and the experts was 92.21%. One inspector was also assigned to check 10% of the reviewed charts in each hospital.

In addition, we asked the surveyed hospitals whether they had implemented the CP for CAP in their own hospitals and whether they provided CP training, initiated quality control for CP implementation and utilized incentive mechanisms for CP implementation.

Data analysis
In the study, the compliance rate for the timely use of initial antibiotics reflected the proportion of inpatients who received initial antibiotics within 8 h after hospital admission, the compliance rate for the use of recommended antibiotics reflected the proportion of inpatients who received the recommended categories of antibiotics, the compliance rate for the use of the recommended antibiotic combination reflected the proportion of inpatients who received the recommended combination of antibiotics, and the overall compliance rate reflected the proportion of inpatients who received initial antibiotics from recommended categories and recommended combinations within 8 h [27]. Antibiotic use in emergency departments, outpatient departments or at home were not considered in the study because the national CP for CAP in China considers only inpatient care. For each indicator, the auditors judged whether a patient received recommended or non-recommended antibiotics and then assigned a code of "1" or "0", respectively.

In the study, the patients with severe CAP were classified mainly by the hospital physicians in medical records or by the auditors according to the information in medical records and the criteria in the CAP guideline of China (2006) when the classification was not made by the hospital physicians. Severe CAP is defined in the CAP guideline of China (2006) as: a) having disturbance of consciousness; b) with ≥30 breaths per minute; c) with $PaO_2 < 60$ mmHg, $PaO_2/FiO_2 < 300$ and/or mechanical ventilation needed; d) with arterial systolic pressure < 90 mmHg; e) with septic shock; f) bilateral or multiple pulmonary lobes involved and/or expanded lesion area ≥ 50% within 48 h of hospital admission shown in chest X-ray radiograph; or g) with oliguria (urine volume < 20 ml per hour or < 80 ml per 4 h), or acute renal failure requiring dialysis [6].

Chi-square tests and the t-test were used to compare differences in inpatient characteristics, antibiotic administration

and compliance rates for antibiotic use between the hospitals that implemented the CP for CAP (CP group) and those that did not (non-CP group). A multivariate logistic analysis was used to test whether CP implementation in the hospitals influenced their overall compliance rates for antibiotic use while controlling for hospital (level and location) and inpatient characteristics (sex, age, number of comorbidities and CAP severity).

Results
Characteristics of the surveyed hospitals and CAP cases
In the 18 surveyed hospitals, the numbers of hospital beds in secondary and tertiary hospitals ranged from 249 to 910 and from 502 to 3283 in 2014, respectively. Among those hospitals, 12 hospitals implemented the CP for inpatients with CAP and conducted training and quality control for CP implementation. In addition, 9 hospitals that implemented the CP for inpatients with CAP also had incentives for CP implementation (Additional file 1: Table S1).

A total of 534 CAP cases were enrolled in the study, including 66.29% from the 12 hospitals that implemented the CP for CAP (CP group) and 33.71% from the 6 hospitals that did not implement the CP for CAP (non-CP group). Among the surveyed cases, the elderly (aged 60 years or older), males and patients with at least one comorbidity accounted for 46.63%, 48.13% and 61.42% of the sample, respectively. No significant differences were found in age, sex and the number of comorbidities between the patients in the CP and non-CP groups. However, the percentage of cases classified as severe CAP was higher in the non-CP group (19.38%) than in the CP group (7.26%) ($p < 0.0001$) (Table 1).

Timely administration of initial antibiotics
The study showed that 84.18% of inpatients with CAP received initial antibiotics within 4 h of hospital admission, including 89.49% in the CP group and 73.74% in the non-CP group ($p < 0.0001$). According to the requirement of the CP for inpatients with CAP, 85.69% of the inpatients with CAP received initial antibiotics in a timely manner (within 8 h of hospital admission); this compliance rate was substantially higher in the CP group (90.63%) than in the non-CP group (75.98%) ($p < 0.0001$) (Table 2).

Use of recommended antibiotics
A total of 18 categories of antibiotics (796 antibiotics) were administered to 531 inpatients with CAP from the 18 surveyed hospitals. Regarding the antibiotics administered to the inpatients with CAP, respiratory quinolones, β-lactam/β-lactamase inhibitors, 2nd-generation cephalosporins, macrolides and recommended 3rd-generation cephalosporins (ceftriaxone and cefotaxime) were among the top 5 most utilized antibiotics (accounting for

Table 1 Patient demographics in the CP and non-CP groups

Items	Total ($n = 534$)	CP group ($n = 354$)	Non-CP group ($n = 180$)	p-value[a]
Age (years)				
mean	56.31	55.47	57.96	0.147
SD	18.79	19.09	18.11	
Male				
n	257	174	83	0.506
%	48.13	49.15	46.11	
Comorbidities				
No comorbidity				
n	206	146	60	
%	38.58	41.24	33.33	
1 comorbidity				
n	141	87	54	0.176
%	26.40	24.58	30.00	
≥ 2 comorbidities				
n	187	121	66	
%	35.02	34.18	36.67	
Severe CAP [b]				
n	53	22	31	< 0.0001
%	11.45	7.26	19.38	

[a]The t-test was used to compare the age of the inpatients with CAP and Chi-square tests were used to compare the other characteristics between the CP group and the non-CP group;
[b]Condition severities were not assessed for 71 inpatients

79.52% of the administered antibiotics) and were recommended in the CP for CAP in China. In addition, respiratory quinolones accounted for 32.79% of the antibiotics used in the inpatients with CAP, which was the most prescribed antibiotic in both the CP group (32.82%) and the non-CP group (32.72%), with no significant difference ($p = 0.98$) (Fig. 1). Approximately 79.52% of the 796 antibiotics administered to inpatients with CAP were the recommended antibiotics of the national CP.

The study also showed that 70.81% of the inpatients with CAP received the recommended antibiotics and that the compliance rate for the recommended antibiotics was much higher in the CP group (80.11%) than in the non-CP group (52.51%) ($p < 0.0001$) (Table 2).

Use of the recommended combination of antibiotics
A total of 45.95% of the inpatients with CAP received combined antibiotics. The compliance rate for use of the recommended antibiotic combination was 57.38%, but it was much higher in the CP group (66.46%) than in the non-CP group (38.75%) ($p = 0.001$). In addition, the compliance rate for use of the recommended antibiotic combination (57.38%) was much lower than that for use of the recommended antibiotics for inpatients with CAP who received only one category of antibiotics (83.28%) (Table 2).

Overall compliance with the CP
The overall compliance rate for inpatients with CAP was 43.69%; the overall compliance rate was much higher in the CP group (51.14%) than in the non-CP group (29.05%) ($p < 0.0001$) (Table 2).

Factors influencing antibiotic use
A multivariate logistic model for the overall compliance among inpatients with CAP showed that the hospitals in the CP group had greater overall compliance than those in the non-CP group (odds ratio [OR] = 1.76; 95% confidence interval [CI] = 1.16–2.71) after controlling for hospital (level and location) and inpatient characteristics (sex, age, the number of comorbidities and severity). In addition, the hospitals in the Hubei and Gansu provinces had lower overall compliance (OR = 0.31, 95% CI = 0.20–0.48; OR = 0. 26, 95% CI = 0. 16–0.41) than those in Shanghai (Table 3).

Table 2 Comparison of compliance rates for antibiotic use between the CP and non-CP groups

Items	Total ($n = 531$)		CP group ($n = 352$)		Non-CP group ($n = 179$)		p-value
	n	%	n	%	n	%	
Timely administration of antibiotics	455	85.69	319	90.63	136	75.98	< 0.0001
Use of recommended antibiotics	376	70.81	282	80.11	94	52.51	< 0.0001
One category of antibiotics used	239	83.28 [a]	176	93.62	63	63.64	< 0.0001
Use of recommended combination of antibiotics	140	57.38	109	66.46	31	38.75	0.001
Overall compliance[b]	232	43.69	180	51.14	52	29.05	< 0.0001

[a]Compliance rates for the use of recommended antibiotics in inpatients with CAP who used only one antibiotic were significantly different from the compliance rates for the use of recommended combinations of antibiotics ($p < 0.0001$);
[b]Overall compliance applied to cases that met the requirements of timely use of initial antibiotics (≤ 8 h), use of recommended antibiotics and use of the recommended antibiotic combination

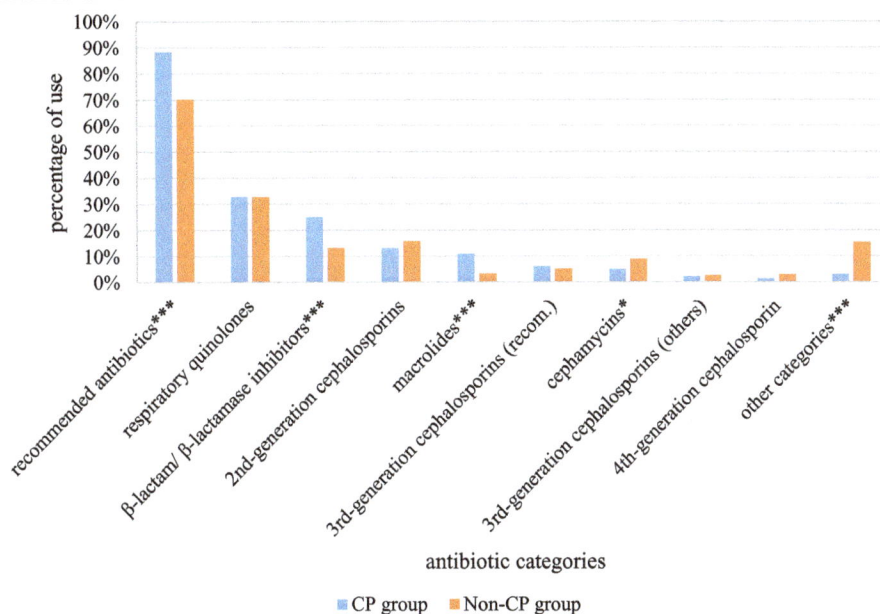

Fig. 1 Distribution of antibiotic use in the CP and non-CP groups
[a]Recommended antibiotics include respiratory quinolones, β-lactam/β-lactamase inhibitors, 2nd-generation cephalosporins, macrolides and the recommended 3rd-generation cephalosporins (ceftriaxone and cefotaxime). $*p < 0.05$, $***p < 0.001$.

Discussion

This study found that CP implementation for patients with CAP has a positive influence on antibiotic utilization. However, some social and economic factors may affect CP compliance, which led to differences in CP compliance among hospitals in different regions of China.

Relatively higher compliance with timely use of antibiotics

Timely initial use of antibiotics may lead to a lower risk of a fatal outcome in patients with CAP [28]. Our study found that antibiotic use in the inpatients with CAP was timely in most cases (84.18% received antibiotics within 4 h of hospital admission) and mostly followed the national CP (85.69% compliance rate). In the United States, the rates of administration of an initial dose of antibiotic within 4 and 8 h of admission were 78% and 93%, respectively [29]. However, the compliance rate for timely antibiotic use among inpatients with CAP was much higher in the CP group (90.63%) than in the non-CP group (75.98%). This discrepancy suggests that timely antibiotic use can be further improved if hospitals implement the CP for inpatients with CAP.

Large gap in compliance with recommended antibiotics

To reach the goal of anti-infective therapy, appropriate antibiotics must be selected. In our study, we found that 796 antibiotics within 18 antibiotic categories were administered to inpatients with CAP. Respiratory quinolones, β-lactam/β-lactamase inhibitors, 2nd-generation

cephalosporins, macrolides and 3rd-generation cephalosporins (ceftriaxone and cefotaxime), which were recommended in the CP for CAP in China, were among the top 5 utilized antibiotics (approximately 80% of the antibiotics used in inpatients with CAP).

In particular, respiratory quinolones accounted for approximately one-third of the antibiotics used in both the CP and non-CP groups in the study, which may be attributed to their effective antibacterial activity, less prominent cross-drug resistance, low protein-binding rate and high capacity for tissue penetration [30]. In China, a number of epidemiological studies have found that mycoplasma pneumoniae and streptococcus pneumoniae are important pathogens of adult CAP [31–35]. Furthermore, mycoplasma pneumoniae is highly resistant to macrolides but is sensitive to doxycycline or minocycline and quinolones [36, 37], which may be one of the reasons that in China, respiratory quinolones are the recommended medications in the CAP guidelines [6, 38]. In fact, respiratory quinolones are also generally recommended for non-ICU hospitalized CAP patients in the guidelines of many other countries [3, 5, 39]. However, respiratory quinolones are broad-spectrum antibiotics, and the use of them in initial treatments for CAP patients may lead to a delay in the discovery of and implementation of appropriate therapy for pulmonary tuberculosis [40–43]; therefore, caution should be employed when respiratory quinolones are used as an initial therapy for CAP.

In addition, the study revealed that 70.81% of the inpatients with CAP were administered the recommended

Table 3 Multivariate logistic analysis of overall compliance with antibiotic use [a]

Parameters	OR Estimates	95% CI [b]		p-value
		Lower	Upper	
Intercept				0.760
Regions (comparison = Shanghai)				
Hubei province (1 = yes, 0 = no)	0.31	0.20	0.48	< 0.0001
Gansu province (1 = yes, 0 = no)	0.26	0.16	0.41	< 0.0001
Tertiary hospital (1 = yes, 0 = no)	0.73	0.50	1.07	0.108
Male (1 = yes, 0 = no)	0.93	0.64	1.35	0.699
Age (years)	1.01	1.00	1.02	0.184
No. of comorbidities (comparison = 0)				
1 comorbidity (1 = yes, 0 = no)	0.83	0.54	1.29	0.410
2 comorbidities (1 = yes, 0 = no)	1.05	0.60	1.83	0.871
Non-severe CAP (1 = yes, 0 = no)	0.85	0.54	1.32	0.463
Hospital implementation of CP (1 = yes, 0 = no)	1.76	1.16	2.71	0.009

[a]The dependent variable was overall compliance with antibiotic use in inpatients with CAP (1: overall compliance; 0: overall non-compliance), and $\chi^2_{likelihood\ ratio} = 67.66$, $p < 0.001$;
[b]CI: Confidence interval

antibiotics, which was lower than the rate in the United States (81%) [29]. A large gap existed in compliance with the use of recommended antibiotics between the CP (80.11%) and non-CP groups (52.51%).

Low compliance with the recommended combination of antibiotics

Appropriate antibiotic use can improve antibacterial effectiveness and can reduce side effects in inpatients with CAP [44]; therefore, appropriate antibiotic use also includes the appropriate use of combined antibiotics. Our study revealed that 45.95% of the inpatients with CAP received combined antibiotics in hospitals in China and that the compliance rate for the use of the recommended combination of antibiotics was much lower than that in the inpatients who received non-combined antibiotics (57.38% vs. 83.28%). This finding suggested that many inpatients with CAP did not receive appropriate combined antibiotics according to the recommendations in the national CP. Inappropriate use of combined antibiotics in China was also found in one study of primary healthcare facilities in China [11].

Facilitation of CP implementation for better antibiotic utilization

Our study demonstrated a large gap between evidence-based recommended therapy and actual clinical practice [45, 46]. The overall compliance rate in China (43.69%) was much lower than the 75–80% compliance rates reported for antibiotic prescriptions for CAP patients in some previous studies [29, 47, 48]. Inappropriate antibiotic utilization can not only impact the effectiveness and safety of medical care for CAP patients but can also easily create multidrug-resistant bacterial strains [48].

Adherence to CAP guidelines has been shown to improve clinical outcomes, including reductions in the length of hospital stay, morbidity and mortality [49, 50]. The CP for CAP in China is based on CAP guidelines; therefore, antibiotic use consistent with the CP can theoretically result in more effective and safer patient care. This study showed that inpatients with CAP in the CP group received antibiotics more concordantly with the CP (51.14% vs. 29.05% overall compliance). The multivariate logistic analysis also found that the hospitals that implemented the CP had greater overall compliance than the hospitals that did not (OR = 1.76) after controlling for hospital and inpatient characteristics. Our study indicated that facilitation of CP implementation improved antibiotic utilization, including initial antibiotic administration, antibiotic selection and the use of combined antibiotics.

Although the 12 hospitals that implemented the CP for inpatients with CAP in our study had training and quality control for CP implementation, 3 hospitals did not have incentives for CP implementation. Many articles have discussed the effects of social, organizational, cognitive and/or motivational factors on the implementation of clinical practice guidelines (CPGs) or CPs [51–53]. Other factors, such as CP quality, which is mainly related to whether the CP is applied in complex clinical practice in a timely, effective and accurate manner, and internal and external support from the hospital, may also affect CP implementation.

Associations of local social and economic statuses with antibiotic use

According to the findings from the multivariate logistic analysis, the hospitals in Shanghai, which is one of the most developed cities in China, had a higher overall compliance rate for antibiotic use than those in the Hubei and Gansu provinces, suggesting that external social and economic statuses affected antibiotic use. One probable reason for this result was greater awareness of the negative impacts of inappropriate antibiotic use on patient outcomes among hospitals, physicians and the local population and strict monitoring of antibiotic use by the local government in Shanghai [54, 55]. Another possible reason is that hospital regions with higher social and economic levels tend to allocate more resources towards improving antibiotic utilization (including more education on the proper use of antibiotics and the construction of health information systems to provide antibiotic information, authorize antibiotic prescriptions, warn against unusual utilization and provide real-time monitoring) and providing financial incentives for proper antibiotic use based on related assessments [56–58].

Conclusions

In China, the overall compliance rate with the national CP for inpatients with CAP was low, but the inpatients in the hospitals of the CP group received antibiotics more concordantly with the national CP. Adherence to evidence-based care has been shown to improve clinical outcomes but requires internal and external support from hospitals to facilitate CP implementation for inpatients with CAP and governmental commitment, hospital input and population involvement to improve antibiotic utilization.

Abbreviations

CAP: Community-acquired pneumonia; CGs: Clinical guidelines; CI: Confidence interval; CP: Clinical pathway; CPG: Clinical practice guidelines; ICD-10: International Statistical Classification of Diseases and Related Health Problems10th Revision; ICU: Intensive care unit; IDSA: Infectious Diseases Society of America; NHC: National Health Commission; OR: Odds ratio; WHO: World Health Organization

Acknowledgements

We gratefully acknowledge the significant contributions of Fei Bai, Hongbo Zhu, Huiqin Tang, Xuefeng Wei, Ping Zhou, Minqi Li and other students and colleagues in designing this study, gathering information, analysing data and/or sharing their views with us during the research process. The authors also acknowledge all of the hospitals and the Health and Family Planning Commissions at the provincial and district levels that provided assistance with data collection for this research project.

Funding

This research project was funded by a grant from the National Natural Science Foundation of China (grant number 71473047). The funder was not involved in the design of the study, in the collection, analysis and interpretation of the data, or in writing the manuscript.

Authors' contributions

DX, JB and YC conceived of and designed the study. JB, YC and DX performed the investigation. LZ and JB conducted the statistical analyses and interpreted the data. LZ drafted the manuscript. DX revised the manuscript. All authors have read and approved the manuscript and have approved the submitted version of the manuscript.

Author information

Jie Bai was a PhD student at the School of Public Health, Fudan University from September 2014 to July 2017 and is a staff member of the Pudong Institute for Health Development.

Consent for publication

Since we used chart reviews of medical records in this study, and the data extracted from the medical records did not include any information identifying patients, no informed consent from patients was required in this study.

Competing interests

The authors declare that they have no competing interests.

Author details

[1]NHC Key Laboratory of Health Technology Assessment (Fudan University), Department of Hospital Management, School of Public Health, Fudan University, Shanghai, People's Republic of China. [2]School of Public Health, Lanzhou University, Lanzhou, People's Republic of China.

References

1. Prina E, Ranzani OT, Torres A. Community-acquired pneumonia. Lancet. 2015;386:1097–108. Available from: http://linkinghub.elsevier.com/retrieve/pii/S0140673615607334
2. José RJ, Periselneris JN, Brown JS. Community-acquired pneumonia. Current opinion in pulmonary medicine. 2015;21(3):212–8. Available from: https://www.ncbi.nlm.nih.gov/pubmed/25775050
3. Mandell LA, Wunderink RG, Anzueto A, Bartlett JG, Campbell GD, Dean NC, et al. Infectious Diseases Society of America/American Thoracic Society consensus guidelines on the Management of Community-Acquired Pneumonia in adults. Clin Infect Dis. 2007;44:S27–72. Available from: https://academic.oup.com/cid/article-lookup/doi/10.1086/511159
4. National Institute for Health Excellence. Pneumonia in adults: diagnosis and management. NICE guidelines, 2014. 2014 [cited 2017 Sep 5]. Available from: https://www.nice.org.uk/guidance/cg191
5. Woodhead M, Blasi F, Ewig S, Garau J, Huchon G, Ieven M, et al. Guidelines for the management of adult lower respiratory tract infections - full version. Clin Microbiol Infect. 2011;17:E1–59. Available from: http://linkinghub.elsevier.com/retrieve/pii/S1198743X1461404X.
6. Chinese Medical Association for respiratory diseases. Guidelines for diagnosis and treatment of community acquired pneumonia. Chinese Journal of tuberculosis and respiratory diseases. 2006;29:651–5.
7. Chinese Medical Association. Guideline of clinical therapy for respiratory diseases. Beijing: People's Medical Publishing House; 2009.
8. Sedrak A, Anpalahan M, Luetsch K. Enablers and barriers to the use of antibiotic guidelines in the assessment and treatment of community-acquired pneumonia-a qualitative study of clinicians' perspectives. Int J Clin Pract. 2017;71(6):e12959. Available from:. https://doi.org/10.1111/ijcp.12959.
9. World Health Organization. Antimicrobial resistance: global report on surveillance. 2014. Available from: http://www.searo.who.int/thailand/publications/2013/9789241564748/en/.

10. McGowan JE. Economic impact of antimicrobial resistance. Emerging infectious diseases. 2001;7(2):286–92. Available from: http://www.ncbi.nlm.nih.gov/pubmed/11294725.

11. Li YB, Xu J, Wang F, Wang B, Liu LQ, Hou WL, et al. Overprescribing in China, driven by financial incentives, results in very high use of antibiotics, injections, and corticosteroids. Health affairs (Millwood). 2012;31(5):1075–82. Available from: https://www.healthaffairs.org/doi/abs/10.1377/hlthaff.2010.0965?url_ver=Z39.88-2003&rfr_id=ori:rid:crossref.org&rfr_dat=cr_pub%3dpubmed.

12. Li CH, Wu AH, Wen XM, Ren N. National health care-associated infection surveillance system point-prevalence trend of antibacterial use in Chinese hospitals 2001-2010. Chinese J hospital infection. 2012;22(21):4859–61. Available from: http://g.wanfangdata.com.cn/details/detail.do?_type=perio&id=zhyygrxzz201221079.

13. Heddini A, Cars O, Qiang S, Tomson G. Antibiotic resistance in China—a major future challenge. Lancet. 2009;373(9657):30. Available from: http://linkinghub.elsevier.com/retrieve/pii/S014067360861956X.

14. Davey P, Sneddon J, Nathwani D. Overview of strategies for overcoming the challenge of antimicrobial resistance. Expert review of clinical pharmacology. 2010;3(5):667–86. Available from: https://www.ncbi.nlm.nih.gov/pubmed/22111749.

15. Wiegand PN, Nathwani D, Wilcox MH, Stephens J, Shelbaya A, Haider S. Clinical and economic burden of Clostridium difficile infection in Europe: a systematic review of healthcare-facility-acquired infection. Journal of Hospital Infection Elsevier Ltd. 2012;81(1):1–14. Available from: https://www.ncbi.nlm.nih.gov/pubmed/?term=22498638.

16. Kuijper EJ, Coignard B, Tüll P, ESCMID Study Group for Clostridium difficile; EU Member States; European Centre for Disease Prevention and Control. Emergence of Clostridium difficile-associated disease in North America and Europe. Clinical Microbiology and Infection. 2006;12(Suppl 6):2–18. Available from: http://linkinghub.elsevier.com/retrieve/pii/S1198743X15300124.

17. Owens RC, Fraser GL, Stogsdill P, Society of Infectious Diseases Pharmacists. Antimicrobial stewardship programs as a means to optimize antimicrobial use. Insights from the Society of Infectious Diseases Pharmacists. Pharmacotherapy. 2004;24(7):896–908. Available from: http://www.ncbi.nlm.nih.gov/pubmed/15303453.

18. Barlam TF, Cosgrove SE, Abbo LM, MacDougall C, Schuetz AN, Septimus EJ, et al. Implementing an antibiotic stewardship program: guidelines by the Infectious Diseases Society of America and the Society for Healthcare Epidemiology of America. Clin Infect Dis. 2016;62(10):e51–77. Available from: https://academic.oup.com/cid/article-lookup/doi/10.1093/cid/ciw118.

19. Owens RC. Antimicrobial stewardship: concepts and strategies in the 21st century. Diagn Microbiol Infect Dis. 2008;61(1):110–28. Available from: https://www.ncbi.nlm.nih.gov/pubmed/?term=18384997.

20. Rotter T, Kinsman L, James EL, Machotta A, Gothe H, Willis J, et al. Clinical pathways: effects on professional practice, patient outcomes, length of stay and hospital costs. Cochrane database of systematic reviews. 2010; No.: CD006632. Available from: http://doi.wiley.com/10.1002/14651858.CD006632.pub2.

21. Scott SD, Grimshaw J, Klassen TP, Nettel-Aguirre A, Johnson DW. Understanding implementation processes of clinical pathways and clinical practice guidelines in pediatric contexts: a study protocol. Implementation Science BioMed Central Ltd. 2011;6:133. Available from: http://www.implementationscience.com/content/6/1/133.

22. Morrissey D. Guidelines and pathways for clinical practice in Tendinopathy: their role and development. J Orthop Sports Phys Ther. 2015;45(11):819–22. Available from: http://www.jospt.org/doi/10.2519/jospt.2015.0111.

23. Notification of the National Health and Family Planning Commission on the implementation of clinical pathways for related diseases. General Office of the National Health and Family Planning Commission of People's Republic of China; 2016 [cited 2017 Mar 20]. Available from: http://www.nhfpc.gov.cn/yzygj/s7659/201612/e02b9324fc344f45979b6c20d7497b71.shtml.

24. Marr JJ, Moffet HL, Kunin CM. Guidelines for improving the use of antimicrobial agents in hospitals: a statement by the Infectious Diseases Society of America. J infectious diseases. 1988;157(5):869–76. Available from: https://academic.oup.com/jid/article-abstract/157/5/869/2190562?redirectedFrom=fulltext.

25. Tian GL, Ding ZH. Effect of clinical pathway on antimicrobial prophylaxis in patients with hip joint replacement. Chinese J Infection Control. 2013;12(5):367–9. Available from: http://g.wanfangdata.com.cn/details/detail.do?_type=perio&id=zggrkzzz201305012.

26. Duan XC, Yin J, Yu J, Ji HM, Ma JH. Effect of chronic subdural hematoma clinical pathway on the rational usage of antimicrobial agents. Chin J Neurosurg Dis Res. 2014;13(4):341–3. Available from: http://g.wanfangdata.com.cn/details/detail.do?_type=perio&id=zhsjwkjbyjzz201404014.

27. National Health Commission of the People's Republic of China. Clinical pathway of community acquired pneumonia (2009). 2009 [cited 2016 Dec 31]. Available from: http://www.nhfpc.gov.cn/zhuz/xzqq/200912/45417.shtml.

28. Tacconelli E. Antimicrobial use: risk driver of multidrug resistant microorganisms in healthcare settings. Curr Opin Infect Dis. 2009;22(4):352–8. Available from: https://insights.ovid.com/pubmed?pmid=19461514.

29. Dudas V, Hopefl A, Jacobs R, Guglielmo BJ. Antimicrobial selection for hospitalized patients with presumed community-acquired pneumonia: a survey of nonteaching US Community hospitals. Ann Pharmacother. 2000;34(4):446–52. Available from: http://journals.sagepub.com/doi/10.1345/aph.19174.

30. YM LI, JZ MIU. Rational use of antimicrobial agents in community-acquired pneumonia. Chinese General Practice. 2008;11(16):1423–5. Available from: http://g.wanfangdata.com.cn/details/detail.do?_type=perio&id=zgqkyx200816001.

31. Tao LL, Hu BJ, He LX, Wei L, Xie HM, Wang BQ, et al. Etiology and antimicrobial resistance of community-acquired pneumonia in adult patients in China. Chin med J (Engl). 2012;125(17):2967–72. Available from: http://med.wanfangdata.com.cn/Paper/Detail?id=PeriodicalPaper_zhcmj201217002 .

32. Liu YF, Gao Y, Chen MF, Cao B, Yang XH, Wei L. Etiological analysis and predictive diagnostic model building of community-acquired pneumonia in adult outpatients in Beijing. China BMC Infect Dis. 2013;13:309. Available from: https://www.ncbi.nlm.nih.gov/pmc/articles/PMC3728139/ .

33. Cao B, Ren LL, Zhao F, Gonzalez R, Song SF, Bai L, et al. Viral and mycoplasma pneumoniae community-acquired pneumonia and novel clinical outcome evaluation in ambulatory adult patients in China. Eur J Clin Microbiol Infect Dis. 2010;29(11):1443–8. Available from: https://www.ncbi.nlm.nih.gov/pubmed/?term=10.1007%2Fs10096-010-1003-2.

34. Bao ZY, Yuan XD, Wang L, Sun YL, Dong XQ. The incidence and etiology of community-acquired pneumonia in fever outpatients. Exp Biol Med (Maywood). 2012;237(11):1256–61. Available from: https://www.ncbi.nlm.nih.gov/pubmed/23239436.

35. Liu YN, Chen MJ, Zhao TM, Wang H, Wang R, Liu QF, et al. A multicenter study on the pathogenic agents in 665 adult patients with community-acquired pneumonia in cities of China. Chin J Tuberc Respir Dis. 2006;29(1):3–8. Available from: https://www.ncbi.nlm.nih.gov/pubmed/?term=16638292.

36. Yin YD, Cao B, Wang H, Wang RT, Liu YM, Gao Y, et al. Survey of macrolide resistance in mycoplasma pneumoniae in adult patients with community-acquired pneumonia in Beijing. China Chin J Tuberc Respir Dis. 2013;36(12):954–8. Available from: http://g.wanfangdata.com.cn/details/detail.do?_type=perio&id=zhjhhhx201312021.

37. Liu Y, Ye XY, Zhang H, Xu XG, Li WH, Zhu DM, et al. Antimicrobial susceptibility of mycoplasma pneumoniae isolates and molecular analysis of macrolide-resistant strains from shanghai, China. Antimicrob Agents Chemother. 2009;53(5):2160–2. Available from: https://www.ncbi.nlm.nih.gov/pubmed/?term=10.1128%2FAAC.01684-08.

38. Chinese Medical Association for respiratory diseases. Guidelines for diagnosis and treatment of adult community-acquired pneumonia in China (2016 edition). Chin J Tuberc Respir Dis. 2016;39(4):253–79. Available from: http://g.wanfangdata.com.cn/details/detail.do?_type=perio&id=zhjhhhx201604005.

39. Kaysin A, Viera AJ. Community-Acquired Pneumonia in Adults: Diagnosis and Management. Am Fam Physician. 2016;94(9):698–706. Available from: https://www.ncbi.nlm.nih.gov/pubmed/27929242.

40. Dooley KE, Golub J, Goes FS, Merz WG, Sterling TR. Empiric treatment of community-acquired pneumonia with fluoroquinolones, and delays in the treatment of tuberculosis. Clinical Infectious Diseases. 2002;34(12):1607–12. Available from: https://academic.oup.com/cid/article/34/12/1607/349210 .

41. Yoon YS, Lee HJ, Yoon HI, Yoo CG, Kim YW, Han SK, et al. Impact of fluoroquinolones on the diagnosis of pulmonary tuberculosis initially treated as bacterial pneumonia. International Union Against Tuberculosis and Lung Disease. 2005;9(11):1215–9. Available from: https://www.ncbi.nlm.nih.gov/pubmed/?term=16333927.

42. Wang JY, Hsueh PR, Jan IS, Lee LN, Liaw YS, Yang PC, et al. Empirical treatment with a fluoroquinolone delays the treatment for tuberculosis and is associated with a poor prognosis in endemic areas. Thorax. 2006;61(10):903–8. Available from: https://www.ncbi.nlm.nih.gov/pubmed/?term=16809417.

43. Golub JE, Bur S, Cronin WA, Gange S, Sterling TR, Oden B, et al. Impact of empiric antibiotics and chest radiograph on delays in the diagnosis of tuberculosis. International Union Against Tuberculosis and Lung Disease. 2005;9(4):392–7. Available from: https://www.ncbi.nlm.nih.gov/pubmed/?term=15832463.

44. Tang KM, Xiang QZ, Zhu JJ. Application analysis of antibacterial drugs in inpatients with CAP. Chinese Journal of Drug Application and Monitoring. 2008;5(5):31–4. Available from: http://g.wanfangdata.com.cn/details/detail.do?_type=perio&id=zgywyyyjc200805011.

45. Grol R. Successes and failures in the implementation of evidence-based guidelines for clinical practice. Medical care. 2001;39(8 Suppl 2):II46–54. Available from: http://www.ncbi.nlm.nih.gov/pubmed/11583121.

46. Davis D, Evans M, Jadad A, Perrier L, Rath D, Ryan D, et al. The case for knowledge translation: shortening the journey from evidence to effect. BMJ. 2003;327(7405):33–5. Available from: https://www.ncbi.nlm.nih.gov/pubmed/?term=12842955.

47. Mortensen EM, Restrepo M, Anzueto A, Pugh J. Effects of guideline-concordant antimicrobial therapy on mortality among patients with community-acquired pneumonia. Am J Med. 2004;117(10):726–31. Available from: http://linkinghub.elsevier.com/retrieve/pii/S0002934304005224.

48. Kong XM. Rational use of antimicrobial agents in community-acquired pneumonia. Chinese Rural Health Service Administration. 2012;32(6):593–6. Available from: http://g.wanfangdata.com.cn/details/detail.do?_type=perio&id=zgncwssygl201206021.

49. Spoorenberg V, Hulscher MEJL, Akkermans RP, Prins JM, Geerlings SE. Appropriate antibiotic use for patients with urinary tract infections reduces length of hospital stay. Clin Infect Dis. 2014;58(2):164–9. Available from: https://academic.oup.com/cid/article-lookup/doi/10.1093/cid/cit688.

50. South M, Royle J, Starr M. A simple intervention to improve hospital antibiotic prescribing. Med j Australia. 2003;178(5):207–9. Available from: http://www.ncbi.nlm.nih.gov/pubmed/12603182.

51. Abrahamson KA, Fox RL, Doebbeling BN. Facilitators and barriers to clinical practice guideline use among nurses. Am j nursing. 2012;112(7):26–35. quiz 46,36. Available from: https://www.ncbi.nlm.nih.gov/pubmed/22705494.

52. McConnell T, O'Halloran P, Porter S, Donnelly M. Systematic realist review of key factors affecting the successful implementation and sustainability of the Liverpool care pathway for the dying patient. Worldviews Evid-Based Nurs. 2013;10(4):218–37. Available from: http://doi.wiley.com/10.1111/wvn.12003.

53. Hulscher ME, Grol RP, van der Meer JW. Antibiotic prescribing in hospitals: a social and behavioural scientific approach. lancet infectious diseases. 2010; 10(3):167–75. Available from: http://www.ncbi.nlm.nih.gov/pubmed/20185095.

54. Antibiotic Utilization Reduces by Half and Proper Antibiotic Utilization in Population Increases to 89.7%. Shanghai Municipal Commission of Health and Family Planning; 2013 [cited 2017 Sep 7]. Available from:http://www.wsjsw.gov.cn/jtyx/20180526/41854.html .

55. Zhang YX. Guideline for standardized clinical application of antibiotics: shanghai issues rules for its implementation. Shanghai Medical & Pharmaceutical J. 2007;28(3):101–3. Available from: http://g.wanfangdata.com.cn/details/detail.do?_type=perio&id=shyy200703001.

56. Shu W, Ren SH, Jiang J, Liu JY, Li J, Xu JL, et al. Analysis of antibiotics application in five hospitals in our district before and after the implementation of measures for the Management of Clinical use of antibiotics. China Pharmacy. 2015;26(17):2314–8. Available from: http://kns.cnki.net/KCMS/detail/detail.aspx?dbcode=CJFQ&dbname=CJFDLAST2015&filename=ZGYA201517004&uid=WEEvREcwSlJHSldRa1FhdkJkVWI0UTAvaXVBUmpjVjRVT2F5aXYxQ2Ridz0.

57. Guo YJ. Research on enhancing hospital culture construction under new situation. 2014 [cited 2017 Sep 7]. Available from: http://www.wsjsw.gov.cn/llyt/20180525/25463.html.

58. Yuan KJ, Yang WH, Suo ZL, Ni YX, Yuan JY, Fang J, et al. Effect and practice of the information system in the management and monitoring of hospital clinical antibacterials. Shanghai Med Pharma J. 2012;33(11):32–4. Available from: http://g.wanfangdata.com.cn/details/detail.do?_type=perio&id=shyy201211012.

20

Clinical, immunological and bacteriological characteristics of H7N9 patients nosocomially co-infected by *Acinetobacter Baumannii*

William J. Liu[1,2†], Rongrong Zou[1†], Yongfei Hu[3†], Min Zhao[3], Chuansong Quan[2], Shuguang Tan[3], Kai Luo[1], Jing Yuan[1], Haixia Zheng[1], Jue Liu[4], Min Liu[4], Yuhai Bi[1,3,6], Jinghua Yan[3], Baoli Zhu[3], Dayan Wang[2], Guizhen Wu[2], Lei Liu[1], Kwok-Yung Yuen[5], George F. Gao[1,2,3,6*] and Yingxia Liu[1*]

Abstract

Background: Bacterial co-infection of patients suffering from influenza pneumonia is a key element that increases morbidity and mortality. The occurrence of *Acinetobacter baumannii* co-infection in patients with avian influenza A (H7N9) virus infection has been described as one of the most prevalent bacterial co-infections. However, the clinical and laboratory features of this entity of H7N9 and *A. baumannii* co-infection have not been systematically investigated.

Methods: We collected clinical and laboratory data from laboratory-confirmed H7N9 cases co-infected by *A. baumannii*. H7N9 patients without bacterial co-infection and patients with *A. baumannii*-related pneumonia in the same hospital during the same period were recruited as controls. The antibiotic resistance features and the corresponding genome determinants of *A. baumannii* and the immune responses of the patients were tested through the respiratory and peripheral blood specimens.

Results: Invasive mechanical ventilation was the most significant risk factor for the nosocomial *A. baumannii* co-infection in H7N9 patients. The co-infection resulted in severe clinical manifestation which was associated with the dysregulation of immune responses including deranged T-cell counts, antigen-specific T-cell responses and plasma cytokines. The emergence of genome variations of extensively drug-resistant *A. baumannii* associated with acquired polymyxin resistance contributed to the fatal outcome of a co-infected patient.

Conclusions: The co-infection of H7N9 patients by extensively drug-resistant *A. baumannii* with H7N9 infection is an important issue which deserves attention. The dysfunctions of immune responses were associated with the co-infection and were correlated with the disease severity. These data provide useful reference for the diagnosis and treatment of H7N9 infection.

Keywords: Avian influenza A(H7N9) virus, *Acinetobacter baumannii*, Extensively drug-resistant bacteria, Nosocomial infection, Pneumonia, Immune responses

* Correspondence: gaofu@chinacdc.cn; yingxialiu@hotmail.com
[†]William J. Liu, Rongrong Zou and Yongfei Hu contributed equally to this work.
Kwok-Yung Yuen, George F. Gao and Yingxia Liu jointly supervised this work.
[1]Shenzhen Key Laboratory of Pathogen and Immunity, State Key Discipline of Infectious Disease, Shenzhen Third People's Hospital, Shenzhen 518112, China

Background

Although influenza viruses by itself can cause highly fatal primary influenza pneumonia, the excess mortality rates during influenza pandemics is mainly caused by secondary bacterial pneumonia [1]. Epidemiologic evidence suggests that 95% and 70% of deaths during the influenza pandemic of 1918–19 and 1957–58, respectively, were due to bacterial pneumonia [2]. During the first season (between May 2009 and August 2009) of 2009 pandemic H1N1 influenza, 29% of fatal cases in the United States were associated with a secondary bacterial infection, which was also correlated with the severity of the pneumonia [3]. In hospitalized patients with seasonal influenza, sepsis with or without bacteremia were one of the severe complications, and associated with increased duration of hospitalization days and the requirement of intensive care [4]. The secondary bacterial pneumonia was also observed in patients infected by avian influenza viruses including H5N1 and H7N9 [5]. However, the frequency of secondary bacterial respiratory infection and its effect on the disease severity of avian influenza virus-infected human cases were still lacking.

Acinetobacter baumannii is one of the major opportunistic pathogens that have been implicated in various nosocomial infections [6]. The most frequent clinical manifestation of nosocomial *A. baumannii* infection is ventilator-associated pneumonia [7]. Although the clinical impact of nosocomial *A. baumannii* infection has been a matter of continuing debate as many patients with severe influenza had major underlying diseases [8], it has been concluded that *A. baumannii* infection was associated with an increase in attributable mortality, ranging from 7.8 to 23% [9]. *A. baumannii* is attracting much attention owing to the increase in antimicrobial resistance and occurrence of strains that are resistant to virtually all available drugs [10]. The rapid global emergence of multidrug-resistant *A. baumannii* (MDR-AB) strains resistant to all β-lactams, including carbapenems, illustrated the potential of this organism to respond swiftly to changes in selective environmental pressure [11]. Though it is still very rare, recently, resistance to polymyxins has also been described [12], which leads to a pandrug-resistant *A. baumannii* (PDR-AB) that can be fully refractory to the currently available antimicrobial armamentarium.

From March 2013, hundreds of human cases infected by avian influenza A (H7N9) virus with a mortality of 40% were reported and the epidemic situation seems more severe currently with over 100 new cases within December 2016 (http://www.who.int/influenza). Among the H7N9 patients complicated by bacterial infections, MDR-AB was the most common etiology for secondary bacterial pneumonia revealed by independent descriptive studies. Herein, we studied the occurrence of secondary infection by *A. Baumannii* in these severe H7N9 patients. We sought to investigate the role of dysfunctional immunity in the pathogenesis of severe pneumonia in H7N9 patients nosocomially co-infected with *A. baumannii*. Our study may improve the understanding of the high pathogenicity of H7N9 in humans and provide useful recommendations for the clinical diagnosis and treatment.

Methods

The patients

From December 2013 to April 2014, 24 patients hospitalized for H7N9 influenza in the Shenzhen Third People's Hospital, Guangdong, China, which is the designated for H7N9 patients in Shenzhen. The laboratory confirmation of H7N9 virus infection were performed using the protocols as described previously [13, 14]. Briefly, the H7N9 infections of patients were confirmed by real-time RT-PCR assay using influenza subtype-specific primers. Real-time RT-PCR experiments were performed using the RNA which was extracted from the samples using the RNeasy Mini Kit (QIAGEN, Germany). The patients who were diagnosed in other hospitals in Shenzhen were also transferred to our hospital. Meanwhile, we made a surveillance of *A. baumannii* in the hospital. The diagnosis of nosocomial pneumonia by *A. baumannii* was based on the clinical signs of the patients and confirmed by sputum culture and (or) blood culture according to standard microbiological criteria [15]. The patients without typical clinical manifestations were excluded as bacterial colonization of *A. baumannii*. Among the 24 H7N9 patients, 9 patients were diagnosed as secondary infection by *A. baumannii* (H7N9-*A. baumannii* or H7N9-AB case group). Thirteen H7N9 patients without secondary bacterial infection with complete clinical data were termed as H7N9 controls. Fifteen patients with hospital acquired pneumonia due to *A. baumannii*, but H7N9 negative in the same period of our hospital, were also recruited as *A. baumannii* controls. The Declaration of Helsinki was strictly followed. The methods were carried out in accordance with the approved guidelines. We obtained written informed consent from all of the participants or their guardians.

Clinical data investigation

Data collection (including information prior to and during hospitalization until discharge or death) started immediately after admission and continued on a daily basis. The clinical data were integrated by two independent inputs and checked and verified by the third party. Antimicrobial resistance was determined according to National Committee for Clinical Laboratory Standards guidelines [16].

The meta-analyses

We screened the previous studies on the clinical descriptions of H7N9 patients published from April 2013 to December 2016, through the US National Library of Medicine National Institutes of Health (www.ncbi.nlm.nih.gov). Eleven publications which described the secondary bacterial infections of H7N9 patients were summarized (Table 1).

Inflammatory mediator tests

We collected the plasma of H7N9-*A. baumannii* co-infected cases and H7N9 controls on the first day of hospitalization and every seven days afterwards. The levels of different cytokines and chemokines were measured with the Bio-Plex ProTM Human Cytokine Array Kits on a Luminex200TM (Luminex®Multiplexing Instrument, Merck Millipore) following the manufacturers' instructions. The raw data were analyzed using xPONENT 3.1 software (Merck Millipore). Plasmas from seven healthy individuals were used as controls.

H7N9-specific T cell response tests

The CTL epitope-specific response was measured by performing IFN-γ ELISPOT assays as described previously [17]. Previously identified HLA class I-restricted epitopes (8–11 residues) of influenza virus were retrieved from published data [17, 18]. Conserved peptides between H7N9 and 2009pH1N1 were mixed into a conserved peptide pool as described in reference (JID reference) [19]. Mutated HLA class I-restricted peptides between H7N9 and 2009pH1N1 were considered as H7N9-specific peptide pools (JID reference). The number of spots was determined using an automatic ELISPOT reader and image analysis software (Cellular Technology Limited).

A. baumannii genome sequencing and analyzing

The genomes of the *A. baumannii* isolates SMGC-AB1 and SMGC-AB2 were sequenced by Illumina HiSeq sequencing platform according to manufacturer's instructions. The 150-bp length pair-end raw reads were first filtered to remove low-quality reads using the Dynamic-Trim and LengthSort Perl scripts within SolexaQA [20] and then assembled and gap closed using SOAPdenovo2 program (http://soap.genomics.org.cn) [21]. The comparative genome analysis and SNP calling were performed using Mauve software [22]. The draft genomes were annotated using the RAST program (rapid annotation using subsystem technology) [23]. For SNP-based phylogenetic analysis, the whole-genome alignment and SNP calling were performed using Mugsy [24]. The antibiotic resistance gene information was first summarized based on the Subsystem subcategory "Resistance to antibiotics and toxic compounds" according to RAST annotation. Then, the Comprehensive Antibiotic Resistance Database (CARD) [25] was used for the further searching of resistance genes in the sequenced *A. baumannii* genomes.

Accession codes

The Whole Genome Shotgun projects of patient B4-derived original extensively drug-resistant (XDR) *A. baumannii* SMGC-AB1 and subsequently polymyxin resistant, i.e. a pandrug-resistant isolate (PDR) named *A. baumannii* SMGC-AB2 have been deposited at DDBJ/ENA/GenBank under the accessions NIBI00000000 and NIBH00000000, respectively.

Statistics

The Student's *t*-test or χ2-test was used to determine differences between two groups. The Pearson correlation coefficient and Spearman rank correlation coefficient were used for linear correlation analysis. We calculated

Table 1 Mutation information in *A. baumannii* SMGC-AB2 isolated from H7N9 patient B4[a]

No.	Gene Annotation	ORF length	position (NT)	mutation (NT)	AA length	position (AA)	substitute (AA)
1	putative permease, YjgP/YjgQ family protein	1101 bp	164	G → A	366	55	Arg → His
2	histidine kinase; PmrB	1335	704	C → T	444	235	Thr → Ile
3	Lipid A phosphoethanolamine transferase, associated with polymyxin resistance, PmrC	1647	1598	A → C	548	533	Lys → Thr
4	NAD-dependent aldehyde dehydrogenase	1575	421	C → T	524	141	Leu → Leu
5	Large repetitive protein, type I secretion C-terminal target domain protein	6657	547	A → G	2218	183	Val → Ile
6	Large repetitive protein, type I secretion C-terminal target domain protein	6657	874	G → A	2218	292	Val → Ile
7	Large repetitive protein, type I secretion C-terminal target domain protein	6657	876	T → C	2218	292	Val → Ile
8	Contig C497	8383 (position)		C → T		Non-coding region	

[a]The reference sequence is *A. baumannii* SMGC-AB1 isolated from H7N9 patient B4 isolated on Day 21 after disease onset. *A. baumannii* SMGC-AB2 was isolated from this patient B4 on Day 26 after disease onset

receiver operating characteristic curves for predictive analysis. Logistic regression was used for multivariate analysis of the risk factors. These statistical analyses were performed with SPSS 16.0 for Windows (SPSS, Inc.). A P-value < 0.05 was considered statistically significant.

Results

The incidence of A. baumannii in H7N9 patients

We have done the meta analyses of the previous studies on the clinical descriptions of H7N9 patients (Additional file 1: Table S1). We found the overall incidence of *A. baumannii* among the reported H7N9 patients was 19.0% (37/195). For the 11 *A. baumannii* cases whose outcome were available, 10 patients (90.9%) was reported fatal, much higher than the crude mortality rate of 32.9% (56/170) amongst H7N9 patients. Most of the identified *A. baumannii* were MDR-AB, and with one case of PDR-AB.

From December 2013 to April 2014, 24 patients infected by H7N9 virus were hospitalized in the Shenzhen Third People's Hospital, Guangdong, China. We found that there were two peaks of hospital admission for H7N9 patients (Fig. 1a, Additional file 2: Table S2 and Additional file 3: Table S3). One is from the late December 2013 to early February 2014 and the second peak is from the early March to early April 2014. Meanwhile, we made a surveillance of positive *A. baumannii* isolation in our hospital and found that the weekly incidence of *A. baumannii* was correlated with the hospitalization of H7N9 patients (Fig. 1b). Among the 24 H7N9 patients, 9 patients (37.5%) were diagnosed as secondary bacterial pneumonia caused by *A. baumannii* (H7N9-*A. baumannii* group) during the hospitalization or on retrospective testing (Fig. 1c). Meanwhile, in the same Infectious Disease Unit which was specially designated for H7N9 admission, none of the other 353 patients

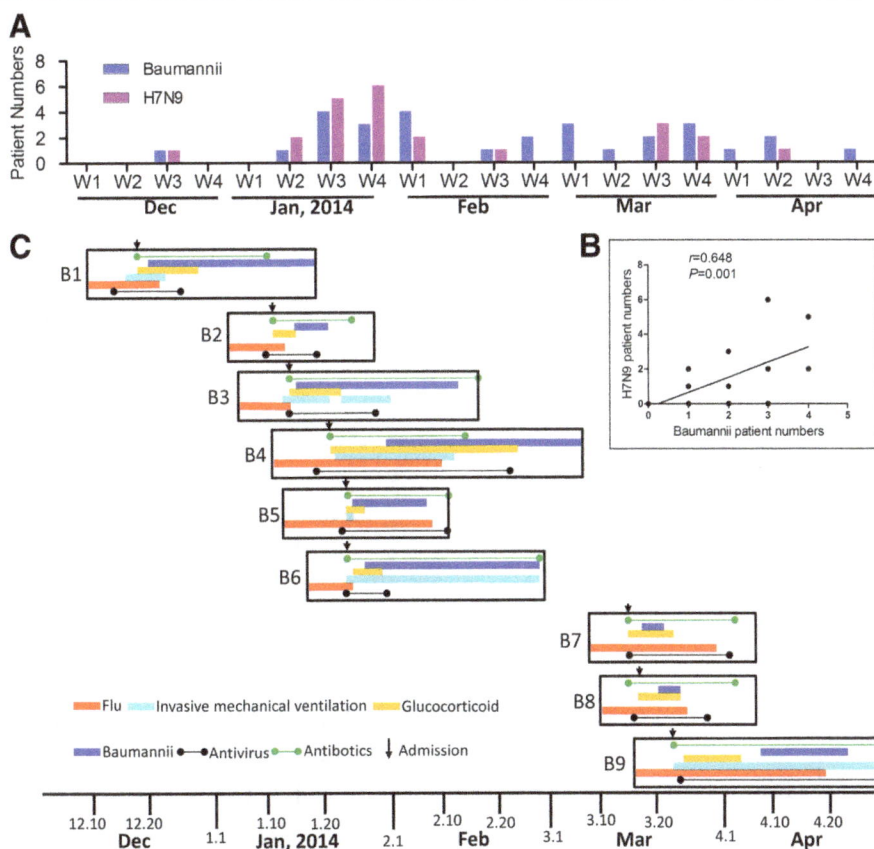

Fig. 1 The occurrence of nosocomial *A. baumannii* infection in H7N9 patients during the timeline of the 2013–2014 H7N9 epidemic wave in the hospital. **a**. The weekly reported cases infected by H7N9 and *A. baumannii*, respectively, from December 2013 to April 2014 in Shenzhen Third People's Hospital, Guangdong China. The first week to the fourth week of each month were denoted as W1 to W4. **b**. The linear correlation of weekly reported numbers of H7N9 patients and *A. baumannii* patients. **c**. The timeline of the laboratory test and clinical treatment of the H7N9 and *A. baumannii* co-infected patients. The corresponding dates for timeline were shown below as the horizontal axis. Flu: The persistent period for positive result of H7N9 RNA detected by RT-PCR; Baumannii: The period for *A. baumannii* positive; Admission: the date for the admission of the patient; Antivirus: the period for the anti-influenza drug therapy; Antibiotics: the period for the antibiotic use; Glucocorticoid: the period for glucocorticiod pulse therapy; Invasive mechanical ventilation: the period for the manipulation of invasive mechanical ventilation

without H7N9 were diagnosed as *A. baumannii* infection. This may exclude the possibility that any poor infection control led to a high frequency of this *A. baumannii* infection in H7N9 patients.

The risk factors for *A. baumannii* co-infection in H7N9 patients

The median duration from admission to the detection of *A. baumannii* was three days. Based on the time line of the clinical interventions, we found that most of the *A. baumannii* co-infection with H7N9 occurred after the application of invasive mechanical ventilation, antibiotics and broad-spectrum immune intervention drugs such as glucocorticoid (methylprednisolone). Furthermore, the risk factors for the secondary infection of *A. baumannii* in the H7N9 patients were analyzed. We found that the H7N9-*A. baumannii* co-infected patients have a significantly longer duration of invasive mechanical ventilation (Fig. 2a), antibiotics use (Fig. 2b) and glucocorticoid use (Fig. 2c) compared to the 13 H7N9 patients without secondary bacterial infection (H7N9 group, the clinical data for the left two patients are not completed). The total dosages of glucocorticoid and globulin were also higher among H7N9 patients co-infected by *A. baumannii* compared to other H7N9 patients without secondary bacterial infection (Fig. 2d). The multivariate analysis

considering the mutual effects of different risk factors showed that invasive mechanical ventilation was still the risk factor for the *A. baumannii* coinfection in H7N9 patients (Additional file 4: Table S4 and Additional file 5: Table S5).

The clinical impact of *A. baumannii* on H7N9 infection

The basic demographic characteristics of H7N9 patients co-infected with *A. baumannii* are similar to H7N9 control patients without secondary infection (Additional file 2: Table S2). The average age of H7N9-*A. baumannii* co-infection group was higher than the H7N9 controls but without significance (61.8 ± 18.3 vs 48.2 ± 14.9, $P > 0.05$). No significant differences were found for the clinical manifestations at the time of admission of H7N9-*A.baumannii* cases compared to the H7N9 controls, including the oxygenation index (PaO_2/FiO_2) (136.3 ± 60.0 vs 217.3 ± 145.0, $P > 0.05$) (Additional file 3: Table S3 and Fig. 3a). However, the lowest oxygenation index was lower and the time for the restoring of oxygenation index was longer during the hospitalization process of the H7N9-*A. baumannii* cases than the H7N9 controls (66.8 ± 31.5 vs 163.9 ± 122.1) (Fig. 3b). Furthermore, the recovered times for the abnormal oxygenation indexes in H7N9-*A. baumannii* cases were longer than the H7N9 controls (Fig. 3c), indicating a more severe pulmonary ventilation

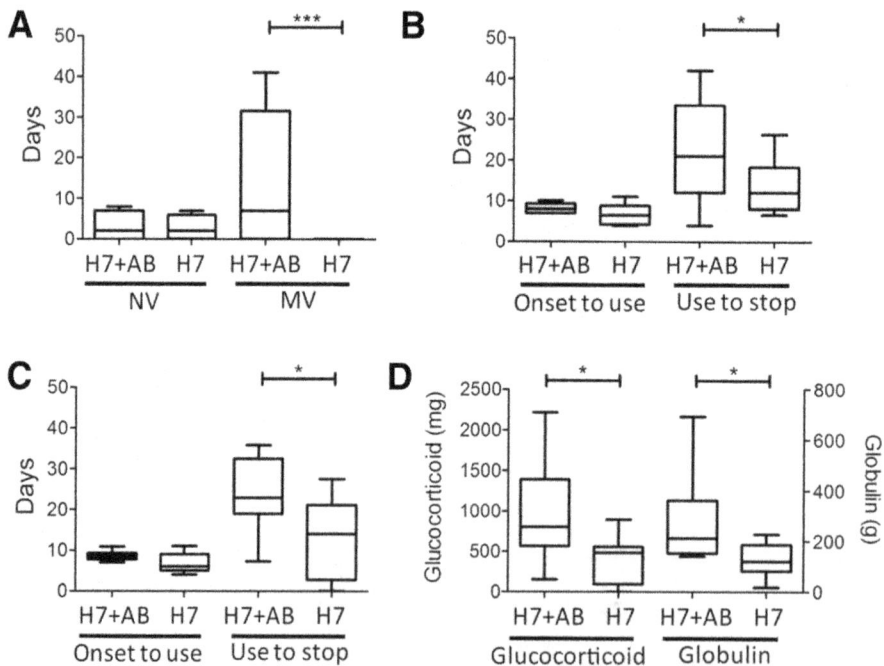

Fig. 2 The risk factors for H7N9-*A. baumannii* co-infection. **a**. The comparison of the manipulation of non-invasive ventilation (NV) and invasive mechanical ventilation (MV) between H7N9-*A. baumannii* co-infected cases (H7N9 + AB) and H7N9 control patients without bacterial co-infection (H7N9). **b**. The time from the disease onset to the use of antibiotics (Onset to use) and the total time for the antibiotic use (Use to stop) is compared between H7N9 + AB cases and H7N9 controls. **c**. The time from the disease onset to the use of glucocorticoid (Onset to use) and the total time for the glucocorticoid use (Use to stop) is compared between H7N9 + AB cases and H7N9 controls. **d**. The total dosages for glucocorticoid and gamma globulin compared between between H7N9 + AB cases and H7N9 controls

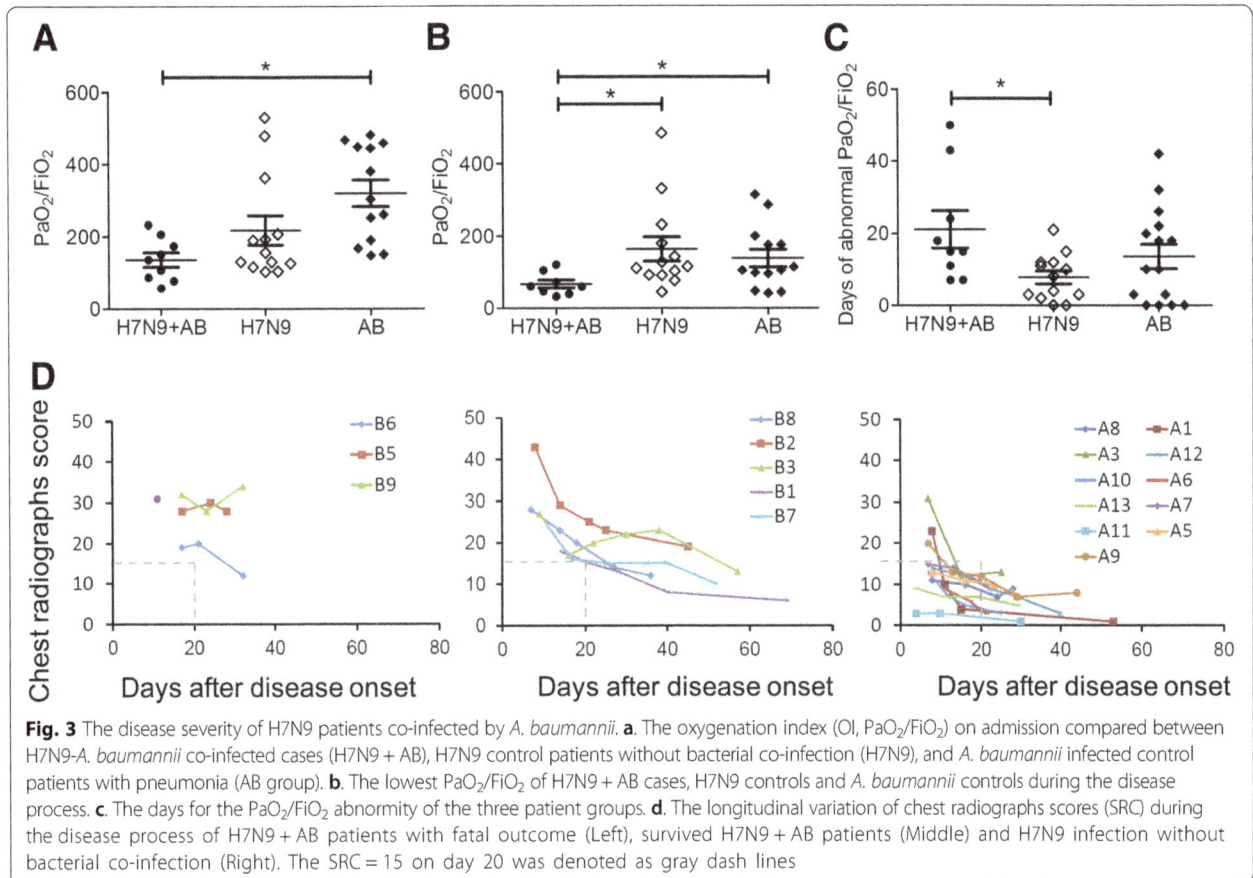

Fig. 3 The disease severity of H7N9 patients co-infected by *A. baumannii*. **a.** The oxygenation index (OI, PaO₂/FiO₂) on admission compared between H7N9-*A. baumannii* co-infected cases (H7N9 + AB), H7N9 control patients without bacterial co-infection (H7N9), and *A. baumannii* infected control patients with pneumonia (AB group). **b.** The lowest PaO₂/FiO₂ of H7N9 + AB cases, H7N9 controls and *A. baumannii* controls during the disease process. **c.** The days for the PaO₂/FiO₂ abnormity of the three patient groups. **d.** The longitudinal variation of chest radiographs scores (SRC) during the disease process of H7N9 + AB patients with fatal outcome (Left), survived H7N9 + AB patients (Middle) and H7N9 infection without bacterial co-infection (Right). The SRC = 15 on day 20 was denoted as gray dash lines

disorder of the H7N9-*A. baumannii* cases after onset of co-infection by *A. baumannii*. The evaluation of chest radiograph score (SRC) which reflects the lung injury during the infection indicates a prolonged high SRC in the H7N9-*A. baumannii* cases (Fig. 3d). All the SRC of the H7N9-*A. baumannii* cases are still > 15 on day 20 after disease onset, while the SRC of most H7N9 controls without co-infection decreased to < 15 on day 20 after disease onset. The H7N9-*A. baumannii* cases had longer time for fever duration (14.3 ± 9.2 vs 8.1 ± 2.5) and the length of hospital are also longer than the H7N9 controls without co-infection (30.0 ± 11.2 vs 15.5 ± 7.1). All H7N9 controls without co-infection survived, but four of the nine (44.4%) H7N9-*A. baumannii* patients died. In the H7N9-*A. baumannii* cases, the patients who died had persistent abnormal oxygenation index compared to that of a gradual improvement in the survivors (Additional file 6: Figure S1).

Dysfunctional immunity in co-infected patients
IL-6 and IL-8 are two major representative cytokines which can reflect the disease severity during the acute phase of H7N9 as reported previously [26]. Furthermore, the cytokines IL-6 and IL-8 among H7N9 patients without *A. baumannii* presented a decreasing trend during

the disease course (Fig. 4a and b). In contrast, both the IL-6 and IL-8 among the plasma of the H7N9-*A. baumannii* patients increased in the third week after disease onset and remained higher than the H7N9 patients until the fifth week after disease onset or death.

The T-cell counts correlated with the lung function of the H7N9 patients (Additional file 7: Figure S2). We next investigated the T-cell subgroups of the H7N9-*A. baumannii* cases. We found that the patients who had co-infection by *A. baumannii* have fewer CD4⁺ and CD8⁺ T-cells, compared to H7N9 controls without co-infection, and also lower than the *A. baumannii* controls without H7N9 infection (Fig. 4c-f). Generally, the normalization time for the CD4⁺ T-cell count among the H7N9-*A. baumannii* cases are also longer than those of the H7N9 controls and *A. baumannii* controls (Fig. 4e). For the longitudinal profile of the lymphocyte count, fatal patients with H7N9-*A. baumannii* co-infection had a consistently low level of both CD4⁺ and CD8⁺ T-cell counts, while the survived H7N9-*A. baumannii* patients have gradual normalization of T-cell counts but still much slower than the H7N9 controls without co-infection (Additional file 8: Figure S3).

We performed biostatistical analyses to further identify correlations between immune factors as of H7N9-*A.*

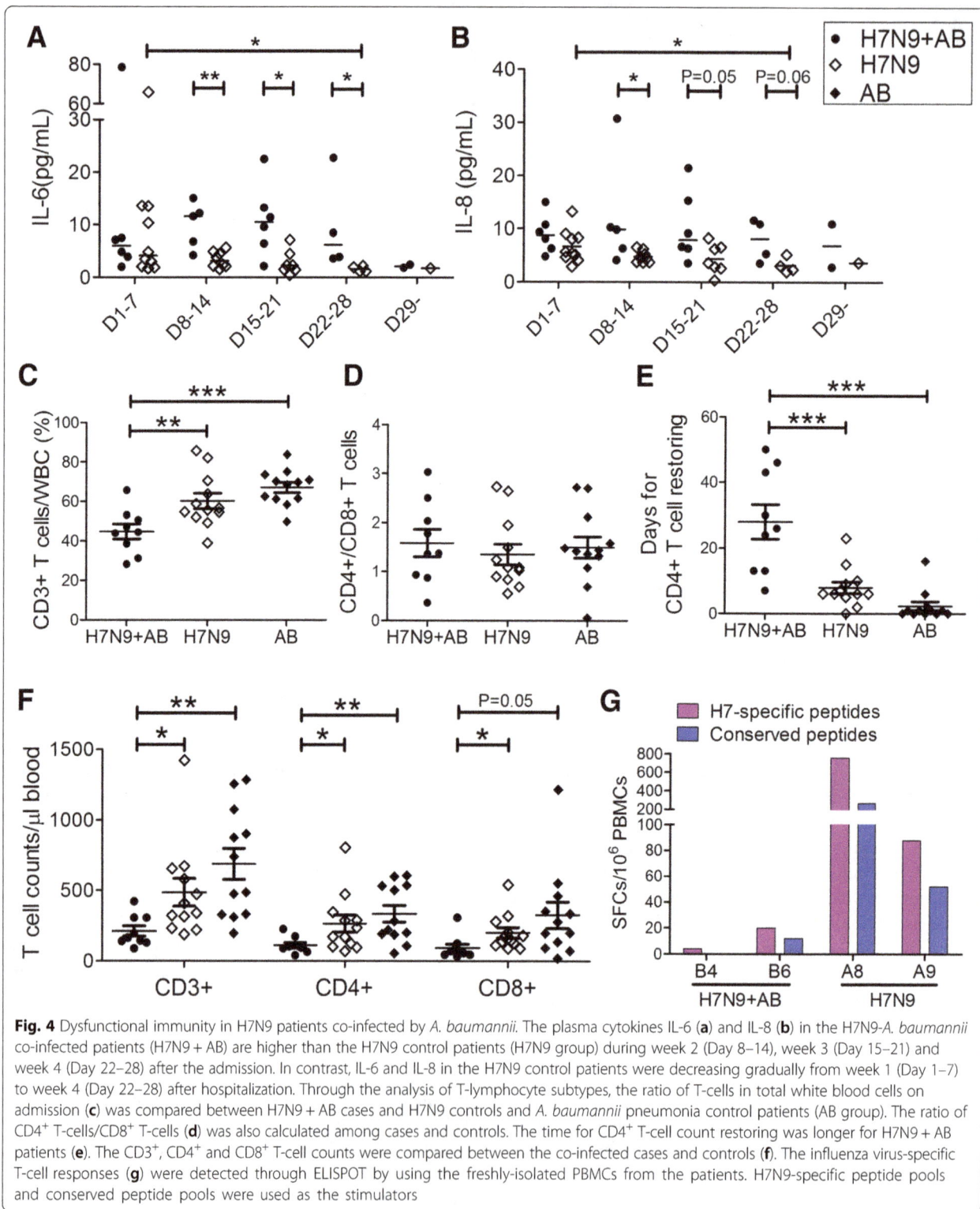

Fig. 4 Dysfunctional immunity in H7N9 patients co-infected by *A. baumannii*. The plasma cytokines IL-6 (**a**) and IL-8 (**b**) in the H7N9-*A. baumannii* co-infected patients (H7N9 + AB) are higher than the H7N9 control patients (H7N9 group) during week 2 (Day 8–14), week 3 (Day 15–21) and week 4 (Day 22–28) after the admission. In contrast, IL-6 and IL-8 in the H7N9 control patients were decreasing gradually from week 1 (Day 1–7) to week 4 (Day 22–28) after hospitalization. Through the analysis of T-lymphocyte subtypes, the ratio of T-cells in total white blood cells on admission (**c**) was compared between H7N9 + AB cases and H7N9 controls and *A. baumannii* pneumonia control patients (AB group). The ratio of CD4$^+$ T-cells/CD8$^+$ T-cells (**d**) was also calculated among cases and controls. The time for CD4$^+$ T-cell count restoring was longer for H7N9 + AB patients (**e**). The CD3$^+$, CD4$^+$ and CD8$^+$ T-cell counts were compared between the co-infected cases and controls (**f**). The influenza virus-specific T-cell responses (**g**) were detected through ELISPOT by using the freshly-isolated PBMCs from the patients. H7N9-specific peptide pools and conserved peptide pools were used as the stimulators

baumannii co-infection. We first used SPSS software to calculate its predictive value for co-infection. The area under the curve (AUC) of plasma IL-6 and IL-8 levels were 0.927 and 0.850 respectively during the second week of hospitalization among H7N9-infected patients, and were 0.881 and 0.833 during the third week (Additional file 9: Figure S4). In addition, the CD3$^+$ T-cell counts (AUC: 0.846), CD8$^+$ T-cell counts (AUC: 0.812) on admission and the restoring time for the abnormal CD4$^+$ T-cell counts (AUC: 0.876) were all predictive for the H7N9-*A.*

baumannii co-infection. Additionally, the traditional biomarkers of bacterial infection, procalcitonin and C-reactive protein levels in blood fluctuated during the disease process, but the two indicators of fatal cases with H7N9-*A. baumannii* co-infection remained at a higher level during a longer period compared to survived cases (Additional file 10: Figure S5 and Additional file 11: Figure S6). We also used multivariate analysis in logistic regression to further analyze the independent predictor for *A. baumannii* co-infection among patients with H7N9 infections (Additional file 4: Table S4 and Additional file 5: Table S5). CD4$^+$ T-cell counts in blood harvested on the day of admission were found to be an independent indicator among the clinical parameters of H7N9-infected patients including procalcitonin and C-reactive protein.

Lower virus-specific T-cell responses amongst H7N9-*A. baumannii* co-infected patients

The influenza virus-specific T-cell tests through the ELI-POST assays by the stimulation of H7N9-derived peptides or conserved peptides, indicated that H7N9-*A. baumannii* patients had a weak CD8$^+$ T-cell responses to H7N9 virus compared to H7N9 controls without co-infection (Fig. 4g).

The antibiotic resistance features of the *A. baumannii* noscomially acquired by H7N9 patients

After an average time of 6 days of invasive ventilation, the H7N9 patients were detected to be *A. baumannii* positive. According to standard drug resistance definition [27], the original isolates from six patients were identified as extensively drug-resistant (XDR). As the *A. baumannii* strains were susceptible to polymyxin, the patients were then treated with polymyxin B with an average total dosage of 14.7 million units for an average 10.5 days. Notably, for patient B4, after polymyxin treatment for five days, the original XDR isolate SMGC-AB1 became polymyxin resistant, i.e. a pandrug-resistant isolate (PDR) named SMGC-AB2 (Table 1, Additional file 12: Table S6).

Rapid emergence of a pandrug-resistant isolate featured by candidate polymyxin resistance-associated mutations

To gain insights into the genetic features of the H7N9 patient infected with *A. baumannii*, the whole genomes of both SMGC-AB1 and SMGC-AB2 were sequenced. SNP-based phylogenic analysis showed that SMGC-AB1 was clustered into the European clone (EC) II group, including MDR-ZJ06, MDR-TJ, BJAB0868 and BJAB07104 from Mainland China, TYTH-1 and TCDC-AB0715 from China Taiwan and AB1656–2 from Korean (Additional file 13: Figure S7). The SMGC-AB1 genome harbored a total of 57 genes belonging to Subsystem subcategory "Resistance to antibiotics and toxic compounds" according to RAST annotation (Additional file

14: Figure S8). Notably, SMGC-AB1 encodes 6 β-lactamases and 2 aminoglycoside adenylyl-transferases.

When comparing the genome of SMGC-AB1 with its polymyxin resistance descendant, SMGC-AB2, only 8 nucleotide point mutations were identified in SMGC-AB2, 7 of which were located in coding regions and 6 lead to nonsynonymous mutation (Table 1). The 1st mutation was located in a putative permease protein encoding gene belonging to YjgP/YjgQ family (now LptF/LptG), which has been identified to be a component of ABC transporter for lipopolysaccharide transport to the cell surface [28]. Notably, the 2nd and 3rd mutations were located in the *pmrCAB* operon, a gene cluster encoding the PmrC phosphoethanolamine phosphotransferase involved in polymyxin resistance [29]; mutations in genes of *pmrB* and *pmrC* leading to Thr → Ile (T235I) and Lys → Thr (L533 T) substitution, respectively. The 5th to 7th mutations causing Val → Ile (V183I and V292I) are all located in a large repetitive protein harboring type I secretion C-terminal target domain. The 4th mutation resulting in no amino acid substitution appeared in a gene encoding NAD-dependent aldehyde dehydrogenase, and the 8th lies in the non-coding region.

Discussion

It is known that secondary bacterial pneumonia during influenza virus infection is a major cause for high mortality of severe or fatal cases. Compared with the dominant bacterial infection of *Streptococcus pneumoniae* and *Staphylococcus aureus* in other influenza virus pandemics [30], *A. baumannii* is the most commonly encountered pathogen in sputum or endotracheal samples in the H7N9 virus infected clinical cases [31]. Here, we presented a typical cohort of the H7N9 patients confected by *A. baumannii* and elucidated their dysfunctional immune responses. Furthermore, the genome features of the *A. baumannii* and particularly the genome variations contributed to the acquired polymyxin resistance which might have led to the fatal outcome of this patient.

The role of the hospital environment as a reservoir for *A. baumannii* has been well defined [32]. Hospital equipment, especially the medical equipment for invasive mechanical ventilation, is one of the important risk factors that predispose individuals to the acquisition of, and infection with, *A. baumannii* [6]. Other risk factors include prior antibiotic use and prior use of broad-spectrum drugs [33]. In our study, H7N9 patients co-infected by *A. baumannii* have a longer use of antibiotics, glucocorticoid, and the invasive mechanical ventilation, all of which may predispose to the occurrence of the *A. baumannii* co-infection in these patients.

In fact, influenza virus infection itself also enhances the susceptibility of the patients to secondary bacterial infection by its impacts on the inflammatory signals and function of early innate immune defense [34]. It is known that levels of inflammatory mediators such as IL-6 and IL-18 were higher in the patients with co-infection of influenza virus and bacteria than in patients with bacterial pneumonia or influenza virus infection alone [35]. Concordantly, in our study, the IL-6 and IL-8 increased to a higher level in the H7N9-*A. baumannii* co-infected patients compared to H7N9 patients without bacterial infection.

Influenza A infection could also increase susceptibility to secondary bacterial pneumonia by dysregulation of different innate immune cells. The influenza virus can inhibit Th17 immunity by the induction of type I IFNs [36] and IL-27 [37], and also can inhibit neutrophil attraction through the mediation of protein Setdb2 [38] and the production of IL-10 [39]. In our study, we found that the H7N9 patients with a persistently low level of CD8+ and CD4+ T-cell population, especially hyporesponsive antigen-specific T-cell responses, are susceptible to the *A. baumannii* infection and the subsequent fatal outcome. This may indicate a T-cell anergy after the avian H7N9 influenza virus infection as previously defined in severe H1N1 infected patients [40].

It is surprising that SMGC-AB1 quickly acquired resistance to polymyxin, an antibiotic that is considered to be the last hope to cope with MDR and or XDR gram-negative bacteria. Polymyxins are cyclic cationic peptides with a long hydrophobic tail that interact with the lipid A moiety of lipopolysaccharide (LPS) to disrupt the integrity of outer membranes of gram-negative bacteria. Three major resistance mechanisms to polymyxin in bacteria have been identified: modification of the bacterial outer membrane lipopolysaccharide, proteolytic cleavage of the drug and activation of broad-spectrum efflux pumps, among which modification of lipid A of LPS regulated by the two-component regulatory system PmrAB has been frequently reported in *A. baumannii* [41]. It is reported that a single mutation in *pmrB* gene causing T235I amino acid substitution can lead to 16-fold increases in polymyxin B MIC in *A. baumannii* [29]. In this study, we found that the SMGC-AB2 harbors a mutation in *pmrB* gene exactly resulting in T235I amino acid substitution; we believe that this mutation plays a decisive role for this isolate to resist polymyxin. As demonstrated, mutations in the *pmrA* or *pmrB* genes usually result in the constitutive expression of *pmrC*, thus leading to LPS modification and reduction of the affinity of polymyxins [42]. In clinical resistant isolates, similar mutations have also been found in *pmrC* gene. However, in SMGC-AB2, the mutation located at the end of the C-terminus of pmrC protein (L533 T), beyond the functional

sulfatase domain (aa 237–532), may not contribute to the resistance. It is reported that *A. baumannii* can also develop resistance to polymyxin by mutating genes responsible for LPS production [43]. Though no mutations were found in the biosynthesis pathway of LPS in SMGC-AB2, a mutation appeared in a pupative permease (Table 1, mutation No. 1) that probably functions in LPS transport. We speculate that this mutation may cause the decrease of LPS production, thus leading to the decrease of the drug target, which may also play a secondary role in the resistance phenotype of SMGC-AB2. Finally, we also found three mutations in a large repetitive protein harboring type I secretion C-terminal target domain leading to two amino acid substitutions (Val → Ile); whether and how this protein and the mutations are involved in the polymyxin resistance in SMGC-AB2 needs further investigations.

In conclusion, we described the occurrence of secondary infection of *A. baumannii* and its impacts on the disease severity in H7N9 patients. The dysfunctional immunity in the H7N9 patients correlated to the *A. baumannii* co-infection. Furthermore, the genome variations of *A. baumannii* contributed to the acquired polymyxin resistance in the patient with fatal outcome. We suggest that the enhancement of the anti-nosocomial infection measures for the prevention of *A. baumannii* in the H7N9 patients with risk factors for secondary infections, and the early administration of appropriate antibiotic regimen when such co-infection is detected by frequent microbiological testing.

Conclusions

Invasive mechanical ventilation is the most significant risk factor for the nosocomial *A. baumannii* co-infection in in patients with avian influenza A (H7N9) virus infection. The occurrence of H7N9 co-infection with *A. baumannii* is a key factor for the severity of the patients, with a manifestation of lower oxygenation indexes and chest radiograph scores. Dysregulation of immune responses in the H7N9 patients correlates to the susceptibility of *A. baumannii* co-infection and severe clinical manifestation. Novel polymyxin resistance-associated genome variations of *A. baumannii* could quickly emerge during the disease process and may contribute to fatal outcome of the H7N9-*A. baumannii* co-infected patients. Both the immune and bacterial features in the patients may contribute to and act as biomarkers for the severe pneumonia and fatal outcome of the co-infection. These conclusions shed light on the pathomechanism, diagnosis and treatment of H7N9 and bacterial co-infections.

Additional files

Additional file 1: Table S1. The meta analyses of *A. baumannii* infection in H7N9 patients.

Additional file 2: Table S2. Basic characters of the patients.

Additional file 3: Table S3. Clinical presentation and main lab-findings on admission.

Additional file 4: Table S4. The multivariate analysis of the risk factors of H7N9 patients co-infected by A. baumannii (*n* = 13) compared to H7N9 control patients (*n* = 9).

Additional file 5: Table S5. The multivariate analysis of the clinical risk factors and indicators of H7N9 patients co-infected by *A. baumannii* (*n* = 13) compared to the group (*n* = 24) combined of H7N9 control and *A. baumannii* control patients.

Additional file 6: Figure S1. The longitudinal variation of oxygenation index (PaO_2/FiO_2) in the H7N9 patients co-infected by *A. baumannii*.

Additional file 7: Figure S2. The association of T-cell counts with oxygenation index (PaO_2/FiO_2) in the H7N9 patients.

Additional file 8: Figure S3. The longitudinal trends of $CD3^+$ T-cell counts, $CD4^+$ T-cell counts and $CD8^+$ T-cell counts among the H7N9 patients.

Additional file 9: Figure S4. ROC curve of the plasma levels of cytokines and T-cell characteristics in H7N9 patients.

Additional file 10: Figure S5. The longitudinal variation of PCT in the H7N9 patients co-infected by *A. baumannii*.

Additional file 11: Figure S6. The longitudinal variation of CRP in the H7N9 patients co-infected by *A. baumannii*.

Additional file 12: Table S6. Antibiotic susceptibility profiles for *A. baumannii* SMGC-AB1 and SMGC-AB2.

Additional file 13: Figure S7. Phylogenetic position of *A. baumannii* SMGC-AB1 and its polysaccharide antigen gene clusters. (PDF 624 kb)

Additional file 14: Figure S8. Comparison of gene distribution in Subsystem subcategory "Resistance to antibiotics and toxic compounds".

Acknowledgements
We thank Dr. Jianfang Zhou and Dr. Hui Li for their helpful suggestions.

Funding
This study was supported by grants from National Natural Science Foundation of China (81373141, 81330082 and 81401312), the Intramural Special Grant for Influenza Virus Research from the Chinese Academy of Science (KJZD-EW-L15), the Shenzhen Science and Technology Research and Development Project (JCYJ20160427151920801) and the National Key Research and Development Program of China (2016YFC1200800). GFG is a leading principal investigator of the National Natural Science Foundation of China Innovative Research Group (81621091). YH is a member of the Youth Innovation Promotion Association of Chinese Academy of Sciences (2015069). The funding sources had no role in the study design, data collection and analysis, decision to publish, or preparation of the manuscript.

Authors' contributions
WJL, GFG, YL designed research studies; WL, YH, MZ, CQ, ST conducted the experiments; RZ, KL, JY, HZ JL, ML collected and analyzed the clinical data; YB, JY, BZ, DW, GW, LL supported the materials; WJL, YH, K-YY, GFG, YL wrote the paper. All authors read and approved the final manuscript.

Consent for publication
Not applicable.

Competing interests
The authors declare that they have no competing interests.

Author details
[1]Shenzhen Key Laboratory of Pathogen and Immunity, State Key Discipline of Infectious Disease, Shenzhen Third People's Hospital, Shenzhen 518112, China. [2]NHC Key Laboratory of Medical Virology and Viral Diseases, National Institute for Viral Disease Control and Prevention, Chinese Center for Disease Control and Prevention, Beijing, China. [3]CAS Key Laboratory of Pathogenic Microbiology and Immunology, Institute of Microbiology, Chinese Academy of Sciences (CAS), Beijing, China. [4]Department of Epidemiology and Biostatistics, School of Public Health, Peking University, Beijing, China. [5]State Key Laboratory for Emerging Infectious Diseases, The University of Hong Kong, Special Administration Region, Hong Kong, China. [6]Center for Influenza Research and Early-Warning (CASCIRE), Chinese Academy of Sciences, Beijing, China.

References
1. Kash JC, Taubenberger JK. The role of viral, host, and secondary bacterial factors in influenza pathogenesis. Am J Pathol. 2015;185(6):1528–36.
2. Morens DM, Taubenberger JK, Fauci AS. Predominant role of bacterial pneumonia as a cause of death in pandemic influenza: implications for pandemic influenza preparedness. J Infect Dis. 2008;198(7):962–70.
3. Weinberger DM, Simonsen L, Jordan R, Steiner C, Miller M, Viboud C. Impact of the 2009 influenza pandemic on pneumococcal pneumonia hospitalizations in the United States. J Infect Dis. 2012;205(3):458–65.
4. Dawood FS, Chaves SS, Perez A, Reingold A, Meek J, Farley MM, Ryan P, Lynfield R, Morin C, Baumbach J, et al. Complications and associated bacterial coinfections among children hospitalized with seasonal or pandemic influenza, United States, 2003-2010. J Infect Dis. 2014;209(5): 686–94.
5. Yuen KY, Chan PK, Peiris M, Tsang DN, Que TL, Shortridge KF, Cheung PT, To WK, Ho ET, Sung R, et al. Clinical features and rapid viral diagnosis of human disease associated with avian influenza a H5N1 virus. Lancet. 1998; 351(9101):467–71.
6. Garnacho-Montero J, Ortiz-Leyba C, Fernandez-Hinojosa E, Aldabo-Pallas T, Cayuela A, Marquez-Vacaro JA, Garcia-Curiel A, Jimenez-Jimenez FJ. Acinetobacter baumannii ventilator-associated pneumonia: epidemiological and clinical findings. Intens Care Med. 2005;31(5):649–55.
7. Trouillet JL, Chastre J, Vuagnat A, Joly-Guillou ML, Combaux D, Dombret MC, Gibert C. Ventilator-associated pneumonia caused by potentially drug-resistant bacteria. Am J Respir Crit Care Med. 1998;157(2):531–9.
8. Garnacho J, Sole-Violan J, Sa-Borges M, Diaz E, Rello J. Clinical impact of pneumonia caused by Acinetobacter baumannii in intubated patients: a matched cohort study. Crit Care Med. 2003;31(10):2478–82.
9. Falagas ME, Rafailidis PI. Attributable mortality of Acinetobacter baumannii: no longer a controversial issue. Crit Care. 2007;11(3):134.
10. Perez F, Hujer AM, Hujer KM, Decker BK, Rather PN, Bonomo RA. Global challenge of multidrug-resistant Acinetobacter baumannii. Antimicrob Agent Chemother. 2007;51(10):3471–84.
11. Wu W, He Y, Lu J, Lu Y, Wu J, Liu Y. Transition of blaOXA-58-like to blaOXA-23-like in Acinetobacter baumannii clinical isolates in southern China: an 8-year study. PLoS One. 2015;10(9):e0137174.
12. Li J, Rayner CR, Nation RL, Owen RJ, Spelman D, Tan KE, Liolios L. Heteroresistance to colistin in multidrug-resistant Acinetobacter baumannii. Antimicrob Agent Chemother. 2006;50(9):2946–50.
13. Gao R, Cao B, Hu Y, Feng Z, Wang D, Hu W, Chen J, Jie Z, Qiu H, Xu K, et al. Human infection with a novel avian-origin influenza a (H7N9) virus. New Engl J Med. 2013;368(20):1888–97.
14. Li J, Yu X, Pu X, Xie L, Sun Y, Xiao H, Wang F, Din H, Wu Y, Liu D, et al. Environmental connections of novel avian-origin H7N9 influenza virus infection and virus adaptation to the human. Sci China Life Sci. 2013;56(6):485–92.
15. Calandra T, Cohen J. International Sepsis forum definition of infection in the ICUCC: the international sepsis forum consensus conference on definitions of infection in the intensive care unit. Crit Care Med. 2005;33(7):1538–48.
16. Patel JB, Cockerill FR, Bradford PA, Eliopoulos GM, Hindler JA, Jenkins SG, Lewis JS, Limbago B, Miller LA, Nicolau DP et al: Performance standards for antimicrobial susceptibility testing; twenty-fourth informational supplement. CLSI Standard Antimicrob Suscep Test 2015, 35(3):231.

17. Liu J, Wu B, Zhang S, Tan S, Sun Y, Chen Z, Qin Y, Sun M, Shi G, Wu Y, et al. Conserved epitopes dominate cross-CD8+ T-cell responses against influenza a H1N1 virus among Asian populations. Eur J Immunol. 2013;43(8):2055–69.

18. Vita R, Zarebski L, Greenbaum JA, Emami H, Hoof I, Salimi N, Damle R, Sette A, Peters B. The immune epitope. database 2.0. Nucleic Acid Res. 2010; 38(Database issue):D854–62.

19. Liu WJ, Tan S, Zhao M, Quan C, Bi Y, Wu Y, Zhang S, Zhang H, Xiao H, Qi J, et al. Cross-Immunities against Avian Influenza H7N9 Virus in the Healthy Population Affected by Antigenicity-Dependent Substitutions. J Infect Dis. 2016;214:1937-46.

20. Cox MP, Peterson DA, Biggs PJ. SolexaQA: at-a-glance quality assessment of Illumina second-generation sequencing data. BMC Bioinformatics. 2010;11:485.

21. Luo R, Liu B, Xie Y, Li Z, Huang W, Yuan J, He G, Chen Y, Pan Q, Liu Y, et al. SOAPdenovo2: an empirically improved memory-efficient short-read de novo assembler. Gigascience. 1(1):18.

22. Darling AC, Mau B, Blattner FR, Perna NT. Mauve: multiple alignment of conserved genomic sequence with rearrangements. Genome Res. 2004; 14(7):1394–403.

23. Aziz RK, Bartels D, Best AA, DeJongh M, Disz T, Edwards RA, Formsma K, Gerdes S, Glass EM, Kubal M, et al. The RAST server: rapid annotations using subsystems technology. BMC Genomics. 2008;9:75.

24. Angiuoli SV, Salzberg SL. Mugsy: fast multiple alignment of closely related whole genomes. Bioinformatics. 2011;27(3):334–42.

25. McArthur AG, Waglechner N, Nizam F, Yan A, Azad MA, Baylay AJ, Bhullar K, Canova MJ, De Pascale G, Ejim L, et al. The comprehensive antibiotic resistance database. Antimicrob Agent Chemother. 2013;57(7):3348–57.

26. Guo J, Huang F, Liu J, Chen Y, Wang W, Cao B, Zou Z, Liu S, Pan J, Bao C, et al. The serum profile of Hypercytokinemia factors identified in H7N9-infected patients can predict fatal outcomes. Sci Rep. 2015;5:10942.

27. Magiorakos AP, Srinivasan A, Carey RB, Carmeli Y, Falagas ME, Giske CG, Harbarth S, Hindler JF, Kahlmeter G, Olsson-Liljequist B, et al. Multidrug-resistant, extensively drug-resistant and pandrug-resistant bacteria: an international expert proposal for interim standard definitions for acquired resistance. Clin Microbiol Infect. 2012;18(3):268–81.

28. Ruiz N, Gronenberg LS, Kahne D, Silhavy TJ. Identification of two inner-membrane proteins required for the transport of lipopolysaccharide to the outer membrane of Escherichia coli. Proc Natl Acad Sci U S A. 2008;105(14):5537–42.

29. Arroyo LA, Herrera CM, Fernandez L, Hankins JV, Trent MS, Hancock RE. The pmrCAB operon mediates polymyxin resistance in Acinetobacter baumannii ATCC 17978 and clinical isolates through phosphoethanolamine modification of lipid a. Antimicrob Agent Chemother. 2011;55(8):3743–51.

30. McCullers JA. Insights into the interaction between influenza virus and pneumococcus. Clin Microbiol Rev. 2006;19(3):571–82.

31. Gao HN, Lu HZ, Cao B, Du B, Shang H, Gan JH, Lu SH, Yang YD, Fang Q, Shen YZ, et al. Clinical findings in 111 cases of influenza a (H7N9) virus infection. N Engl J Med. 2013;368(24):2277–85.

32. Peleg AY, Seifert H, Paterson DL. Acinetobacter baumannii: emergence of a successful pathogen. Clin Microbiol Rev. 2008;21(3):538–82.

33. Dijkshoorn L, Nemec A, Seifert H. An increasing threat in hospitals: multidrug-resistant Acinetobacter baumannii. Nat Rev Microbiol. 2007;5(12):939–51.

34. McCullers JA. The co-pathogenesis of influenza viruses with bacteria in the lung. Nat Rev Microbiol. 2014;12(4):252–62.

35. Rosseau S, Hocke A, Mollenkopf H, Schmeck B, Suttorp N, Kaufmann SH, Zerrahn J. Comparative transcriptional profiling of the lung reveals shared and distinct features of Streptococcus pneumoniae and influenza a virus infection. Immunology. 2007;120(3):380–91.

36. Li W, Moltedo B, Moran TM. Type I interferon induction during influenza virus infection increases susceptibility to secondary Streptococcus pneumoniae infection by negative regulation of gammadelta T cells. J Virol. 2012;86(22):12304–12.

37. Robinson KM, Lee B, Scheller EV, Mandalapu S, Enelow RI, Kolls JK, Alcorn JF. The role of IL-27 in susceptibility to post-influenza Staphylococcus aureus pneumonia. Respir Res. 2015;16:10.

38. Schliehe C, Flynn EK, Vilagos B, Richson U, Swaminathan S, Bosnjak B, Bauer L, Kandasamy RK, Griesshammer IM, Kosack L, et al. The methyltransferase Setdb2 mediates virus-induced susceptibility to bacterial superinfection. Nat Immunol. 2015;16(1):67–74.

39. van der Sluijs KF, van Elden LJ, Nijhuis M, Schuurman R, Pater JM, Florquin S, Goldman M, Jansen HM, Lutter R, van der Poll T. IL-10 is an important mediator of the enhanced susceptibility to pneumococcal pneumonia after influenza infection. J Immunol. 2004;172(12):7603–9.

40. Agrati C, Gioia C, Lalle E, Cimini E, Castilletti C, Armignacco O, Lauria FN, Ferraro F, Antonini M, Ippolito G, et al. Association of profoundly impaired immune competence in H1N1v-infected patients with a severe or fatal clinical course. J Infect Dis. 2010;202(5):681–9.

41. Adams MD, Nickel GC, Bajaksouzian S, Lavender H, Murthy AR, Jacobs MR, Bonomo RA. Resistance to colistin in Acinetobacter baumannii associated with mutations in the PmrAB two-component system. Antimicrob Agent Chemother. 2009;53(9):3628–34.

42. Beceiro A, Llobet E, Aranda J, Bengoechea JA, Doumith M, Hornsey M, Dhanji H, Chart H, Bou G, Livermore DM, et al. Phosphoethanolamine modification of lipid a in colistin-resistant variants of Acinetobacter baumannii mediated by the pmrAB two-component regulatory system. Antimicrob Agent Chemother. 2011;55(7):3370–9.

43. Moffatt JH, Harper M, Harrison P, Hale JD, Vinogradov E, Seemann T, Henry R, Crane B, St Michael F, Cox AD, et al. Colistin resistance in Acinetobacter baumannii is mediated by complete loss of lipopolysaccharide production. Antimicrob Agent Chemother. 2010;54(12):4971–7.

The association between serum magnesium levels and community-acquired pneumonia 30-day mortality

Roni Nasser[1*†], Mohammad E. Naffaa[2†], Tanya Mashiach[3], Zaher S. Azzam[1,4] and Eyal Braun[4,5]

Abstract

Background: Community acquired pneumonia (CAP) is a common illness affecting hundreds of millions worldwide. Few studies have investigated the relationship between serum magnesium levels and outcomes of these patients. We aimed to study the association between serum magnesium levels and 30-day mortality among patients with CAP.

Methods: Retrospective overview of patients hospitalized with CAP between January 1, 2010 and December 31, 2016. Participants were analyzed retrospectively in order to identify the risk factors for a primary endpoint of 30-day mortality. Normal levels of magnesium levels in our laboratory varies between 1.35 and 2.4 mg/dl.

Results: 3851 patients were included in our cohort. Age > 75 years, blood urea nitrogen (BUN) > 20 mg/dl, hypoalbuminemia, and abnormal levels of magnesium were all associated with increased risk of 30-day mortality. Normal magnesium levels were associated with the lowest mortality rate (14.7%). Notably, within the normal levels, high normal magnesium levels (2–2.4 mg/dl) were correlated with higher mortality rates (30.3%) as compared to levels that ranged between 1.35–2 mg/dl (12.9%). Hypomagnesemia and hypermagnesemia were both associated with excess of 30-day mortality, 18.4 and 50%, respectively.

Conclusion: Hypomagnesemia and hypermagnesemia on admission were associated with an increased rate of 30-day mortality among adult patients hospitalized with CAP. Interestingly, magnesium levels within the upper normal limits were associated with higher mortality.

Keywords: Pneumonia, Hypomagnesemia, Hypermagnesemia, Mortality

Background

Community acquired pneumonia (CAP) is a common illness affecting hundreds of millions worldwide, with increasing hospital admissions throughout the years mainly due to the aging population. It is a major cause of mortality and morbidity in all age groups, especially elderly, despite the effectiveness of the diverse antibiotic treatment [1–3].

The prognostic scores used in the clinical settings, such as CURB 65 and Pneumonia Severity Index (PSI) are acknowledged as tools to estimate the mortality rates and thus determine the treatment setting, either outpatient or inpatient [2, 4].

Magnesium (Mg) is the second most profound intracellular mineral in the human body. It is essential for energy production, mainly by binding ATP; synthesis of DNA, RNA and proteins. Mg also plays a role in the active transport of calcium and potassium ions across cell membranes, and thus has an essential role for maintaining proper function of the neuromuscular and cardiovascular systems [5].

Magnesium deficiency has been associated with a number of clinical manifestations such as arrhythmias, cardiac insufficiency, sudden death, muscle weakness, bronchospasm, tetany, seizures, as well as hypokalemia, hypocalcaemia, hyponatremia, and hypophosphatemia [6, 7]. Several studies demonstrated that hypomagnesemia at admission or during ICU stay was associated with guarded prognosis [8, 9], and magnesium supplementation was associated with a lower mortality rate [8].

* Correspondence: roni.nasser@gmail.com
†Roni Nasser and Mohammad E. Naffaa contributed equally to this work.
[1]Department of Internal Medicine "B", Ramabm Health Care Campus, HaAliya HaShniya St 8, 3109601 Haifa, Israel

Hypermagnesemia, which is less frequent than hypomagnesemia, commonly occurs due to excessive administration of magnesium salts or magnesium-containing drugs, especially in patients with reduced renal function. It may be caused, also, by rapid mobilization from soft tissues in patients with sepsis or trauma, adrenal insufficiency and hypothyroidism. Hypermagnesemia may cause severe symptomatic hypotension, bradycardia and ECG changes like wide QRS [5, 10]. Hypermagnesemia was associated with highest rates of death in critically ill patients [11].

We recently showed that hyperphosphatemia and hypophosphatemia were independently associated with increased 30-days mortality rates in patients with CAP [12].

In this study, we aimed to examine the association between serum magnesium levels on admission and the 30-day mortality in patients with CAP.

Methods
Study design
Retrospective overview of patients who were admitted to Rambam Health Care Campus (RHCC), Haifa, Israel, between January 2010 and 31 December 2016. RHCC is a 1000 bed teaching hospital. The patient population is diverse, as RHCC is the major tertiary medical center for all of Northern Israel, serving more than two million residents. According to hospital records, there are 140,000 emergency department visits every year and about 90,000 inpatient admissions. The Rambam Hospital Institutional Review Board approved the study. The approval number is 0597–16-RMB. The need for informed consent was waived because of the retrospective, medical record-based design of the study. The study population included patients 18 years or older with CAP. The diagnosis of pneumonia was based upon the primary diagnosis of pneumonia on the discharge report, within the first twenty-four hours from admission. Exclusion criteria included patients younger than 18 years, those who were transferred from another acute care facilities, hospitalization during the month prior to admission, hospital-acquired pneumonia (HAP) or partial antibiotic treatment.

Patients' data was retrieved and analyzed using Prometheus, RHCC integrated electronic medical records system. The 30-day mortality data were retrieved from Prometheus and the ministry of health. The retrieved data included age, gender; vital signs including blood pressure (BP), systolic and diastolic, heart rate (HR), Oxygen saturation (SO2) respiratory rate (RR), temperature; Comorbidities: history of prior or current malignancies (solid or hematologic), lung disease, smoking status, cardiovascular diseases, kidney diseases, immune deficiency conditions, HIV status, diabetes mellitus, liver cirrhosis, prior neurologic damage, alcohol abuse, intravenous drug abuse and nursing house residence smoking history. The Charlson's comorbidity score was calculated based on data collected; laboratory values (first values within 48 h): Hemoglobin (Hb), White blood cell count (WBC), red blood cell distribution width (RDW), pH, partial pressure of carbon dioxide (pCO2), Serum glucose, serum creatinine, sodium, calcium, phosphorus, magnesium, blood urea nitrogen (BUN), and serum albumin.

Hematological values were measured using the Advia 120 Hematology Analyzer (Siemens Healthcare Diagnostics Deerfield, Illinois, USA). Serum glucose, serum creatinine, sodium, calcium, phosphorus, magnesium, blood urea nitrogen (BUN), and serum albumin were measured on admission Using "Dimension" (Siemens Healthcare Diagnostics Deerfield, Illinois, USA). PH, bicarbonate, partial pressure of CO2 and lactate were measured using GEM premier 3500.

The normal serum magnesium range in our laboratory is 1.35–2.4 mg/dl.

Statistical analysis
Statistical analysis was performed by using the SPSS statistical package (SPSS, Inc., Chicago, USA) version 21.0.

Quantitative variables are expressed as mean ± SD. Qualitative variables are expressed as values and percentages. The odds ratio (OR) with 95% confidence interval (CI) was computed using bivariate logistic regression analysis. The correlation between patients' characteristics and 30-day mortality were evaluated by P values derived from bivariate analysis. Multivariate forward stepwise logistic regression was used to evaluate the relation between patients' features, co-morbidities, laboratory parameters, and 30-day mortality.

Parameters with notable level of significance ($P < 0.1$) of the bivariate association with 30-day mortality were chosen for the multivariate analysis. Bootstrap multivariate analysis was used to evaluate the accuracy of the parameters in the model by estimating standard error, confidence intervals, and bias. The area under curve (AUC) was applied in the model to assess the prognostic value of magnesium. P values equals or less than 0.05 was acknowledged as statistically significant.

Results
Between January 1, 2010 and December 31, 2016, 4708 patients were diagnosed with CAP at discharge. 3851 patient had magnesium levels within 48 h. Fifty five percent were males. Median age was 72 years old. The 30-day mortality was 15.2% (587 patients) and almost the same each year during the study.

Hypomagnesemia (≤1.35 mg/dl) was detected in 240 patients (6%) and hypermagnesemia (≥2.4 mg/dl) in 26 patients (1%), while 3581 patients (93%) were normomagnesemic (1.35–2.4 mg/dl).

Table 1 shows bivariate analysis of the association between patients' characteristics, laboratory parameters and 30-day mortality.

Figure 1 demonstrates that hypomagnesemia and hypermagnesemia were associated with higher 30-day mortality rates (18.4%, OR 1.52, CI 1.13–2.03 and 50% OR 5.78, CI 2.66–12.53 respectively) compared to normomagnesemic group (14.8%). Thirty-day mortality rate was significantly higher (30.3%, OR 2.92, CI 2.27–3.75) in patients with magnesium levels within the upper normal limit (2–2.4 mg/dl) compared to the levels 1.35–2 mg/dl which has mortality rate of 12.9%.

Relationship between phosphorous levels, magnesium levels and 30-day mortality

As shown in Table 2, abnormal magnesium levels were associated with high mortality rates regardless of all phosphorus levels.

Relationship between blood urea nitrogen (BUN), magnesium, albumin, age and mortality

As shown in Fig. 2, the association between serum magnesium levels and 30-day mortality due to community acquired pneumonia outcome was maintained after adjustment for BUN, albumin and age.

Multivariate analysis of factors associated with 30-day mortality

As shown in Table 3, in multivariate regression analysis, variables associated with increased risk of 30-day mortality include age > 75 years, BUN > 20 mg/dl, albumin < 3 g/dl, inorganic phosphorus levels > 4.5 mg/dl and abnormal levels of magnesium (hypermagnesemia, including high normal levels and hypomagnesemia).

In bootstrap multivariate analysis we show that all variables, including magnesium, which were significant in multivariate analysis were also significant in the model. The

Table 1 Bivariate analysis of parameters associated with 30 days mortality

| | | Total | | | 30 day mortality | | | | 95%CI | |
		Number	Percent (%)		Number	Percent %	P value	OR	lower	Upper
	Total patients	3851			587	15.2%				
Age (years)	< 65	1215	32%		81	6.7%	0.000	1.00	0.00	0.00
	65–69	354	9%		31	8.8%	0.180	1.34	0.87	2.07
	70–79	947	25%		156	16.5%	0.000	2.76	2.08	3.67
	80–85	545	14%		114	20.9%	0.000	3.70	2.73	5.03
	> 85	790	21%		205	25.9%	0.000	4.91	3.72	6.47
Gender	Male	2136	55%		339	15.9%	0.226	1.12	0.93	1.33
	Female	1715	45%		248	14.5%	0.000	1.00	0.00	0.00
Albumin (g/dl)	3.5–4	374	10%		8	2.1%	0.000	1.00	0.00	0.00
	3–3.4	728	19%		39	5.4%	0.016	2.59	1.20	5.60
	2–3	2649	69%		303	14.2%	0.000	7.59	3.73	15.46
	< 2	520	14%		220	42.3%	0.000	33.55	16.30	69.05
BUN (mg/dl)	< 20	1690	44%		108	6.4%	0.000	1.00	0.00	0.00
	20–39	1479	38%		239	16.2%	0.000	2.82	2.22	3.59
	40–59	438	11%		130	29.7%	0.000	6.18	4.66	8.20
	≥60	244	6%		110	45.1%	0.000	12.03	8.74	16.54
RDW (%)	< 14.5	1647	43%		128	7.8%	0.000	1.00	0.00	0.00
	≥14.5	2204	57%		459	20.8%	0.000	3.12	2.54	3.84
Phosphorus (mg/dl)	1.51 < IP < 3.99	2841	74%		339	11.9%	0.000	1.00	0.00	0.00
	≤1.5	49	1%		14	28.6%	0.001	2.95	1.57	5.54
	4–4.49	479	12%		79	17.2%	0.002	1.53	1.16	2.01
	≥4.5	482	13%		155	32.2%	0.000	3.50	2.80	4.37
Magnesium (mg/dl)	1.35–2	3136	81%		406	12.9%	0.000	1.00	0.00	0.00
	≤1.35	342	9%		63	18.4%	0.005	1.52	1.13	2.03
	2–2.4	347	9%		105	30.3%	0.000	2.92	2.27	3.75
	≥2.4	26	1%		13	50%	0.000	6.72	3.10	14.61

Abbreviations: *OR* odds ratio, *CI* confidence interval, *BUN* blood urea nitrogen, *RDW* Red blood cell distribution width

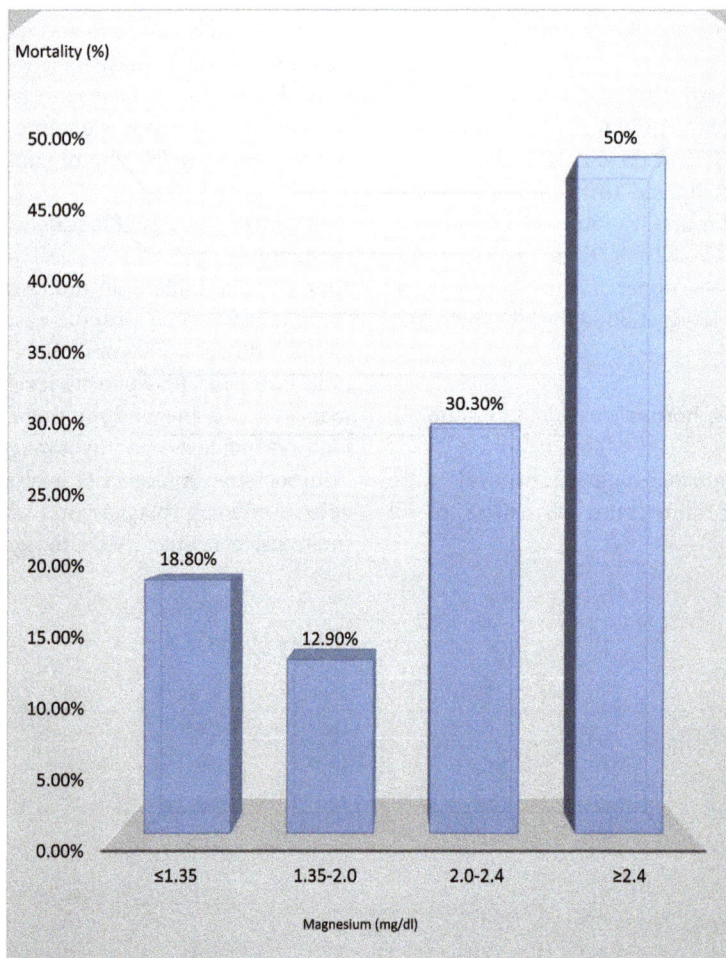

Fig. 1 30 days mortality according to magnesium levels

area under the curve for magnesium was 0.806 (95% CI 0.787–0.825).

Discussion

In this retrospective study we studied the association between magnesium levels on admission and 30-day mortality in patients with community acquired pneumonia.

We found different 30-day mortality rates within the different magnesium levels: 18.8% in hypomagnesemia, 50% in hypermagnesemic, and 14.8% in normomagnesemic patients. This association was maintained even after adjustment for several parameters including albumin, BUN and age. Notably, magnesium levels within the upper normal limit, namely (2–2.4 mg/dl), were also associated with higher rates of 30-day mortality (30.3%).

Magnesium is an intracellular cation that possesses various physiological functions. It functions as a co-factor in intracellular enzymatic activities especially by chelating intracellular anionic ligands. Magnesium also competes with calcium in binding sites on proteins and membranes. It is involved in other cell cycle related processes including

DNA and RNA synthesis, cell growth and reproduction, membrane structure, signal transduction modulation, and fat and protein synthesis [5, 13–15].

Magnesium deficiency is a common underdiagnosed problem in the ICU. Several studies have demonstrated high incidence of magnesium disturbances in ICU patients. Low Magnesium levels have been reported in approximately 50 % of ICU patients. The morbidity and mortality rates were significantly higher in these patients compared to patients with normal magnesium rates [16–20]. Rubeiz et al. [18] reported a 46% mortality rates in patients with hypomagnesemia in ICU. Conceivably, there were two-fold increase in mortality rates among patient with hypomagnesemia as compared to those with normal levels. Thus, the conclusion was that patients admitted with hypomagnesemia in ICU have an excess mortality rates.

It is interesting to assume that supplementation of magnesium to CAP may improve outcome. Therefore, it is conceivable to plan a prospective study to examine magnesium as a therapeutic modality in addition to the accepted treatment of CAP.

Table 2 The association between the different phosphorus and magnesium levels with 30-day mortality

		Total		30 day mortality				95%CI	
		Number	Percent (%)	Number	Percent %	P value	OR	lower	Upper
Phosphorus (mg/dl)	Magnesium (mg/dl)	3851							
1.51–3.99	1.35–2	2370	62%	245	10.3	0.000	1.00	0.00	0.00
	≤1.35	256	7%	45	17.6	0.001	1.85	1.31	2.62
	≥2	215	6%	49	22.8	0.000	2.56	1.81	3.62
	Other	1010	26%	248	24.6	.	.	.	.
≤1.5	1.35–2	34	1%	9	26.5	0.726	1.00	0.00	0.00
	≤1.35	13	0%	5	38.5	0.424	1.74	0.45	6.71
	≥2	2	0%	0	0.0	0.999	0.00	0.00	0.00
	Other	3802	99%	573	15.1	.	.	.	.
≥4	1.35–2	698	18%	148	21.2	0.000	1.00	0.00	0.00
	≤1.35	68	2%	13	19.1	0.687	0.88	0.47	1.65
	≥2	153	4%	69	45.1	0.000	3.05	2.12	4.40
	Other	2932	76%	357	12.2	.	.	.	.
≥4.5	1.35–2	354	9%	101	28.5	0.002	1.00	0.00	0.00
	≤1.35	34	1%	9	26.5	0.799	0.90	0.41	2.00
	≥2	94	2%	45	47.9	0.000	2.30	1.44	3.67
	Other	3369	87%	432	12.8				

Abbreviations: OR-odds ratio, CI–confidence interval, IP-Inorganic Phosphorus, MG - Magnesium

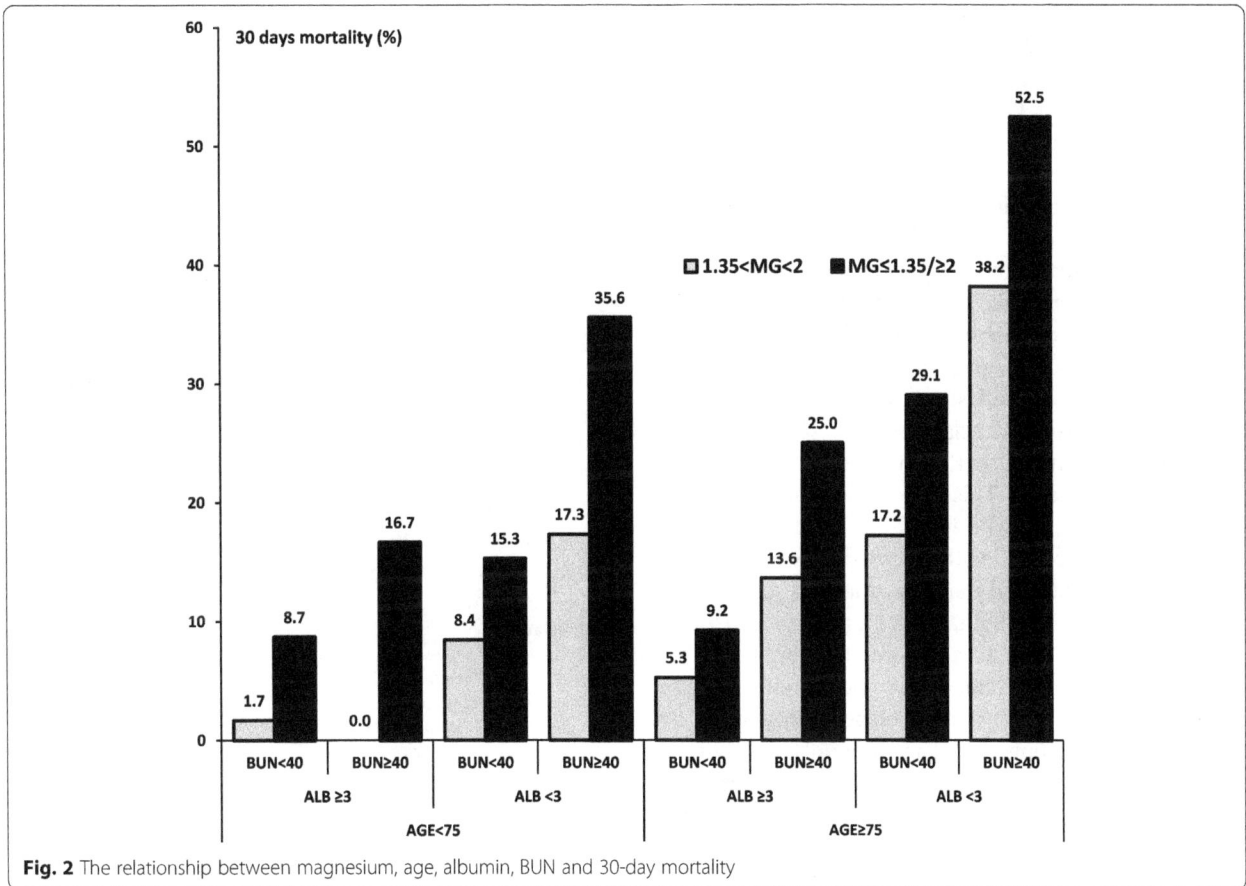

Fig. 2 The relationship between magnesium, age, albumin, BUN and 30-day mortality

Table 3 Multivariate analysis of parameters associated with 30-day mortality

Variables		Coeff. B	P value	Adjusted OR	Bootstrap for variable in equation						
					95% C.I.for OR		Bias	Std. Error	P value	95% CI of B	
					Lower	Upper				Lower	Upper
Albumin (g/dl)	>3		0.00								
	2–3	1.13	0.00	3.10	2.24	4.29	−0.03	0.18	0.010	0.83	1.53
	<2	2.59	0.00	13.32	9.31	19.05	0.03	0.19	0.010	2.22	3.01
BUN (mg/dl)	≤20		0.00								
	20–39	0.57	0.00	1.77	1.37	2.29	0.02	0.14	0.010	0.28	0.92
	40–59	1.05	0.00	2.86	2.09	3.92	0.03	0.15	0.010	0.79	1.36
	≥60	1.28	0.00	3.61	2.49	5.24	0.01	0.20	0.010	0.97	1.72
Age (years)	≥75	0.93	0.00	2.53	1.98	3.22	−0.00	0.11	0.010	0.60	1.18
Magnesium (mg/dl)	≥2/≤1.35	0.63	0.00	1.87	1.42	2.48	−0.01	0.11	0.010	0.27	0.91
Inoraganic phosphorous (mg/dl)	≥4.5	0.83	0.00	2.29	1.77	2.96	0.00	0.11	0.010	0.58	1.18

Abbreviations: *OR* odds ratio, *CI* confidence interval, *BUN* blood urea nitrogen

Hypermagnesemia, less frequently reported than hypomagnesemia, is found in 6–11% of patients admitted to ICU. It can also lead to cardiovascular and neuromuscular manifestations. The development of hypermagnesemia during the ICU stay is associated with higher morbidity and mortality rates and might be the direct result of prolonged disease, or sepsis [11, 21]. *Celi* et al. found that hypermagnesemic patients had a 2.5-fold greater likelihood of receiving intravenous vasopressors during the first 24 hours of ICU care, due to lower systemic blood pressure [22].*Guerin* et al. found that hypermagnesemia is associated with higher fatalities than hypomagnesemia [11]. Cheungpasitporn et al. found that respiratory diseases were associated with hypermagnesemia. This finding was probably attributed to magnesium mediated airway relaxation, immunomodulation and anti-inflammatory effects. Magnesium as an adjunctive therapy has been advocated for patients with moderate to severe airway diseases such as asthma despite inconclusive evidence of its benefit [23].

Magnesium is often given as a treatment of cardiac rhythm disturbances and status asthmaticus or for prevention of seizures and eclampsia [24, 25]. In the past, magnesium treatment was thought to be beneficial in treating ICU patients. This hypothesis was investigated by Broman et al. [13] who found that mild hypermagnesemia was associated with markedly worse survival parameters compared to normomagnesemic controls.

Our study has some limitations. First, is the retrospective nature of the study. It is important to emphasize that we did not have any influence on blood tests including magnesium levels which were taken according to the discretion of the treating physician. Secondly, our primary endpoint was all cause mortality. We did not have data regarding the specific cause of 30-day mortality. Third, data regarding that exact antibiotic agents prior to admission was missing in many patients. Therefore, we decided to exclude patients with prior antibiotic therapy. Fourth, data dealing with permanent medications were not available for many patients, with special emphasis on Proton Pump Inhibitors (PPI), a group of medication increasingly reported as a cause of hypomagnesemia. Fifth, the high mortality rates noticed in the study were due to selection bias since only hospitalized patients with pneumonia were included in the study.

Conclusion

In conclusion, in this cohort study of patients with CAP, we demonstrated that abnormal magnesium levels on admission may be associated with increased 30-day mortality rates, compared to normal levels. Being a simple and readily available blood test, we believe that magnesium levels on admission in patients with CAP may play, in conjugation with other scores such as PASI or CURB65, a valuable role in stratifying these patients on the basis of 30-day mortality. Prospectively, well-designed, comprehensive studies are necessary to validate our findings before making any practical conclusions. Whether magnesium disturbances play a causative role in 30-day mortality in patients with CAP, or just being a surrogate marker, is a question to be answered by prospective interventional studies designed to examine to effect of correcting these disturbances on the final outcome.

Abbreviations
AUC: Area Under Curve; BP: Systolic and diastolic blood pressure; BUN: Blood Urea Nitrogen; CAP: Community acquired pneumonia; CI: Confidence intervals; Hb: Hemoglobin; HR: Heart rate; Mg: Magnesium; OR: Odds ratios; pCO2: Partial pressure of carbon dioxide; PSI: Pneumonia Severity Index; RDW: Red blood cell distribution width; RHCC: Rambam Health Care Campus; RR: Respiratory rate; SPSS: Statistics Products Solutions Services; WBC: White blood cell count

Acknowledgements
Not applicable.

Funding
The authors declare they have not accepted any fundings.

Authors' contributions
RN had full access to all of the data in the study and takes responsibility for the content of the manuscript, was involved in the conception, hypotheses delineation, and design of the study, acquisition and analysis of the data, in writing the article and in its revision prior to submission. MN, RN, TN, ZSA and EB were involved in the design of the study, hypotheses delineation, acquisition and analysis of the data, in writing the article and in its revision prior to submission. All authors have read and approved the final version of the manuscript.

Consent for publication
Not applicable – this study does not contain any patient personal details.

Competing interests
The authors declare they have no competing interests.

Author details
[1]Department of Internal Medicine "B", Ramabm Health Care Campus, HaAliya HaShniya St 8, 3109601 Haifa, Israel. [2]Rheumatology unit, Galilee Medical Center, Nahariya, Israel. [3]Epidemiology and Biostatistics Unit, Rambam Health Care Campus, Haifa, Israel. [4]The Rappaport's Faculty of Medicine, The Technion Institute, Haifa, Israel. [5]Department of Internal Medicine "H", Ramabm Health Care Campus, Haifa, Israel.

References

1. Trotter CL, Stuart JM, George R, Miller E. Increasing hospital admissions for pneumonia, England. Emerg Infect Dis. 2008;14(5):727–33 PubMed PMID: 18439353. Pubmed Central PMCID: 2600241. Epub 2008/04/29. eng.
2. Prina E, Ranzani OT, Torres A. Community-acquired pneumonia. Lancet. 2015;386(9998):1097–108 PubMed PMID: 26277247. Epub 2015/08/19. eng.
3. Regunath H, Oba Y. Pneumonia, community-acquired. 2017. PubMed PMID: 28613500. Epub 2017/06/15. eng.
4. Renaud B, Labarere J, Coma E, Santin A, Hayon J, Gurgui M, et al. Risk stratification of early admission to the intensive care unit of patients with no major criteria of severe community-acquired pneumonia: development of an international prediction rule. Crit Care. 2009;13(2):R54 PubMed PMID: 19358736. Pubmed Central PMCID: 2689501. Epub 2009/04/11. eng.
5. Swaminathan R. Magnesium metabolism and its disorders. Clin Biochem Rev. 2003;24(2):47–66 PubMed PMID: 18568054. Pubmed Central PMCID: 1855626. Epub 2008/06/24. eng.
6. Altura BM, Altura BT. Role of magnesium in patho-physiological processes and the clinical utility of magnesium ion selective electrodes. Scand J Clin Lab Invest Suppl. 1996;224:211–34 PubMed PMID: 8865438. Epub 1996/01/01. eng.
7. al-Ghamdi SM, Cameron EC, Sutton RA. Magnesium deficiency: pathophysiologic and clinical overview. Am J Kidney Dis. 1994;24(5):737–52 PubMed PMID: 7977315. Epub 1994/11/01. eng.
8. Dabbagh OC, Aldawood AS, Arabi YM, Lone NA, Brits R, Pillay M. Magnesium supplementation and the potential association with mortality rates among critically ill non-cardiac patients. Saudi Med J. 2006;27(6):821–5 PubMed PMID: 16758043. Epub 2006/06/08. eng.
9. Safavi M, Honarmand A. Admission hypomagnesemia--impact on mortality or morbidity in critically ill patients. Middle East J Anaesthesiol. 2007;19(3):645–60 PubMed PMID: 18044292. Epub 2007/11/30. eng.
10. Sanders GT, Huijgen HJ, Sanders R. Magnesium in disease: a review with special emphasis on the serum ionized magnesium. Clin Chem Lab Med. 1999;37(11–12):1011–33 PubMed PMID: 10726809. Epub 2000/03/22. eng.
11. Guerin C, Cousin C, Mignot F, Manchon M, Fournier G. Serum and erythrocyte magnesium in critically ill patients. Intensive Care Med. 1996;22(8):724–7 PubMed PMID: 8880238. Epub 1996/08/01. eng.
12. Naffaa ME, Mustafa M, Azzam M, Nasser R, Andria N, Azzam ZS, et al. Serum inorganic phosphorus levels predict 30-day mortality in patients with community acquired pneumonia. BMC Infect Dis. 2015;15:332 PubMed PMID: 26268323. Pubmed Central PMCID: 4535260. Epub 2015/08/14. eng.
13. Broman M, Hansson F, Klarin B. Analysis of hypo- and hypermagnesemia in an intensive care unit cohort. Acta Anaesthesiol Scand. 2018;16 PubMed PMID: 29341068.
14. Huijgen HJ, Soesan M, Sanders R, Mairuhu WM, Kesecioglu J, Sanders GT. Magnesium levels in critically ill patients. What should we measure? Am J Clin Pathol. 2000;114(5):688–95 PubMed PMID: 11068541.
15. Escuela MP, Guerra M, Anon JM, Martinez-Vizcaino V, Zapatero MD, Garcia-Jalon A, et al. Total and ionized serum magnesium in critically ill patients. Intensive Care Med. 2005;31(1):151–6 PubMed PMID: 15605229.
16. Chernow B, Smith J, Rainey TG, Finton C. Hypomagnesemia: implications for the critical care specialist. Crit Care Med. 1982;10(3):193–6 PubMed PMID: 7037303.
17. Reinhart RA, Desbiens NA. Hypomagnesemia in patients entering the ICU. Crit Care Med. 1985;13(6):506–7 PubMed PMID: 3996005.
18. Chen M, Sun R, Hu B. The influence of serum magnesium level on the prognosis of critically ill patients. Zhonghua wei zhong bing ji jiu yi xue. 2015;27(3):213–7 PubMed PMID: 25757972.
19. Thongprayoon C, Cheungpasitporn W, Erickson SB. Admission hypomagnesemia linked to septic shock in patients with systemic inflammatory response syndrome. Ren Fail. 2015;37(9):1518–21 PubMed PMID: 26335852.
20. Upala S, Jaruvongvanich V, Wijarnpreecha K, Sanguankeo A. Hypomagnesemia and mortality in patients admitted to intensive care unit: a systematic review and meta-analysis. QJM. 2016;109(7):453–9 PubMed PMID: 27016536.
21. El Said SM, Aly WW. Magnesium levels among critically ill elderly patients; mortality and morbidity correlation. Adv in Aging Res. 2014;Vol. 03(01):6.
22. Celi LA, Scott DJ, Lee J, Nelson R, Alper SL, Mukamal KJ, et al. Association of hypermagnesemia and blood pressure in the critically ill. J Hypertens. 2013;31(11):2136–41 discussion 41. PubMed PMID: 24029865. Pubmed Central PMCID: 5682028.
23. Cheungpasitporn W, Thongprayoon C, Qian Q. Dysmagnesemia in hospitalized patients: prevalence and prognostic importance. Mayo Clin Proc. 2015;90(8):1001–10 PubMed PMID: 26250725.
24. Manrique AM, Arroyo M, Lin Y, El Khoudary SR, Colvin E, Lichtenstein S, et al. Magnesium supplementation during cardiopulmonary bypass to prevent junctional ectopic tachycardia after pediatric cardiac surgery: a randomized controlled study. J Thorac Cardiovasc Surg. 2010;139(1):162–9 e2 PubMed PMID: 19819469.
25. Schuh S, Sweeney J, Freedman SB, Coates AL, Johnson DW, Thompson G, et al. Magnesium nebulization utilization in management of pediatric asthma (MagNUM PA) trial: study protocol for a randomized controlled trial. Trials. 2016;17(1):261 PubMed PMID: 27220675. Pubmed Central PMCID: 4879727.

22

Assessment of factors that influence timely administration of initial antibiotic dose using collaborative process mapping at a referral hospital in Malawi

Chimwemwe Tusekile Mula[1]*(iD), Lyn Middleton[2], Nicola Human[2] and Christine Varga[3]

Abstract

Background: Timely initiation of antibiotics within one hour of prescription is one of the recommended antibiotic stewardship interventions when managing patients with pneumonia in the emergency department. Effective implementation of this intervention depends on effective communication, a well-established coordination process and availability of resources. Understanding what may influence this aspect of care by using process mapping is an important component when planning for improvement interventions. The aim of the study was to identify factors that influence antibiotic initiation following prescription in the Adult Emergency and Trauma Centre of the largest referral hospital in Malawi.

Methods: We conducted a prospective observational case study using process mapping of two purposively selected adult pneumonia patients. One of the investigators CM observed the patient from the time of arrival at the triage area to the time he/she received initial dose of antibiotics. With purposively selected members of the clinical team; we used simple questions to analyze the map and identified facilitators, barriers and potential areas for improvement.

Results: Both patients did not receive the first dose of antibiotic within one hour of prescription. Despite the situation being less than ideal, potential facilitators to timely antibiotic initiation were: prompt assessment and triaging; availability of different expertise, timely first review by the clinician; and blood culture collected prior to antibiotic initiation. Barriers were: long waits, lack of communication/coordinated care and competency gap. Improvements are needed in communication, multidisciplinary teamwork, education and leadership/supervision.

Conclusion: Process mapping can have a significant impact in unveiling the system-related factors that influence timely initiation of antibiotics. The mapping exercise brought together stakeholders to evaluate and identify the facilitators and barriers. Recommendations here focused on improving communication, multidisciplinary team culture such as teamwork, good leadership and continuing professional development.

Keywords: Antimicrobial resistance, Antimicrobial stewardship, Dose optimization, Timely antibiotic initiation, Pneumonia, Process mapping, Health care system, Bottlenecks, Multidisciplinary team

* Correspondence: chimwemula@kcn.unima.mw
[1]Department of Clinical Nursing, Kamuzu College of Nursing, University of Malawi, Blantyre, Malawi
Full list of author information is available at the end of the article

Background

The emergence of drug-resistant organisms is a global health crisis [1]. In response to this threat, antimicrobial stewardship programs (ASPs) have been formed to maximize the benefits of antibiotics while minimizing their unintended consequences [2]. One of the strategies of ASPs is optimizing the dose and timing of antimicrobial agents based on patient and disease [2].

Evidence shows that timely initiation of antibiotics within 4 hours of patient arrival in the emergency department is associated with reduced mortality in patients with community acquired pneumonia [3]. Similarly, timely antibiotic initiation within 3 hours of triage in patients with sepsis is associated with improved outcome [4]. Evidence also demonstrates that rapid initiation of antibiotics within 1 hour of prescription, preferably before a patient leaves the emergency department, is one of the recommended practices for containing pneumonia [5, 6]. In summary, the acceptable time for antibiotic initiation, based on literature, is three to 4 hours after the patient arrives in the emergency department, and within 1 hour of antibiotic prescription.

However, multiple barriers affect these recommendations resulting in delayed administration of the initial dose of antibiotics [7]. In the emergency department, some patients require appropriate attention amidst assessment by multiple providers [8]. In addition, barriers to implementation such as poor collaboration between departments exist [9], overcrowding in the emergency department with high numbers of patients being admitted also affects timely antibiotic administration [10]. This is even more challenging with acute conditions like pneumonia where treatment is largely based on timely prescription of antibiotic therapy [11].

Pneumonia is a common, costly, and potentially fatal illness [12]. At one referral hospital in Malawi, pneumonia was found to be one of the most common admitting diagnoses [13]. In this study setting, antibiotic initiation within 1 hour of prescription is the strategy in practice for patients triaged as priority. The effectiveness of timely antibiotic initiation is determined by timely assessment and triaging; examination by the emergency department physician and then the medical physician; and timely collection of microbiology sample prior to administration of the initial dose. These steps are similar to recommended guidelines in sepsis management [14]. Therefore, as part of an effort to improve timely antibiotic initiation, process mapping was undertaken to identify factors in the environment that affect this care process.

A process map is a diagram of the sequence of major action steps [15] and decisions in a work setting [16]. It is used to track the flow of information, materials, documents, stakeholders and their impact on the process of patient care by clarifying tasks and decisions of actors [17]. It helps to delineate bottlenecks, inefficiencies and redundant steps [18], which can be improved later [19].

Process mapping has been used in various conditions, such as chronic obstructive pulmonary disease [20]; service contexts, such as outpatient attendance [19]; to understand care communication patterns [15]; and to investigate aspects of care requiring improvements for patients coming from other geographical locations such as rural areas [21]. Mapping has also been used to describe the interaction between a clinician, other providers and the endoscopy care process [22]. Mapping can be achieved with case note reviews [23], examinations of protocols [24], observations, patient self-reports and multidisciplinary meetings [22]. There is a dearth of literature about process mapping in the Malawian context and especially for pneumonia patients' antibiotic therapy initiation.

Methods

Aim

The aim of the study was to identify factors that influence timely antibiotic initiation following prescription in the Adult Emergency and Trauma Centre (AETC) of a referral hospital in Malawi and determine areas for improvement. The study seeks to answer the following research question: How do environmental /system related factors affect timely antibiotic initiation?

Design

A case study design [25] was used to study the antibiotic initiation process of patients with pneumonia. We conducted a prospective observation to map the patient journey followed by a meeting with the clinical team to analyze the process. The observation involved observing the pathway firsthand [13] p25 and then discussing the map with the clinical team. The role of the first author, CM, was to shadow (follow) [26] the patients (cases) through each step of the process [21, 22] and map the process as it happened, which resulted in multiple steps [27–29]. The scope of the mapping was from patient arrival at the triage area in the AETC to the time the first dose of antibiotic was given. A similar methodology was used by Johnson [15] to demonstrate how process.

mapping illustrates handover practices between ambulatory and inpatient care settings.

Study population

We used a typical case sampling [30] where we found that pneumonia was the most common medical condition requiring antibiotics in the AETC. In addition, it was observed that timely administration of antibiotics was a challenge.

Therefore, two patient participants, male and female, were recruited with assistance from the nurse in charge. The sample size was adequate because a case study research aims to maximize the lessons learnt, thus one or more cases are considered enough [25]. The inclusion criteria were: clinically diagnosed as having pneumonia, triaged as priority; Which means the patients had a potentially serious but not immediately life-threatening condition and were assigned second priority for treatment and transportation), aged 18 years and above, able to communicate and have had an antibiotic prescribed.

Ethics and consent to participate

All patient participants gave their informed written consent. Written informed consent for the health workers encountered in the mapping was not necessary due to the observational nature of the study. The research presented no more than a minimal risk of harm to the health workers and written consent could not practically be carried out because we could not predict in advance who would be found in the care process during mapping. This is in line with the National Health Sciences Research committee in Malawi: https://www.nhsrc-mw.com

In lieu of the signed consent form, a written statement regarding the research in form of information sheet was provided detailing how the verbal consent was documented. The form contained statement about the research, that no special time will be required from the participants, description of the process mapping, risks and benefits, subjects' rights and contact information of the investigator and COMREC chairperson. Ethics committee approval was granted for verbal consent.Prior to data collection, CM conducted meetings with the nurses and doctors in the AETC and nurses in the two medical wards and used the verbal consent information sheet to ensure team involvement in the improvement process [21]. In addition, we sought verbal consent from the health care worker providing care at the time of mapping. Anonymity was observed by using titles.The study was approved by the University of KwaZulu-Natal Human and Social Sciences Research Ethics Committee (Ref. HSS/0445/015D) and the University of Malawi, College of Medicine Research Ethics Committee (Ref. P03/15/1707).

Data collection

We developed a mapping guide based on hospital protocols and literature (see Additional file 1). The tool had three sections: patient demographics; physical examination findings; and structure/process indicators. We collected data through direct observations supplemented with case note reviews focusing on the four components proposed by McCarthy [31]: Encounters, Tasks, Actors

and Constraints. On both days, CM visited the AETC in the morning and attended the multidisciplinary handover meetings of the previous night's shift as a method of building a rapport with the health care workers. When a patient arrives in the emergency department, he or she is registered using an electronic record system. Depending on the status and severity of the condition, the patient may be referred to the triage area for assessment. The nurse and CM asked the patient what complaints he or she had, and then performed a preliminary identification of the patient for the mapping. After the clinical diagnosis of pneumonia was made, and antibiotic prescribed, CM confirmed with the patient about the patient's willingness to participate and obtained their written consent. None of the participants refused participation. The shadower followed the patient, identifying steps, assessing times and recording the flow of relevant information and actions that related to antibiotic interventions at each step of the process. The shadower documented on post-it notes what transpired and then pasted the notes on the flip chart, which was mounted on the wall in the nearby conference room. Basic flow chart symbols (Fig. 1) were used to identify specific activities and summarize data [19, 29]. Each patient journey was treated as a separate case.

Collaborative analysis of the map

The process mapping involved CM developing an initial understanding of the current process [2], then together with the clinical team, identifying facilitating factors, bottlenecks and solutions to improve the process. The clinical team, that was purposively selected by the first author, comprised the unit matron and deputy registered nurse in charge (coded as 1 and 2 respectively), and male and female doctors (coded as 3 and 4 respectively) from the AETC to participate in analysis of the map. To be more systematic, the team analyzed the map in a structured way using simple questions as guides [15, 16].

Question guides used to analyze data from the map

- What is happening at each step?
- Where is it taking place?
- Who is involved?
- How many steps does the patient have to complete or how many times is the patient passed from one person to another and are they all necessary?
- How quickly do patients move to second line?
- How long does the whole pathway take?
- What are the successes?
- What are the bottlenecks?
- What opportunities for change are there?

Symbol	Description of the symbol
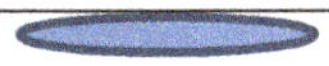 (oval)	Oval: shows the beginning and end of the antibiotic initiation process.
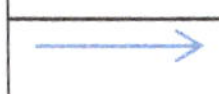 (arrow)	Arrow: shows the movement of the patient or movement to another step in the antibiotic initiation care process.
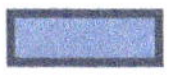 (rectangle)	Rectangle: shows the antibiotic care activity or task that took place at that step.
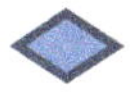 (diamond)	Diamond: shows the antibiotic care decisions that were made or question was asked at that step.
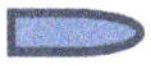 (delay)	Delay: shows sources or the step that contributed to delay in antibiotic initiation.
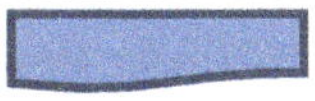 (document)	Document: Shows antibiotic stewardship documentation that was done by a health worker.

Fig. 1 Basic Flowchart Symbols. Is an illustration of basic flow chart symbols that were used to identify specific activities and summarize data. The oval shape shows where the process of antibiotic initiation begun and ended. The arrow shows the direction of patient movement to another step. The rectangle shows the antibiotic care activity or task that took place at that step. The diamond shape shows the antibiotic care decisions that were made at that time. The "D" shape shows the sources or step that contributed to delay in antibiotic initiation. Finally the rectangle with one irregular line shows antibiotic stewardship documentation that was done by a health worker

We discussed what actually occurred (versus what stakeholders would like to occur) during various steps in the patient's journey. We explored the standard practice (what could have happened?).As we discussed, discrepancies started to emerge between what should have happened and what actually happened. We determined the factors (barriers and facilitators) influencing the practice, and located potential areas for improvement based on the clinical team's experience. The discussion took 1 hour 20 minutes and was tape recorded after obtaining verbal consent from the members.

Results

Process mapping was conducted at AETC of the largest referral hospital in the urban setting. On average, a total of 5537 adult patient with emergency medical, surgical and trauma conditions are seen per month.

Following mapping, the researcher wrote the findings as a flowchart diagram for the male and female patients. Figure 2 illustrates the flow chart of a care pathway for the male patient and Fig. 3 for the female patient. The process map shows the actors and actions/decisions at each step. Mapping identified both potential factors that could have influenced timely antibiotic initiation and barriers to timely antibiotic initiation.

Patient characteristics

The first patient mapped was male. He was followed and observed for 4 hours 17 minutes. The second patient was female. She was followed and observed for 7 hours 14 minutes. These patients had clinical manifestations and vital signs that pointed to a potentially serious respiratory problem and were therefore second priority for treatment and transportation to the ward.

Potential facilitating factors

The following are responses from the clinical team to a question about the successes of a patient antibiotic management system which could positively influence timely administration of initial dose:

Timely assessments and triaging, proper chain of procedures were followed

Firstly, assessment of vital signs namely oxygen saturation, pulse rate and temperature followed by triaging took place immediately upon patients' arrival. This was facilitated by the consistent presence of a nurse and student nurses in the triage area. In both cases, the triage nurses acted promptly, this is the recommended practice in the department. Timely checking of vital signs that pointed to the infectious process (i.e. temperature) during the triage and admission in the ward is a potential factor that could have facilitated timely antibiotic

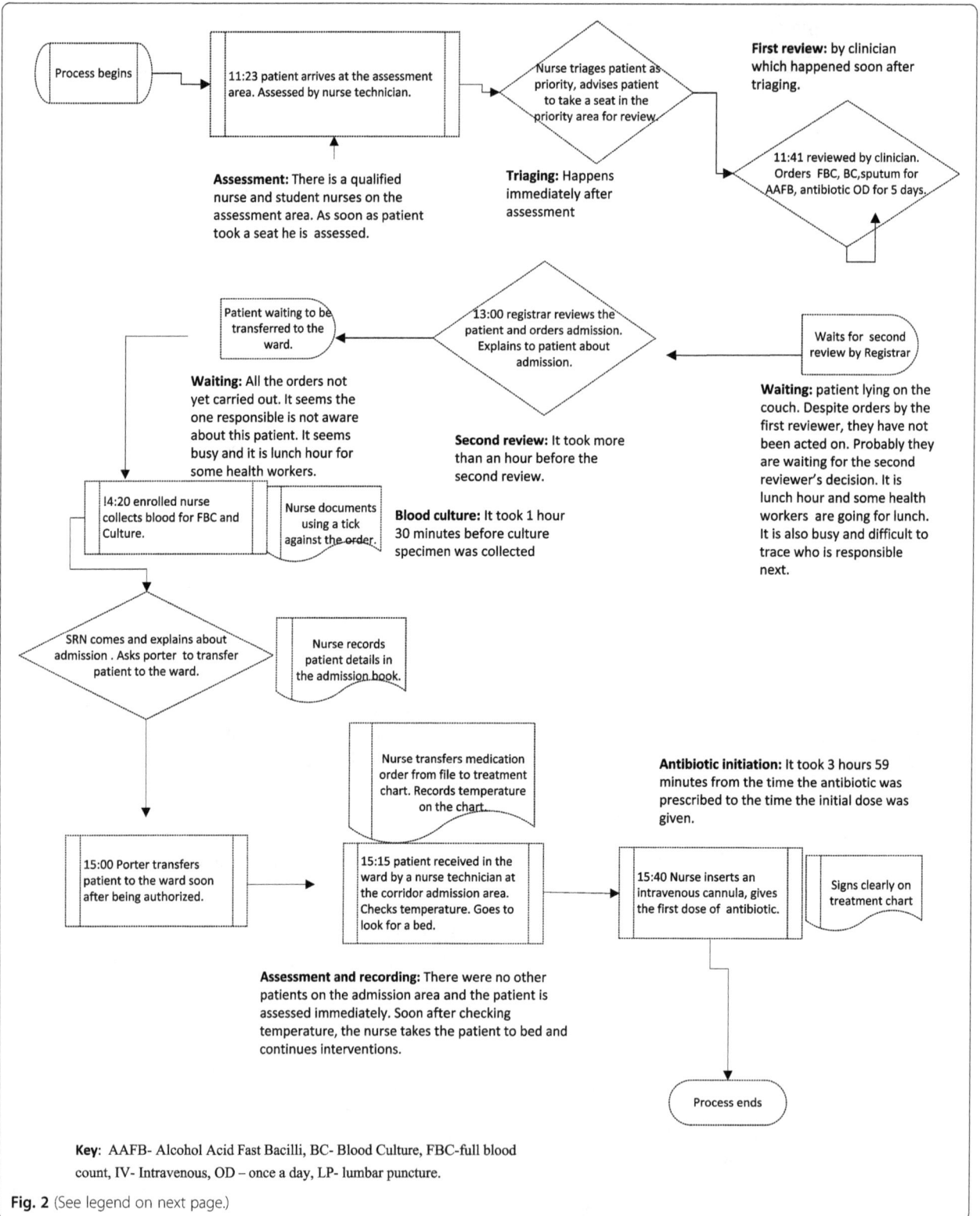

Key: AAFB- Alcohol Acid Fast Bacilli, BC- Blood Culture, FBC-full blood count, IV- Intravenous, OD – once a day, LP- lumbar puncture.

Fig. 2 (See legend on next page.)

Fig. 2 Flowchart of a care pathway in clinical diagnosis and antibiotic initiation of male pneumonia patient. Illustration of the male patient antibiotic initiation data based on direct observation of the process from patient arrival on the assessment area to the time the first dose of antibiotic was given. The observation took 4 h 17 min. Using the relevant symbols; the map shows the actors, actions/ tasks and decisions at each step of the process.Major action steps of the process are highlighted namely assessment, triaging, first review, waiting, second review, blood culture, assessment and recording, and antibiotic initiation. It took 3 h 59 min from the time the antibiotic was prescribed to the time it was given. The potential source of delay in antibiotic initiation was waiting time as shownby the relevant delay symbol. Mapping identified both potential factors that could have influenced timely antibiotic initiation and barriers to timely antibiotic initiation

initiation. One participant during analysis had these positive sentiments about the ward nurse:

> *The nurse admitting patient checked temperature, checked orders and was able to see a gap and administered the antibiotic. (Health worker 2)*

The nurse in the ward checked the patient's temperature (male patient). After identifying a fever and noting that the initial dose of antibiotic was not administered in AETC, she intervened immediately by inserting the cannula and gave the antibiotic. This was a positive action, though the antibiotic was still given after 1 hour of prescription.

First review by clinician and carrying out of orders
Secondly, the clinician reviewed the male patient soon after triaging. This was facilitated by the presence of the AETC clinician and a list of guidelines posted on the wall stipulating these rules. However the female patient was reviewed after an hour of triaging because the priority area was busy. Next, the nurses' presence during clinician review also facilitated timely collection of blood culture specimens in the female patient although the male patient experienced delays. Indeed, nurses are aware that blood cultures should be collected prior to antibiotics.

Second review by doctor
In the male patient, second review by doctor happened after 1 h 14 minutes following first review while in female patient it took 2 h.

Availability of different actors
All required experts were available during the care process. These were AETC clinicians, Medical clinicians, AETC nurses, blood culture nurses and a porter to potentially facilitate timely antibiotic initiation. In addition, student nurses played a role in assessing and triaging patients in the AETC and receiving patients in the ward. Each actor participated in each step of the care pathway, though their efforts were hampered by other factors as will be seen below. As a result, both patients did not receive antibiotics before leaving the AETC. In this case what needs to improve is the care coordination to

ensure that the different actors play their roles optimally hence timely antibiotic initiation would be effected.

Barriers and challenges
The following extracts capture stakeholders' responses when asked what the barriers were to timely antibiotic initiation.

Incomplete actions attributed to material resource challenges

> *This is mainly due to faulty blood pressure machine. (Health worker 2)*

> *A lot of them (nurses) do not have watches so they don't check respirations. (Health worker 3)*

Despite nurses performing timely assessment and triage, it seems they were not able to complete the assessment due to challenges with equipment. For example, in the first action the assessment task is incomplete; both patients did not have their respirations and blood pressure checked even though these are vital parameters when managing a patient with an infectious process.

Long waits attributed to staff shortage and hand offs

> *Initially, we had a clinician allocated to a cubicle (compartment where each patient is assessed) but now clinicians are no longer allocated according to cubicle because now they are less to share the cubicles. (Health worker 4)*

> *A good number of the patients have medical conditions so with one clinician it's a challenge. (Healthworker 2)*

First, the map shows several steps requiring hand offs between one health worker and another. These are tasks such as assessments, triaging, first and second reviews, investigations, and patient transfer. According to the AETC protocol, the patient is reviewed first by the AETC clinician followed by the senior medical clinician to confirm admission. Thus, it took a long time to access the second clinician. The second clinician would be

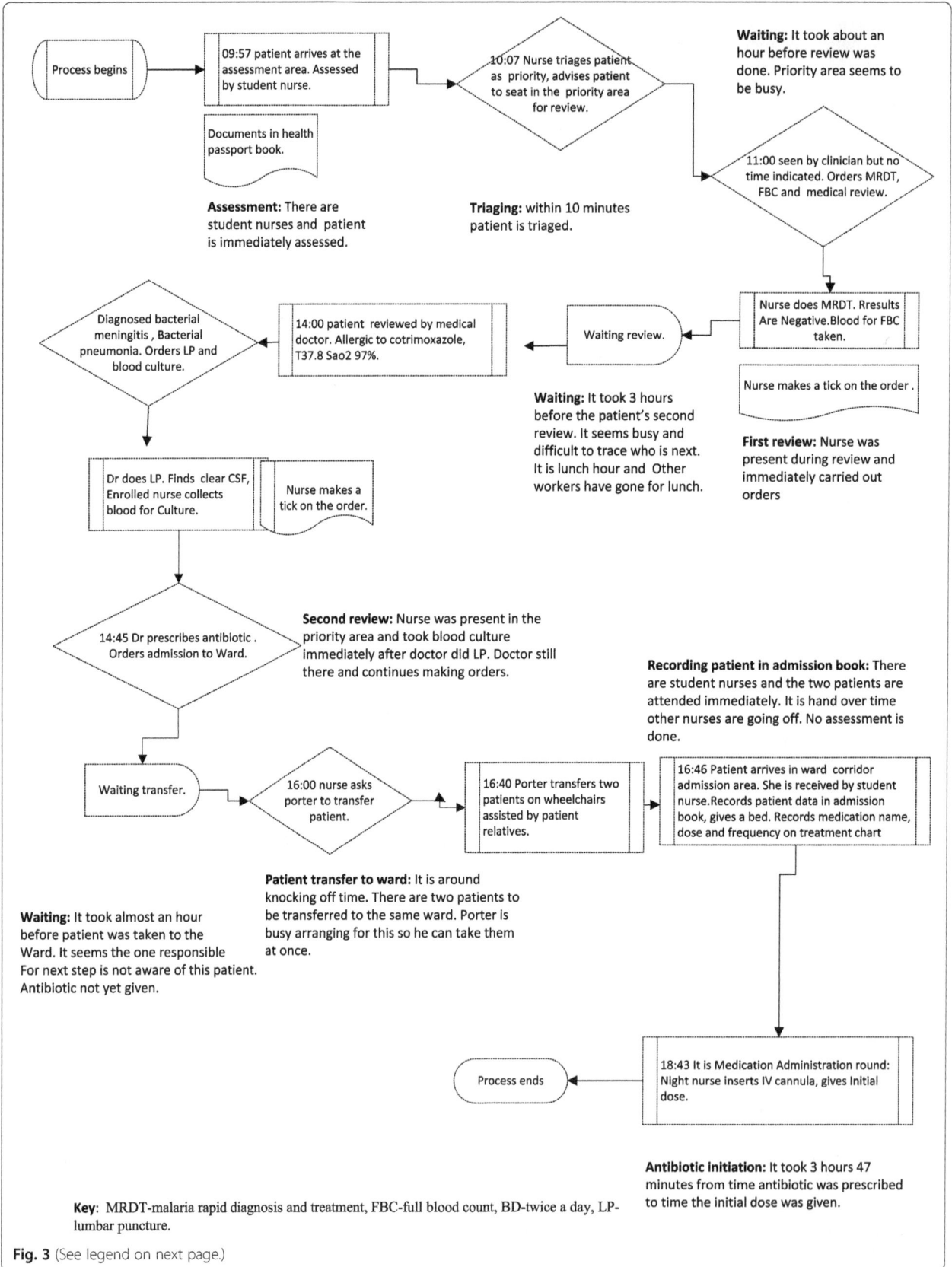

Process begins

09:57 patient arrives at the assessment area. Assessed by student nurse.

Documents in health passport book.

Assessment: There are student nurses and patient is immediately assessed.

10:07 Nurse triages patient as priority, advises patient to seat in the priority area for review.

Triaging: within 10 minutes patient is triaged.

Waiting: It took about an hour before review was done. Priority area seems to be busy.

11:00 seen by clinician but no time indicated. Orders MRDT, FBC and medical review.

Nurse does MRDT. Rresults Are Negative. Blood for FBC taken.

Nurse makes a tick on the order.

First review: Nurse was present during review and immediately carried out orders

Diagnosed bacterial meningitis , Bacterial pneumonia. Orders LP and blood culture.

14:00 patient reviewed by medical doctor. Allergic to cotrimoxazole, T37.8 Sao2 97%.

Waiting review.

Waiting: It took 3 hours before the patient's second review. It seems busy and difficult to trace who is next. It is lunch hour and Other workers have gone for lunch.

Dr does LP. Finds clear CSF, Enrolled nurse collects blood for Culture.

Nurse makes a tick on the order.

14:45 Dr prescribes antibiotic . Orders admission to Ward.

Second review: Nurse was present in the priority area and took blood culture immediately after doctor did LP. Doctor still there and continues making orders.

Recording patient in admission book: There are student nurses and the two patients are attended immediately. It is hand over time other nurses are going off. No assessment is done.

Waiting transfer.

16:00 nurse asks porter to transfer patient.

16:40 Porter transfers two patients on wheelchairs assisted by patient relatives.

16:46 Patient arrives in ward corridor admission area. She is received by student nurse. Records patient data in admission book, gives a bed. Records medication name, dose and frequency on treatment chart

Patient transfer to ward: It is around knocking off time. There are two patients to be transferred to the same ward. Porter is busy arranging for this so he can take them at once.

Waiting: It took almost an hour before patient was taken to the Ward. It seems the one responsible For next step is not aware of this patient. Antibiotic not yet given.

Process ends

18:43 It is Medication Administration round: Night nurse inserts IV cannula, gives Initial dose.

Antibiotic initiation: It took 3 hours 47 minutes from time antibiotic was prescribed to time the initial dose was given.

Key: MRDT-malaria rapid diagnosis and treatment, FBC-full blood count, BD-twice a day, LP-lumbar puncture.

Fig. 3 (See legend on next page.)

(See figure on previous page.)
Fig. 3 Flowchart of a care pathway in clinical diagnosis and antibiotic initiation of female pneumonia patient. Illustration of the female patient antibiotic initiation data based on direct observation of the process from patient arrival on the assessment area to the time the first dose of antibiotic was given. The observation took 7 h 14 min. Using the relevant symbols; the map shows the actors, actions/ tasks and decisions at each step of the process.Major action steps of the process are highlighted namely assessment, triaging, first review, waiting, recording patient data in admission book and antibiotic initiation. It took 3 h 47 min from the time the antibiotic was prescribed to the time it was given. The potential source of delay in antibiotic initiation was waiting time as shown by the relevant delay symbol. Mapping identified both potential factors that could have influenced timely antibiotic initiation such as having different actors (health workers) and barriers (such as waiting)to timely antibiotic initiation

attending to other patients in the resuscitation area or in the same priority area which has six cubicles and sometimes all cubicles could be full of medical patients waiting for the second review.

Challenges with communication/coordinated care
There is minimal direct verbal and written communication especially between nurses and doctors:

Clinicians (after reviewing first patient) may be catching up with other patients (rushing to see the next patient) off they proceed. So communication in the cubicles from both sides is a problem. Documentation is an issue. They can give the antibiotic but they don't document. People have repeated the dose because of no documentation. (Health worker 1)

In our study, we found that there were challenges with direct communication: 1) between the first and second clinicians, 2) between the nurse and the clinician, and 3) among nurses, which resulted in uncoordinated care. Documentation is also a challenge for the nurses.The first clinician may review a patient and write down the orders in the absence of the nurse who might be seeing another patient. As the clinician is trying to work quickly to see other patients, verbal communication does not take place; as a result the nurse is not aware of the orders, which then may not be acted on in time. The AETC department has research nurses responsible for collecting blood cultures (blood culture nurses). After collecting the blood, if the blood culture nurse does not inform the AETC nurse to come and give the antibiotics, this may contribute to the delay. At the same time, when a blood culture is ordered and the blood culture nurse is not present, sometimes the AETC nurse does not collect the specimen and waits for the former.

There were also delays in communication between nurse and porter regarding patient transfer. For example, the male and female patients had to wait for about 40 min and one hour respectively after an admission was ordered, before being transferred to the ward due to poor communication.

Coordination of care was another barrier

During lunch hour, there is a little bit of slow down on activities. Lunch hour is mostly busy, more patients coming, people (health care workers) are tired and others have gone for lunch. (Health worker 1)

Health care delivery during the lunch hour proved to be ineffective as more patients require assistance, yet fewer health care workers are available. Staffing patterns during lunch hour and shift change handoffs affected the process of care.

Competency gap is a barrier to the process
Knowledge gaps, poor attitudes and inexperience were also mentioned as possible barriers influencing delays:

Attitude and to sustain standards is a challenge, unless policing. Lack of knowledge and low confidence level (referring to nurses). Because even before second clinician reviews patient, the nurse is supposed to carry out the emergency orders. (Health worker 1)

Some clinicians clear (review) patients automatically and faster. But it depends; an intern may take longer to see one patient because he has to concentrate as does not have much experience but when with registrar it's faster. So level and also experience matters. (Health worker 3)

First, it seems the sustainability of the standards is a challenge as actors need to be closely monitored for them to comply. This demonstrates knowledge, attitude and supervisory gaps. Secondly, doctors' experience and knowledge affects the process as it takes longer for an inexperienced doctor to complete the same task.

Areas for improvement
The findings about barriers informed our recommendations for improvement.

Team work: Verbal communication/coordination and documentation

A nurse should be there (allocated) already and carry out orders but if the nurse is not there, the clinician is supposed to communicate after review. (Health Worker1)

Both verbal and written communication is an area to improve and collaboration between a clinician and a nurse. This will help to prioritize care. Documentation by ticking against the order after it is carried out (i.e. blood culture) is acceptable considering the volume of work and the urgency in the AETC. (Health Worker3)

There is a need to improve nurse-doctor communication and documentation. Documentation using a tick (√) symbol only is not enough and the team analysing the data agreed that the time the action is taken should be documented in addition to the tick.

AETC clinician should communicate with medical clinician. They are supposed to consult, sometimes depends on clinician. (Health Worker 1)

There is also a need to improve communication amongst clinicians.

Blood Culture nurse could have communicated with AETC nurse after collection of blood culture. But even Blood Culture nurse can insert cannula and give the antibiotic. Mostly after blood culture they administer antibiotics but documentation is an issue. (Health Worker 2)

The AETC and Blood Culture nurses also need to improve their communication and coordination of care.

During patient transfer, nurse is supposed to check again in the file to ensure all is done. Some clever porters may ask if they can take patient or remind nurses. (Health Worker 1)

Similarly, the nurse and the porter need to improve their communication.

Leadership and supervision

Leadership - we cannot run away from it. Spot checking on how things are going should be done. Lead nurse could be checking the priority patients not yet reviewed to ensure patients are reviewed and orders are carried out. (Health Worker1)

Another key issue the participants recommended was leadership. There is a need to spot check to ensure care is delivered in a timely manner. This should be the responsibility of the nurse leader who is assigned to an area on each shift in the AETC to ensure supervision takes place.

Awareness about importance of antibiotics

People (health care workers) need to understand the importance of timely antibiotic initiation, there should be emphasis on this just is the case with those patients that require resuscitation. It should be part of Continuing Professional Development (CPD). (Health worker 3)

If the porter also had some knowledge, to remind the nurse that they have not given the antibiotic prior to transfer. But the challenge is they just transfer the patient with little knowledge. (Health Worker1)

It seems there is a need for CPD so that health workers understand the importance of timely antibiotic initiation. Similarly, the porter responsible for transferring the patient should have some basic knowledge about the patient being transferred.

Discussion

Understanding the process of initiating antibiotics within 1 hour of prescription has implications for the nurses and clinicians to improve practice. Involving stakeholders helped to get a better perspective of the process that was based on their experience. This led to a better interpretation of events [14]. Based on the objective, we identified four themes under the domain 'potential facilitating factors'; five themes from domain 'barriers/bottlenecks'; and three themes from the domain 'areas for improvement'.

Evidence shows that timely assessment facilitates timely antibiotic initiation [32]. However, the results of the mapping show that while there was timely assessment and triage of the patient and that there were different actors in the process as potential facilitating factors to timely antibiotic initiation, waiting time for antibiotic initiation was prolonged. Similarly, adhering to the procedures of timely review and carrying out of microbiology specimen orders as it happened in the male patient could potentially lead to timely identification of the causative organism and timely antibiotic initiation. This is in line with Hatton [33] who states that obtaining appropriate cultures before initiating antimicrobial therapy plays an important role as the chances of identifying the offending microorganism are improved. However this was affected by prolonged waiting times for the female patient.

Antibiotic initiation delays in this study therefore demonstrate poor quality of care. There was variation in the time it took between a male and female patient to get prescribed antibiotic. The male and female patients took 3 hours 59 min and 3 hours 47 min respectively; from prescription to receiving the antibiotic instead of the practice standard of administering it within 1 hour of prescription. In this study, factors in the process contributing to delays were handoffs, staff shortages, control points, poor communication, uncoordinated care and competency gaps.

Excessive handoff is a functional bottleneck as patients are unnecessarily passed from one health worker to another [34]. Staff shortages worsened the delay. Rodriguez et al., [35] assessed processes of care to promote timely antibiotic initiation using surveys and focus group discussions with doctors, pharmacists and radiologists. They identified assessment, shift changes, transportation and communication delays as factors that delayed antibiotic initiation because the steps require handoffs between health care workers. These findings are consistent with the current study.

Valueless steps that delay the process of care are reported. Trebble [22] found valueless steps in the observational mapping study of an endoscopy procedure where five out of the 23 steps added no value to the patient outcome. Similarly, Kainthet al. [36], in a study to determine time taken in the process of management of patient with community acquired pneumonia, found that the longest delay was the process of obtaining a chest x-ray; recommendation was prioritization of chest x-ray by using porters to transfer patients to the radiology department. However, in our study, analysis showed that each step was found to be necessary by the clinical team, except in one step in the female patient. After giving the patient a bed, the nurse was not supposed to wait for the medication rounds to give the initial dose of antibiotic; this waiting for medication round was a valueless step. There is need to prioritize antibiotic initiation irrespective of whether it is medication administration round or not. Nurses need to be educated in this aspect of care and the relevant guidelines and protocols should reflect this.

Related to the handoffs, we noted control points where one health worker needed to provide authorization before the next action [34]. For example, following the review by the AETC clinician, the patient is supposed to be seen by the medical clinician to authorize admission or confirm prescription orders. Similarly, following admission authorization by the medical clinician; the nurse is supposed to authorize the porter to transfer the patient. When the next responsible worker is not aware of the succeeding step or is busy, this delays the process as the following actor cannot act without authorization. This delayed antibiotic initiation further because; for example, if the patient was transferred in time, it would be possible for the ward nurse to give the missed initial dose without further delay.

Similarly, Pinningtonet al., [32] in a quality improvement project found communication barriers that influenced timely treatment in severe sepsis. The communication failures were that staff did not know which nurse/doctor was looking after the patient, there was no communication about the prescribed treatment and staff did not know who was assigned to a specific patient [32]. As a result, interactive multidisciplinary education sessions were identified as important interventions.

Uncoordinated care compounded with staff shortage was another barrier. Spath [37] noted similar findings where there was no correlation between staffing patterns and patient demand and they changed the system for scheduling staff so that working hours reflected predicted levels of demand. Similarly, Watts et al. [38] found that time of the day was a factor affecting timely antibiotic initiation. Therefore, there is a need to increase the staffing levels at the department and consider allocating similar numbers at all times including lunch hours to ensure work is well coordinated.

Competency gap was also evident in this study. There was a lack of awareness of the importance of reduced time to antibiotic initiation as was identified in one study [35]. Though it is suggested that in the AETC, the clinician needs to diagnose rapidly and initiate treatment [39], this may not work well for the less experienced in our study setting, leading to delays.

A common theme throughout discussions about recommendations for improvement has been teamwork. The clinical team analysing data recommended that when a clinician reviews a patient in the absence of a nurse h/she should verbally communicate the orders so the nurse is aware. Clinicians should also consult and communicate whenever a patient on priority is reviewed and requires the review of the second clinician. The same is the case during patient transfer. Before handing over to the porter, the nurse should check the orders to see if the patient has received the antibiotic. Without this care coordination, it is difficult for a multidisciplinary and continuous care to thrive [40]. For example, Downey et al. [41], state that communication between physicians is best done using a formalized process with a consultant contributing in improving the process [42]. There is need for such a formalized process in the current study setting.

The process mapping has shown that synergy is less than optimal, which can lead to poor patient outcomes.

The findings revealed implications for engaging stakeholders who made suggestions for improvement. This concurs with Johnson [15] who states that the value of a process mapping exercise is that it clarifies the process for the actors and builds bridges to engage these actors in future improvement work. Similar to the present study, Martin [43] found that engagement of stakeholders was effective in identifying and explaining sources of delay and aspects that could be improved. Based on these findings, improvement interventions have been done collaboratively with stakeholders.

Strengths and limitations

The map failed to consider the patients' experiences, which is recommended as critical [20, 31] and did not focus on patient-related factors that could have influenced timely antibiotic initiation as was found in one study [44]. For example, patient presentation may determine the urgency of the actions [45]; this was not considered. In addition, the mapping did not consider diagnostic aspect of the care process that could also affect antibiotic initiation.This quality improvement initiative focused mainly on timing of initial antibiotic therapy. While this is a major issue when it comes to the odds of survival, other factors may pay an important role in the outcomes associated with community-acquired pneumonia [46].

Though lacking this integration, the map offers a guide to a solution on the system improvement by answering critical questions. This is in line with the United Kingdom's National Health Service (NHS) Institute for Innovation and Improvement [26], which proposes establishing what is currently happening or how efficient the process is, in order to provide a baseline for solutions.

The two cases are too few to generalize how antibiotic initiation is conducted in this particular context. Based on these results, one may have an impression that all patients do not get the initial dose of antibiotic in time. This is not the case as the sample is small and such generalizations do not apply [25]. The results of the analysis were used to develop other interventions that did not involve designing a map for the department. This was beyond the scope of this study. There is a need therefore to design a map that would guide in timely antibiotic initiation based on the findings.

Conclusion

We have demonstrated that process mapping can have a significant impact in reducing delays in diagnosis and management of pneumonia thus enabling timely administration of initial dose of antibiotic. Evaluating the map

indicates positive issues such as timely assessment, triage and the availability of different actors. From this process map analysis, improvements are needed in communication/coordination, teamwork, leadership and awareness about antibiotic stewardship.

Abbreviations

AETC: Adult Emergency and Trauma Centre; ASPs: Antimicrobial Stewardship Programs; CPD: Continuing Professional Development

Acknowledgements

The authors wish to thank all the patients, health worker participants who contributed to this study and Mr. Humphrey Kumwembe for the graphic work.

Funding

This research received grant and award from the Norwegian Research and Capacity Building for Higher Education (NORHED) and the African Doctoral Dissertation Research Fellowship (ADDRF) respectively.The funders had no role in the design of the study and data collection, analysis, interpretation of data and in writing the manuscript.

Authors' contributions

CM conceptualized, designed and wrote the study protocol. CV reviewed and approved the study protocol. CM, CV, NH, LM analysed the data. CM wrote the manuscript drafts. NH, LM made critical revisions for intellectual content. All authors read and approved the final version.

Ethics approval and consent to participate

We obtained ethical approval from two ethics committees: the university of KwaZulu-Natal Human and Social Sciences Research Ethics Committee (Ref. HSS/0445/015D), where the researcher was a student and the University of Malawi, College of Medicine Research Ethics Committee (Ref. P03/15/1707) where the study was conducted. We obtained written informed consent from the patients prior to participation in the study which was translated into local language. We obtained verbal consent from health workers using the information sheet. This is in line with the National Health Sciences Research committee in Malawi under which College of Medicine Research Ethics Committee falls: https://www.nhsrc-mw.com. The committee adopted the International Ethical Guidelines for Health Related Research Involving Humans [46].

Consent for publication

Consent for publication was not made because the data set present minimal risk to confidentiality of patient participants. This is because place of study (hospital name), dates of data collection related to the patient participants, age, symptoms and specific treatment name are not included. Only two indirect identifiers namely sex and diagnosis have been reported. Reporting of pneumonia diagnosis data was necessary because this is a common medical problem requiring improvement in antibiotic care in the hospital.

Competing interests

The authors declare that they have no competing interests.

Author details

[1]Department of Clinical Nursing, Kamuzu College of Nursing, University of Malawi, Blantyre, Malawi. [2]Department of Pharmacy, School of Health Sciences, University of KwaZulu-Natal, KwaZulu-Natal, South Africa. [3]Ohio State University Wexner Medical Center, Columbus, USA.

References

1. Centre for Disease Control. Core Elements of Hospital Antibiotic Stewardship Programs. 2014. http://www.cdc.gov/getsmart/healthcare/implementation/core-elements.html.d. Accessed Nov 2014.
2. Dellit TH, Owens RC, McGowan JE, Gerding DN, Weinstein RA, Burke JP, et al. Infectious Diseases Society of America and the Society for Healthcare Epidemiology of America guidelines for developing an institutional program to enhance antimicrobial stewardship. Clin Infect Dis. 2007;44:159–77.
3. Houck PM, Bratzler DW, Nsa W, Ma A, Bartlett JG. Timing of antibiotic administration and outcomes for Medicare patients hospitalized with community-acquired pneumonia. Arch Intern Med. 2004;164:637–44.
4. Joo YM, Chae MK, Hwang SY, Jin S-C, Lee TR, Cha WC, et al. Impact of timely antibiotic administration on outcomes in patients with severe sepsis and septic shock in the emergency department. Clin Exp Emerg Med. 2014;1:35–40.
5. ESPAUR SSTF Implementation subgroup. Start Smart Then Focus Antimicrobial Stewardship Toolkit for English Hospitals. PHE publications gateway number: 2014828; 2015.
6. Lim WS, Baudouin SV, George RC, Hill AT, Jamieson C, Le Jeune I, et al. BTS guidelines for the management of community acquired pneumonia in adults: update 2009. Thorax. 2009;64(Suppl 3):iii1–iii55.
7. Bishop BM. Antimicrobial stewardship in the emergency department: challenges, opportunities, and a call to action for pharmacists. J Pharm Pract. 2016;29:556–63.
8. Pines JM. Profiles in patient safety: antibiotic timing in pneumonia and pay-for-performance. AcadEmerg Med. 2006;13:787–90.
9. Phua J, Dean NC, Guo Q, Kuan WS, Lim HF, Lim TK. Severe community-acquired pneumonia: timely management measures in the first 24 hours. Crit Care. 2016;28(20):237.
10. Fee C, Weber EJ, Maak CA, Bacchetti P. Effect of emergency department crowding on time to antibiotics in patients admitted with community-acquired pneumonia. Ann Emerg Med. 2007;50:501–9.
11. Sethi S. Respiratory Infections. CRC Press; 2016.p 340.
12. Scott Obrosky D, Hsu DJ, Meehan TP, Fine JM, Graff LG, Stone RA, et al. Predictors of timely antibiotic Administration for Patients Hospitalized with Community-Acquired Pneumonia from the cluster-randomized EDCAP trial. Am J Med Sci. 2010;339:307–13.
13. SanJoaquin MA, Allain TJ, Molyneux ME, Benjamin L, Everett DB, Gadabu O, et al. Surveillance Programme of IN-patients and Epidemiology [SPINE]: Implementation of an Electronic Data Collection Tool within a Large Hospital in Malawi. PLoS Med. 2013;12(10):e1001400.
14. Dellinger RP, Levy MM, Carlet JM, Bion J, Parker MM, Jaeschke R, et al. Surviving Sepsis campaign: international guidelines for management of severe sepsis and septic shock: 2008. Intensive Care Med. 2008;34:17–60.
15. Johnson JK, Farnan JM, Barach P, Hesselink G, Wollersheim H, Pijnenborg L, et al. Searching for the missing pieces between the hospital and primary care: mapping the patient process during care transitions. BMJ Qual Saf. 2012;21(Suppl 1):i97–105.
16. Barbrow S, Hartline M. Process mapping as organizational assessment in academic libraries. Alice L, Daugherty P, editor. Perform MeasMetr 2015; 16:34–47.
17. CPS Activity Based Costings team. A guide to Process Mapping and Improvement. The Crown Prosecution Service CPS; 2012.
18. Child and Youth Mental Health. Kamloops Patient Journey Mapping Report. 2012. https://divisionsbc.ca/Media/WebsiteContent/8007/PJM%20Report%20-%20November%2028%202011.pdf. Accessed 9 Jan 2017.
19. Francis Report. Use of process mapping in service improvement.Nursing Times. NursPract Res Change Manag. 2013;109:24–6.
20. Jackson K, Oelke ND, Leffelaar D, Besner J, Harrison A. Report on the patient journey study. Edmonton, Alberta. 2008. http://www.albertahealthservices.Ca/Researchers/if-res-hswru-pt-journey-report-2008.pdf. Accessed 23 Nov 2016.
21. Kelly J, Dwyer J, Pekarsky B, MacKean T, McCabe N, Wiseman J, et al. managing two worlds together: stage 3: improving Aboriginal patient journeys -. 2015.
22. Trebble TM, Hansi N, Hydes T, Smith MA, Baker M. Process mapping the patient journey: an introduction. BMJ. 2010;341:c4078.
23. Lee JS, Primack BA, Mor MK, Stone RA, Obrosky DS, Yealy DM, et al. Processes of Care and Outcomes for Community-Acquired Pneumonia. Am J Med. 2011;124:1175 e9–1175.e17.
24. Colligan L, Anderson JE, Potts HW, Berman J. Does the process map influence the outcome of quality improvement work? A comparison of a sequential flow diagram and a hierarchical task analysis diagram. BMC Health Serv Res. 2010;10:1.
25. Yin R K .Case Study Research Design and Methods.Sixth Edition.Vol. 5.SAGE Publications.International Educational and Professional Publisher. Thousand Oaks London New Delhi: SAGE Publications. 1994.
26. NHS Institute for Innovation and Improvement Great Britain., Parliament, House of Commons. NHS Institute for Innovation and Improvement annual report and accounts for the period 1 April 2007 to 31 march 2008. London: TSO; 2008.
27. Ben-Tovim DI, Dougherty ML, O'Connell TJ, McGrath KM. Patient journeys: the process of clinical redesign. Med J Aust. 2008;188:S14.
28. Butterfield S, Stegel C, Maynor. Mapping your Discharge Process and Handoffs.Powerpoint presented at: Quality Improvement Organizations; 2012; New York State Centers for Medicare & Medicaid Services.
29. Arora V, Johnson J. A model for building a standardized hand-off protocol. JtComm J Qual Patient Saf. 2006;32:646–55.
30. Polit DF, Hungler BP. Nursing Research Principles and Methods. 6th ed. Philadelphia: Lippincott William and Wilkins; 1999.
31. McCarthy S, O'Raghallaigh P, Woodworth S, Lim YL, Kenny LC, Adam F. An integrated patient journey mapping tool for embedding quality in healthcare service reform. J Decis Syst. 2016;25(sup1):354–68.
32. Pinnington S, Atterton B, Ingleby S. Making the journey safe: recognizing and responding to severe sepsis in accident and emergency. BMJ Open Qual. 2016;5:u210706.w4335.
33. Hatton RC. Drugs and therapy bulletin. Drug Inf Pharm Resource Cent. 2006;20(10):1–4.
34. Scotland, Health Department, Centre for Change and Innovation. National Health Service in Scotland. A guide to service improvement: measurement, analysis techniques and solutions. Edinburgh: Scottish Executive; 2005.
35. Rodriguez KL, Burkitt KH, Sevick MA, Obrosky DS, Aspinall SL, Switzer GE, et al. Assessing processes of care to promote timely initiation of antibiotic therapy for emergency department patients hospitalized for pneumonia. JtComm J Qual Patient Saf. 2009;35:509–18.
36. Kainth H, Wheeler J, Dainty P. The diagnosis and management of community acquired pneumonia: a quality improvement project. http://www.acutemedicine.org.uk/wp-content/uploads/2014/12/AQI-62- Accessed 29 Nov 2016.
37. Spath P. The Quality-Cost Connection: Improve patient flow by reducing bottlenecks. 2005. https://www.ahcmedia.com/articles/86620-the-quality-cost-connection-improve-patient-flow-by-reducing-bottlenecks. Accessed 5 Jan 2017.
38. Watts SH, Bryan ED. Emergency department pneumonia patients who do not meet the six-hour criteria for antibiotic administration: do they have a different clinical presentation? J Clin Med Res. 2012;4:338.
39. Biomerieux. Emergency Department patient management. 2017.http://www.biomerieux-nordic.com/clinical-diagnostics/solutions/emergency-department-patient-management. Accessed 5 Jan 2017.
40. West Coast District Health Board. Urgent Colonoscopy Pathway Patient Journey Map Final Report and Recommendations; 2007.
41. Downey. What constitutes a good hand offs in the emergency department: a patient's perspective. 2013. https://www.ncbi.nlm.nih.gov/pubmed/24422264-PubMed - NCBI. Accessed 5 Jan 2017.
42. Terris J. Making an impact on emergency department flow: improving patient processing assisted by consultant at triage. Emerg Med J. 2004;21:537–41.
43. Martin M, Champion R, Kinsman L, Masman K. Mapping patient flow in a regional Australian emergency department: a model driven approach. International Emergency Nursing. 2011;19:75–85.
44. Kutz A, Florin J, Hausfater P, Amin D, Amin A, Haubitz S, et al. Predictors for Delayed Emergency Department Care in Medical Patients with Acute Infections – An International Prospective Observational Study. PLOS ONE. 2016;11:e0155363.
45. Rodriguez A, et al. Mortality in ICU patients with bacterial community-acquired pneumonia: when antibiotics are not enough. Intensive Care Med. 2009;35:430–8.
46. International Ethical Guidelines for Health-related Research Involving Humans. Fourth Edition. Geneva. Council for International Organizations of Medical Sciences (CIOMS); 2016.

23

Disseminated extrapulmonary *Legionella pneumophila* infection presenting with panniculitis

Maria N. Chitasombat[1]* ⓘ, Natta Ratchatanawin[2] and Yingluck Visessiri[3]

Abstract

Background: Legionellosis is a well-known cause of pneumonia. Primary cutaneous and subcutaneous infection caused by *Legionella pneumophila* is rare and the diagnosis is challenging.

Case presentation: A 38-year-old Thai woman with systemic lupus erythematosus and myasthenia gravis treated with prednisolone and azathioprine presented to our hospital with low-grade fever, diarrhea, and indurated skin lesions on both thighs. Initial examination showed plaques on both inner thighs. Magnetic resonance imaging showed myositis and swelling of the skin and subcutaneous tissue. Diagnosis of panniculitis due to *L. pneumophila* was carried out by histopathology, Gram stain, and 16S rRNA gene sequencing method of tissue biopsy from multiple sites on both thighs. Myocarditis was diagnosed by echocardiography. The final diagnosis was disseminated extrapulmonary legionellosis. Treatment comprised intravenous azithromycin for 3 weeks and the skin lesions, myositis and myocarditis resolved. Oral azithromycin and ciprofloxacin were continued for 3 months to ensure eradication of the organism. The patient's overall condition improved.

Conclusions: To our knowledge, we report the first case of *L. pneumophila* infection manifesting with panniculitis, possible myositis, and myocarditis in the absence of pneumonia. The diagnosis of extrapulmonary *Legionella* infection is difficult, especially in the absence of pneumonia. A high index of suspicion and appropriate culture with special media or molecular testing are required. Initiation of appropriate treatment is critical because delaying therapy was associated with progressive infection in our patient.

Keywords: *Legionella pneumophila*, Panniculitis, Lupus, Myositis, Myocarditis

Background

Legionella is a well-known cause of pneumonia. Extrapulmonary manifestations of Legionnaires' disease include myocarditis [1, 2], neurological involvement (acute disseminated encephalomyelitis), and multiorgan failure [3, 4]. Legionnaires' disease has been reported together with several types of skin lesions such as maculopapular rash, petechial rash, erythema with focal blister, cellulitis, pustules, abscesses, and subcutaneous masses [5]. Various species of *Legionella*, including *L. pneumophila*, *L. micdadei*, *L. cincinnatiensis*, *L. maceachernii*, and *L. feeleii*, cause skin/soft tissue infection, mostly among immunocompromised patients with pneumonia [6]. Primary cutaneous infection is a rare distinctive feature of direct inoculation of *Legionella* into skin and soft tissue, which occurs as cellulitis necrotizing fasciitis, as a postoperative complication [6–9]. The diagnosis of legionellosis can be challenging in the absence of pneumonia. To the best of our knowledge, this is the first description of panniculitis due to *Legionella*. This report highlights the challenges, pitfalls and importance of diagnosing extrapulmonary *Legionella* infection.

* Correspondence: mchitasombat@gmail.com
[1]Division of Infectious Disease, Department of Medicine, Faculty of Medicine, Ramathibodi Hospital, Mahidol University, 270 Rama VI Road, Ratchathewi District, Bangkok 10400, Thailand

Case presentation

We describe a case of disseminated extrapulmonary legionellosis in an immunocompromised 38-year-old Thai woman. The patient was diagnosed in 2002 with systemic lupus erythematosus (SLE) with fever, polyarthritis, oral ulcer, alopecia, and proteinuria. Since then, she has been treated with prednisolone with azathioprine. She achieved clinical remission but remained on prednisolone (5 mg daily) and azathioprine (50 mg daily) for 13 years. In August 2015, 3 months prior to admission, she suffered from cramping abdominal pain, watery diarrhea two or three times daily, and low-grade fever. She was diagnosed with enteritis and treated with ceftriaxone without clinical improvement. The dose of immunosuppressive medication was increased to prednisolone 45 mg daily and hydroxychloroquine 400 mg daily. In September 2015, 2 months prior to admission, she developed proximal muscle weakness with low-grade fever. She was diagnosed with myasthenia gravis and received treatment with pyridostigmine (Mestinon™) 240 mg daily. She remained weak and lost significant weight because of poor appetite and diarrhea. She was admitted to her local hospital in October 2015 for intravenous fluid hydration and pyridostigmine was discontinued because of diarrhea. As her condition was becoming increasingly compromised with high-grade fever, generalized vesicular rash, and proximal muscle weakness, she was referred to our hospital in November, 2015. She did not recall any exposure to potentially contaminated water or animals. She worked as a school teacher. Upon admission, her temperature was 39 °C, heart rate 100 beats/min, and respiratory rate 20 breaths/min. Blood pressure was 90/60 mmHg. Physical examination revealed a cachectic woman with mild pale conjunctivae and anicteric sclerae. Skin examination showed generalized discrete erythematous papules and macules with dry necrotic crust on the scalp, facial area, trunk and extremities. She also had plaques measuring 15 × 15 cm on both inner thighs (Fig. 1). Abdominal examination showed mild tenderness and distension. The examination did not reveal any cardiac or pulmonary findings. Neurological examination revealed ptosis in both eyes, proximal muscle weakness (grade IV) of all extremities, but normal sensation and tendon reflexes. Laboratory data shown in Table 1. Skin biopsy of the crusted lesion revealed varicella zoster virus from polymerase chain reaction (PCR). She was diagnosed with varicella zoster virus infection. At admission, plasma cytomegalovirus (CMV) viral load (Cobas® Taqman amplicon) was 363,000 copies/mm³. She received intravenous ganciclovir injection with adjuvant granulocyte colony-stimulating factor for leukopenia. The timeline of the patient's illness is illustrated in Additional file 1. She was also treated empirically for skin and soft tissue infection with piperacillin/tazobactam (12 days), and then meropenem

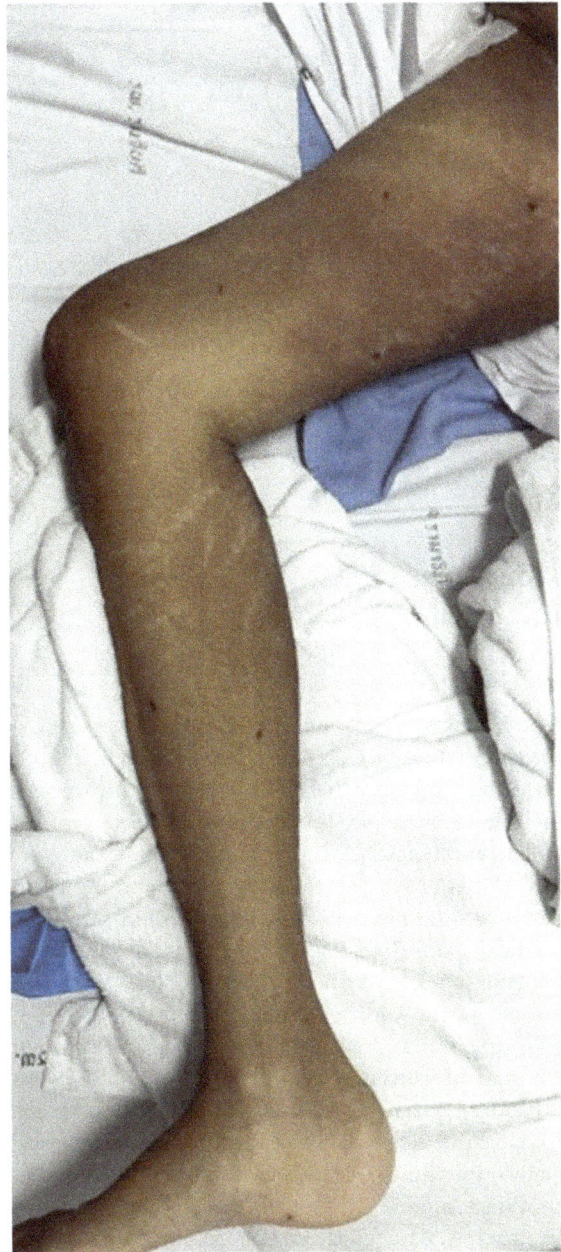

Fig. 1 Multiple erythematous indurated plaques on the proximal right thigh, multiple healed crusted papules on the right lower extremity, and whitish striae (before treatment)

(5 days) and then cefepime (5 days), without any clinical response. Further investigations, computed tomography of the abdomen showed a long segment of jejunal wall thickening and mild rectal wall thickening. Colonoscopy revealed generalized edematous mucosa of the colon without ulceration, and random biopsy was negative. She was diagnosed with CMV syndrome with suspected CMV jejunitis, which later improved with ganciclovir therapy. She was also diagnosed with myasthenia gravis by electromyography, nerve conduction velocity, and presence of acetylcholine

Table 1 Laboratory data on admission

Parameter	Recorded value	Standard value
White blood cell count	1,860 cells/mm^3	4,500–7,500 cells/mm^3
Neutrophils	83 %	
Lymphocytes	14 %	
Hemoglobin	10.8 g/dL	11.3–15.2 g/dL
Hematocrit	32.4 %	36–45 %
Platelet count	179,000 cells/mm^3	130,000–350,000 cells/mm^3
Total protein	33 g/L	69-84 g/L
Albumin	12.3 g/L	39–51 g/L
Total bilirubin	0.6 mg/dL	0.2–1.2 mg/dL
Direct billirubin	0.3 mg/dL	0.1–0.3 mg/dL
Aspartate aminotransferase	23 U/L	11–30 U/L
Alanine aminotransferase	34 U/L	4–30 U/L
Alkaline phosphatase	57 U/L	44–147 U/L
Blood urea nitrogen	9.0 mg/dL	8–20 mg/dL
Creatinine	0.32 mg/dL	0.63–1.03 mg/dL

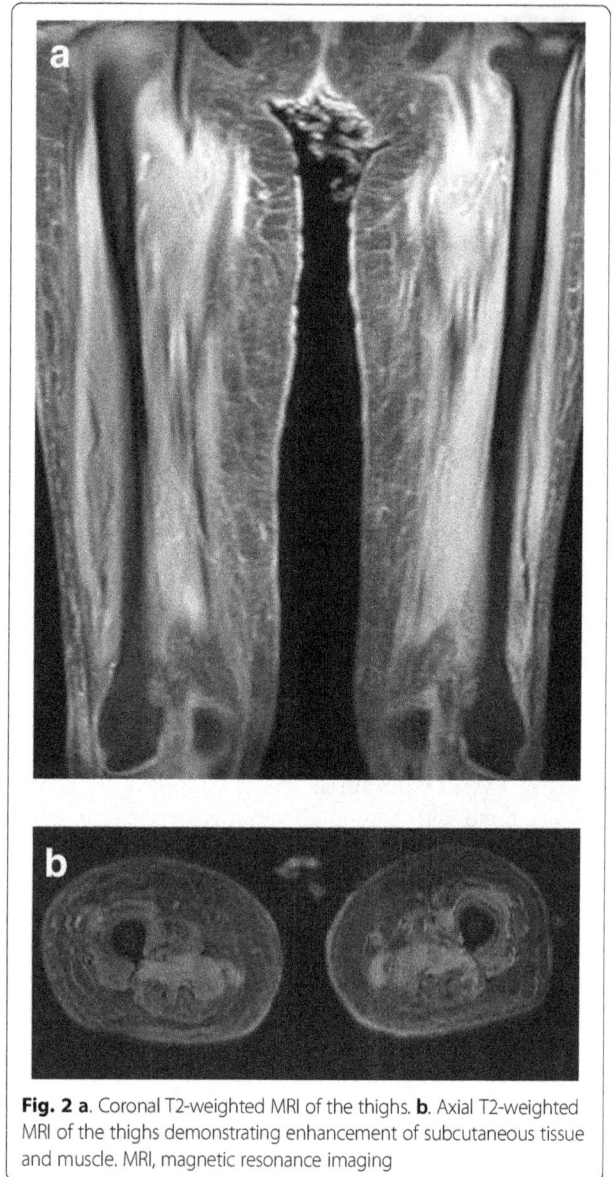

Fig. 2 a. Coronal T2-weighted MRI of the thighs. **b**. Axial T2-weighted MRI of the thighs demonstrating enhancement of subcutaneous tissue and muscle. MRI, magnetic resonance imaging

receptor antibody. Later on, she developed chest pain and shortness of breath. Computed tomography of the chest revealed bilateral pleural effusion and small pericardial effusion. Echocardiography revealed impaired left ventricular systolic function with 40% ejection fraction along with global hypokinesia. She was diagnosed with lupus myocarditis, and treated with a 5-day course of intravenous immunoglobulin (0.4 g/kg/day) and 5 mg/day intravenous dexamethasone. During her hospitalization for 21 days, she remained febrile with a maximum temperature of 38.5–39 °C, despite the previously mentioned therapy. At that time, she had worsening pain in both thighs at the site of the plaques. Magnetic resonance imaging of both lower extremities revealed diffuse enhancing, hyperintense T2 signals in the muscles at the pelvis at both thighs and legs, with diffuse muscle atrophy and swelling of the skin and subcutaneous tissue (Fig. 2a, b). Multiple subcutaneous biopsy specimens were taken from both thighs (site of skin lesions) showed suppurative panniculitis (Fig. 3) and presence of Gram-negative bacilli. Acid-fast and Gomori methenamine stains were negative. Tissue biopsies for aerobic microorganisms showed no growth. Bacterial broad-range 16S ribosomal RNA sequencings revealed *L. pneumophila* (99% similarity to *L. pneumophila* consensus sequence). Culture for fungi and mycobacteria was negative. Her antimicrobial regimen was changed to intravenous azithromycin, and fever subsided within 5 days. Her thigh lesions gradually improved over the first week of therapy (Fig. 4). She was diagnosed with disseminated *L. pneumophila* infection resulting in panniculitis, myositis and myocarditis. She received intravenous

azithromycin for 21 days. Oral azithromycin and ciprofloxacin were continued for 3 months to ensure eradication of the organism from our immunosuppressed patient. She received intravenous ganciclovir until the clearance of CMV viremia (total of 48 days), and then switched to oral valganciclovir maintenance therapy. She underwent physical rehabilitation and was discharged after 64 days hospitalization. Clinically, she is doing well at 1-year follow-up. She did not have any further tests done as follow-up proved successful clinical resolution and eradication of *Legionella* infection.

Discussion

Here, we describe a patient with SLE and myasthenia gravis who suffered multiple infectious complications including varicella, CMV syndrome/jejunitis and *Legionella*

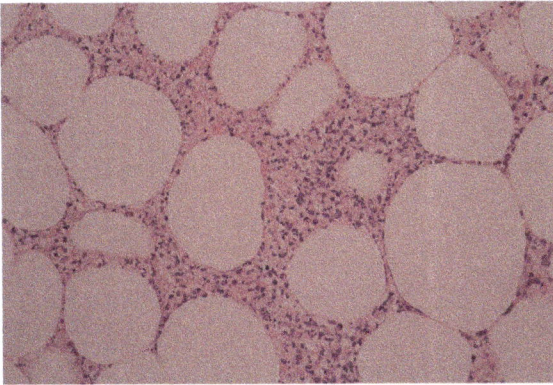

Fig. 3 Histopathology of subcutaneous tissue of right thigh. Photomicrograph revealed neutrophil infiltration in the deep dermis to subcutaneous tissue and fat necrosis (200×, hematoxylin and eosin)

panniculitis with possible dissemination (myositis and myocarditis). Panniculitis cause by *Legionella* has not been reported in the literature. Our initial presumptive diagnosis of panniculitis was lupus panniculitis or CMV related panniculitis. However, our patient did not improve during

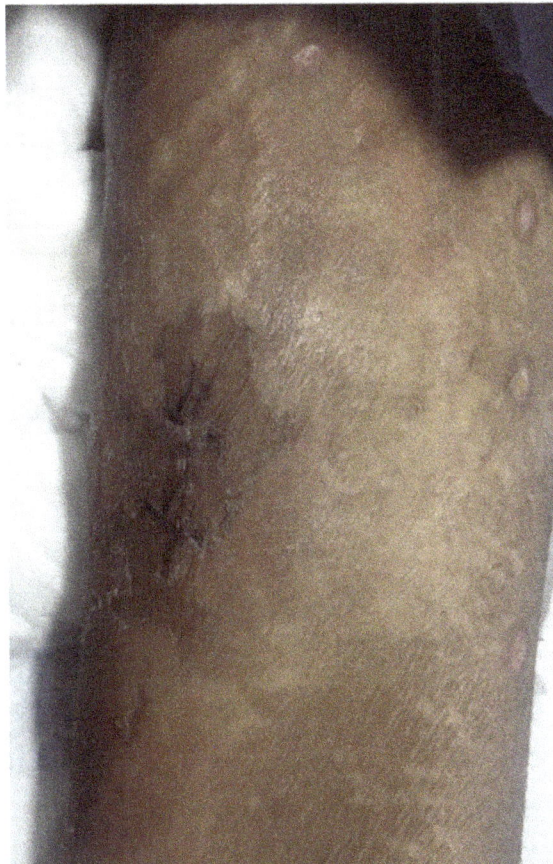

Fig. 4 Proximal right thigh showed resolution of indurated plaque after 8 days of treatment for *Legionella*, biopsy stiches, healed scar of varicella lesions, and whitish striae

the course of treatment for both diseases. The diagnosis of lupus panniculitis should not be assumed in SLE patients, given that immunosuppressive drugs are a predisposing factor for infective panniculitis, and both conditions require different treatment strategies [10]. Infective panniculitis has been described in association with many infectious agents including bacteria (*Nocardia* spp. and *Actinomyces* spp.), mycobacteria, fungi and parasites [11]. Anatomical pathology is the key to distinguishing the etiology of panniculitis by the type of white blood cell infiltrates. Lupus panniculitis presents with lymphocytic infiltrates with or without vasculitis. CMV panniculitis must have evidence of viral cytopathic changes with the characteristic owl's eye inclusion bodies. Our patient had neutrophilic panniculitis that suggested infective panniculitis. Gram staining showed intracellular Gram-negative bacilli that failed to grow on routine culture media, and they were identified as *L. pneumophila* by molecular methods. It was difficult to distinguish whether the panniculitis resulted from primary inoculation or secondary hematogenous spread of *Legionella*. Several features, such as prolonged fever despite broad-spectrum beta-lactam antibiotics, myositis and myocarditis, suggested disseminated *Legionella* infection. Myositis has been reported in one patient with pneumonia [12]. The etiology of myocarditis in our patient remains debatable, and whether it resulted from lupus or *Legionella* infection. Myocardial biopsy was not performed because of the excessive risk in our case, and therapy for both lupus and *Legionella* was initiated at the same time. Follow-up echocardiography showed normal cardiac function. *Legionella* myocarditis has been reported as a complication of Legionnaires' disease [13, 14]. Only one adult patient developed perimyocarditis due to *L. pneumophila* in the absence of respiratory involvement, which resulted in multiorgan failure [1]. The atypical multiorgan involvement of *Legionella* infection in our patient could have resulted from immunosuppression that led to lymphopenia and cell-mediated immunodeficiency. Our patient did not have evidence of pneumonia at any time point before or during hospitalization.

Cutaneous and subcutaneous *Legionella* infection is rare and mostly occurs in immunosuppressed patients, as described previously [5]. Primary extrapulmonary infection of skin/subcutaneous tissue (cellulitis, multiple subcutaneous abscesses, and tenosynovitis) by *L. pneumophila* led to disseminated infection (pneumonia and respiratory failure) in an immunocompromised liver transplant recipient [15]. The diagnosis was made from culture of bronchoalveolar lavage fluid and later, *Legionella* was isolated from the abscesses using special culture media and was confirmed by molecular methods [15]. This highlights the challenging aspect in the diagnosis of *Legionella* infection, as it is a facultative Gram-negative aerobic bacillus that resides within tissue and alveolar macrophages, and it requires specialized media [16]. Non-culture-based diagnostic methods include urinary antigen tests for *L. pneumophila*, which is a rapid diagnostic tool; however, these tests are limited to the detection of *L. pneumophila* serogroup 1, *L. micdadei* and *Legionella longbeachae* [17].

The diagnosis of extrapulmonary *Legionella* infection relies on clinician alertness and a good level of cooperation with the microbiology laboratory, as *Legionella* species must be grown on special media. In our setting we did not have the selective media, *Legionella* urinary antigen and antibody to detect *Legionella*, or direct fluorescent antibody against *Legionella*. The diagnosis in our patient was made by 16S rRNA gene sequencing method. Initiation of appropriate treatment is critical because delay is associated with increased mortality in *Legionella* pneumonia [18]. Effective antimicrobial treatment of legionellosis includes antibiotics that achieve therapeutic intracellular concentrations within macrophages, such as the macrolides, fluoroquinolones, and cyclin families [16]. Azithromycin or levofloxacin are commonly used to treat *Legionella* infection [16, 19]. Optimal treatment duration for cutaneous legionellosis has not been established. Most patients with *Legionella* pneumonia are successfully treated with a 7-to 14-day course of antibiotics. Disseminated legionellosis requires longer duration of therapy, although the duration is not well defined. Immunocompromised patients with cutaneous legionellosis may require 3 weeks of treatment [5, 16].

Conclusion

Legionella infection may cause extrapulmonary manifestations involving skin/subcutaneous and muscle that leads to dissemination, especially in immunocompromised patients. Infective panniculitis caused by *Legionella* should be considered in the differential diagnosis of skin/subcutaneous infection that fails to respond to beta-lactam antibiotics. The diagnosis of extrapulmonary *Legionella* infection is challenging because special culture media are required. In our case, the diagnosis was based on 16S rRNA gene sequencing method. Clinicians should be aware of extrapulmonary manifestation of legionellosis in the absence of pneumonia.

Abbreviations
PCR: Polymerase chain reaction; rRNA: ribosomal ribonucleic acid

Acknowledgements
We are grateful to Siriorn Watcharananan MD for helpful comment, Parawee Chevaisarakul MD for clinical management, Patawee Boontanon MD for providing the picture, Apichart Sudatis MD for data collection, Teerawut Sirikum MD for performing tissue biopsy, and Suthep Jirasuthat MD who gave an opinion on the pathological report. We thank Cathel Kerr, PhD, from Edanz Group (www.edanzediting.com/ac) for editing a draft of this manuscript.

Authors' contributions
MNC drafted the manuscript. MNC and NR and were responsible for the clinical management and therapy. YV performed the histological examination of the tissue biopsy. All authors read and approved the final manuscript.

Consent for publication
The patient gave written consent for publication of her potentially identifying information (including individual details and images).

Competing interests
The authors declare that they have no competing interests.

Author details
[1]Division of Infectious Disease, Department of Medicine, Faculty of Medicine, Ramathibodi Hospital, Mahidol University, 270 Rama VI Road, Ratchathewi District, Bangkok 10400, Thailand. [2]Division of Dermatology, Faculty of Medicine Ramathibodi Hospital, Mahidol University, Bangkok, Thailand. [3]Department of Pathology, Faculty of Medicine Ramathibodi Hospital, Mahidol University, 270 Rama VI Road, Ratchathewi District, Bangkok, Thailand.

References
1. Burke PT, Thabolingam R, Saba S. Suspected *Legionella*-induced Perimyocarditis in an adult in the absence of pneumonia: a rare clinical entity. Tex Heart Inst J. 2009;36(6):601–3.
2. Ishimaru NS, Tokuda Y, Takano T. Severe legionnaires' disease with pneumonia and biopsy-confirmed myocarditis Most likely caused by *Legionella pneumophila* Serogroup 6. Intern Med. 2012;51:3207–12.
3. Bodur H, Savran Y, Koca U, Kilinc O, Albayrak S, Itil O, Akoglu S. *Legionella* pneumonia with acute respiratory distress syndrome, myocarditis and septic shock successfully treated with Drotrecogin alpha (activated). Eur J Anaesthesiol. 2006;23(9):808–10.
4. Sommer JB, Erbguth FJ, Neundorfer B. Acute disseminated encephalomyelitis following *Legionella pneumophila* infection. Eur Neurol. 2000;44(3):182–4.
5. Padrnos LJ, Kusne S, DiCaudo DJ, Mikhael JR. Cutaneous legionellosis: case report and review of the medical literature. Transpl Infect Dis. 2014;16:307–14.
6. Han JH, Harada S, Baddour LM, Edelstein PH, et al. Relapsing *Legionella pneumophila* cellulitis: a case report and review of the literature. J Infect Chemother. 2010;16(6):439–42.
7. Brabender W, Hinthorn DR, Asher M, Lindsey NJ, Liu C. *Legionella pneumophila* wound infection. JAMA. 1983;250(22):3091–2.
8. Kilborn JA, Manz LA, O'Brien M, Douglass MC, Horst HM, Kupin W, Fisher EJ. Necrotizing cellulitis caused by *Legionella micdadei*. Am J Med. 1992;92(1):104_6.
9. Loridant S, Lagier JC, La Scola B. Identification of *Legionella feeleii* cellulitis. Emer Infect Dis. 2011;17(1):145–6.
10. Chan MP. Neutrophilic panniculitis: algorithmic approach to a heterogeneous group of disorders. Arch Pathol Lab Med. 2014;138(10):1337–43.
11. Morrison LK, Rapini R, Willison CB, Tyring S. Infection and panniculitis. Dermatol Ther. 2010;23(4):328–40.
12. Warner CL, Fayad PB, Heffner RR Jr. *Legionella* myositis. Neurology. 1991; 41(5):750–2.
13. Gowani SA, Kumar A, Arora S, Lahiri B. *Legionella pneumonia* complicated by myocarditis and torsades de pointes: a case report and review of literature. Conn Med. 2013;77(6):331–4.
14. Briceno DF, Fernando RR, Nathan S, Loyalka P, Kar B, Gregoric ID. TandemHeart as a bridge to recovery in *Legionella* myocarditis. Tex Heart Inst J. 2015;42(4):357–61.
15. Valve K, Vaalasti A, Anttila VJ, Vuento R. Disseminated *Legionella pneumophila* infection in an immunocompromised patient treated with tigecycline. Scand J Infect Dis. 2010;42(2):152 5.

16. Phin N, Parry-Ford F, Harrison T, Stagg HR, Zhang N, Kumar K, Lortholary O, Zumla A, Abubakar I. Epidemiology and clinical management of legionnaires' disease. Lancet Infect Dis. 2014;14:1011–21.

17. Pierre DM, Baron J, Yu VL, Stout JE. Diagnostic testing for legionnaires' disease. Ann Clin Microbiol Antimicrob. 2017;16:59.

18. Heath CH, Grove DI, Looke DF. Delay in appropriate therapy of *Legionella pneumonia* associated with increased mortality. Eur J Clin Microbiol Infect Dis. 1996;15(4):286–90.

19. Pedro-Botet ML, Yu VL. Treatment strategies for *Legionella* infection. Expert Opin Pharmacother. 2009;10(7):1109–21.

24

Two confirmed cases of severe fever with thrombocytopenia syndrome with pneumonia: implication for a family cluster in East China

Yiyi Zhu[1†], Huanyu Wu[1†], Jie Gao[2], Xin Zhou[1], Renyi Zhu[1], Chunzhe Zhang[1], Hongling Bai[1], Abu S. Abdullah[3,4,5] and Hao Pan[1*]

Abstract

Background: Severe fever with thrombocytopenia syndrome (SFTS) was first reported in China in 2011. Human-to-human transmission of the virus occurred occasionally in family clusters. However, pneumonia as an onset syndrome was not common in most SFTS cases. Our aim is to report a family cluster of SFTS with clinical manifestation of pneumonia in Shanghai.

Methods: Epidemiologic investigations were conducted when a family cluster of severe fever with thrombocytopenia syndrome virus (SFTSV) infection was identified in Shanghai in June 2016. Samples were collected from two secondary cases and two close contacts with fever. SFTSV was detected by Real-Time reverse transcription polymerase chain reaction (RT-PCR).

Results: There were two confirmed STFS cases and one potential index case. The potential index case became ill on 21 May and died on 31 May. Case A had onset from 4 to 23 June and case B from 8 June to 25 June. All the three cases experienced pneumonia at the early stage of SFTSV infection. Three (3) out of thirty two (32) close contacts had symptoms of fever or cough but were detected STFSV negative by real-time RT-PCR. According to epidemiologic investigations, the potential index case had outdoor activities on a nearby hill. A tick bite could have been the reason for the SFTSV infection in the potential index case as ticks were found both in grassland or shrubs on the hill and also found on mice caught in her house. Both cases A and B had provided bedside care for the potential index case without any protection and had contacted with blood and other body fluids.

Conclusion: It was a family cluster of SFTSV infection imported from Jiangsu province located in the east of China. We suggested to become alert to atypical SFTSV infected cases.

Keywords: Severe fever with thrombocytopenia syndrome, New bunyavirus, Human-to-human transmission, Family cluster

Background

An emerging infectious disease, severe fever with thrombocytopenia syndrome (SFTS) was first reported in China in 2011 [1]. A pathogen causing SFTS was simultaneously identified as a novel Bunyavirus, designated SFTSV. Till now, increasing number of new cases have also been reported in Japan, Korea. In Japan, 163 patients with SFTS were confirmed from the autumn of 2012 and October 2015 [2]. Most cases occurred in the western part of Japan. The numbers of SFTS cases also increased annually from 36 (2013), 55 (2014) and 79 (2015) in the Republic of Korea [3]. 5,352 SFTS cases were reported in 23 provinces in China from 2011 to 2014. 99.3% cases were reported from Henan, Shandong, Hubei, Anhui, Liaonin, Zhejiang, and Jiangsu provinces [4]., SFTS cases in China significantly increased from 2013 to October 2016, 7419 cases with 355 deaths. Since 2014, over 1000 SFTS cases were

* Correspondence: panhao@scdc.sh.cn

†Equal contributors

[1]Shanghai Municipal Center for Disease Control and Prevention, Shanghai 200336, China

reported annually in Anhui, Henan, Hubei, and Shandong Provinces [5]. Zhejiang and Jiangsu provinces are both adjacent to Shanghai. A reported case of SFTS in Shanghai was imported from Anhui province, which was historically the only reported SFTS case in Shanghai [6].

Human-to-human transmission of the virus occurred occasionally in family clusters. Several family cluster cases were reported previously in China and Korea [7–12]. Contact with the index patient's blood was significantly associated with development of SFTS. In systematic studies SFTS case fatality rate (CFR) was 12–16% and major clinical features were fever, thrombocytopenia, leucopenia, gastrointestinal symptoms and central nervous system manifestations [13, 14].

We reported a family cluster from Suzhou, Jiangsu Province of China, which was confirmed in Shanghai. Three members of a family presented with high fever and pneumonia were admitted and two of them were detected to be SFTSV positive. Pneumonia was an atypical syndrome for SFTS cases. Epidemiological investigation, clinical syndromes and symptoms, and laboratory testing were described and more evidence of transmission mechanism were provided to further understand SFTS.

Methods
Epidemiological investigation
On June 13, three cases were reported to Shanghai Municipal Center for Disease Control and Prevention (SCDC) and were interviewed immediately by Shanghai local CDC staff. Basic demographic information, clinical manifestation, epidemiological history and timeline of the cluster were collected and analyzed. Exposure to outdoor activities referring to work, live or travel in the regions of hills, forests and mountains in main epidemic season 2 weeks before onset was inquired. Epidemiological investigations were also carried out to obtain information for close contacts, defined as anyone who had contacted with blood, fluid, bloody secretion or excretion of the SFTS patients without any protection. Fourteen-day medical observations among close contacts

were initiated on June 14 [15]. Environmental investigation was carried out immediately to identify ticks around the residential areas of cases. The tick specimens were collected by flagging white cloth on grasslands and also picking from animals' body surface.

Sample collection
The index patient died before the family cluster was identified and therefore there was no sample available for further testing. Two secondary patients and close contacts with fever symptoms during the first week of contact were sampled.

Laboratory analysis
Nucleic acid of SFTS was detected from serum specimens of case A (daughter of the potential index case), B (the son of the potential index case), C (granddaughter of the potential index case), as well as close contacts with fever and other symptoms (Tables 1 and 2). Real-Time Reverse Transcriptase Polymerase Chain Reaction (RT-PCR) [16] was adopted in testing SFTSV in serum. RNA was extracted from serum by Total Nucleic Acid Isolation kit (Roche Diagnostics) according to the manufacturer's instruction. SFTS viral segments were amplified by primers and probes (provided by China CDC). Real-time PCR was performed as follows: 50 °C for 30 min, 95 °C for 10 min. Then 40 cycles of amplification was undertaken: 95 °C for 15 s and 60 °C for 45 s. The cutoff cycle threshold (C_t) value for a positive sample was at 35 cycles. A C_t value less than 35 was judged as positive.

Results
Case A
Case A was a 47-year-old female. On June 4, 2016, she began to feel sick. Next day, she found herself with high fever of 39.9 °C, coughing, sore throat and malaise. She visited local hospitals A and B in Jiangsu Province. Then she was admitted by hospital B and treated with Ticarcillin/Clavulanate Potassium and levofloxacin. No sign of improvement was observed. Laboratory analysis of blood

Table 1 Potential index case and secondary cases in this family cluster of SFTSV

Case	Gender	Age	Relation with index case	Onset date	Onset symptoms	Blood routine testing (admitted)	Liver toxicity Testing (admitted)	Treatments	Real Time RT-PCR	Outcome
Potential index case	Female	73	-	2016/ 5/21	Fever, malaise	WBC1.83 × 10^9/L PLT38 × 10^9/L	ALT220.0 U/L AST805.4 U/L	Cefmetaz	Not available	Deceased
A	Female	47	Daughter	2016/ 6/4	Fever, cough, malaise	WBC2.29 × 10^9/L PLT97 × 10^9/L	ALT 67.0 U/L AST59.0 U/L	Ofloxacin, Methylprednisolone Sodium Succinate, Pantoprazole, Glutamine, Xiyanping	Positive	Cured
B	Male	53	Son	2016/ 6/8	Fever, malaise	WBC1.78 × 10^9/L PLT56 × 10^9/L	ALT 56.0 U/L AST122.0 U/L	Piperacillin, Methylprednisolone Sodium Succinate, Pantoprazole, Glutamine, Xiyanping	Positive	Cured

Table 2 Close contacts with fever and other symptoms in this family cluster of SFTSV

Case	Gender	Age	Relation with the potential index case	Onset date	Onset symptoms	Real time RTPCR detection	Outcome
C	Female	30	Granddaughter	2016/6/1	Fever, cough	Negative	Cured
D	Male	66	Brother-in-law	2016/6/8	Fever	Negative	Cured
E	Male	65	Funeral service	2016/6/9	Fever, malaise	Negative	Cured

revealed leukopenia (white blood cells count 2.29×10^9/L) and thrombocytopenia (platelets count 97×10^9/L). Occult blood (25 + cell/u) and albumin (80 mg/L) were found in urine routine testing. In biochemistry testing, lower total protein (61.5 g/l), pre-albumin (126 mg/l), and elevated blood sugar was detected. Antibiotics, Oseltamivir and Insulin were administrated to control infection and lower the blood sugar. On June 11, blood testing still showed leukopenia (white blood cells count 2.42×10^9/L) and thrombocytopenia (platelets count 68×10^9/L). Mycobacterium tuberculosis (TB), EB virus, Cox A16 virus, EV71 virus, *Chlamydia pneumoniae*, syncytial virus, adenovirus, influenza virus and para-influenza virus were all detected as negative. The case was then transferred to hospital B in Shanghai on the same day. Presenting with the symptoms of coughing and malaise and with chest computerized tomography (CT) of "Left lung patchy shadow, bilateral small amount of pleural effusion, increased width of the longitudinal diaphragm" (Fig. 1), case A was admitted in hospital C. Thrombocytopenia (platelets count 81×10^9/L) continued and white cell counts were normal. Rapid testing for influenza A was negative. Alanine aminotransferase (ALT) and aspartate aminotransferase (AST) were elevated as 67.0 U/L and 59.0 U/L respectively. Ofloxacin Capsules, Methylprednisolone Sodium Succinate, Pantoprazole, Glutamine and Xiyanping (antiviral herbal medicine) were prescribed. Case A's temperature got normal. Cough and muscle soreness were relieved after treatment.

Case B

Case B was case A's elder brother. He was a 53-year-old and became sick since June 8, 2016. Symptoms including fever (38.5 °C), malaise and low lumber soreness appeared early during his illness. He visited hospital B in Jiangsu province on June 9, 2016. He was treated with Reduning (Antiviral herbal medicine), Oseltamivir, Levofloxacin, Ticarcillin/ Clavulanate Potassium and Insulin aspart. Blood routine testing upon admission showed leukopenia (white blood cells count 2.29×10^9/L), erythropenia (red cell count 4.10×10^{12}/L), thrombocytopenia (platelets count 56×10^9/L), occult blood in fecal sample, elevated ALT (56.0 U/L) and AST (122.0 U/L), lowered total protein (59.4 g/L), lowered albumin (38.2 g/L), pre-albumin (163 mg/L), elevated lactate dehydrogenase (LDH) 240 U/L, and elevated blood sugar (12.84 mmol/L). X-ray detection showed increased bronchovascular shadows. He was also screened for other pathogens such as Mycobacterium TB, EB virus, Cox A16 virus, EV71 virus, *Chlamydia pneumoniae*, syncytial virus, adenovirus, influenza virus and para-influenza virus, but all tests were negative. Together with case A, he was transferred to hospital C in Shanghai and was admitted for viral pneumonia and type II diabetes. CT showed two nodular shadows in the left lung and pleural effusion in the right lung (Fig. 1). A Swab was collected and a test for Influenza A showed negative results. Blood routine testing still showed leukopenia (white blood cells count 3×10^9/L) and thrombocytopenia (platelets count 53×10^9/L). Blood gas analysis revealed lowered partial pressure of carbon dioxide (PCO$_2$) (4.2kpa) and total carbon dioxide (TCO$_2$) (22.3 mmol/L). Coagulopathy (activated partial thromboplastin time (APTT) 46.8 s) and elevated creatine phosphate kinase (260 IU/L) was also observed. Whole blood testing was done again on June 13. Leukopenia (white blood cells

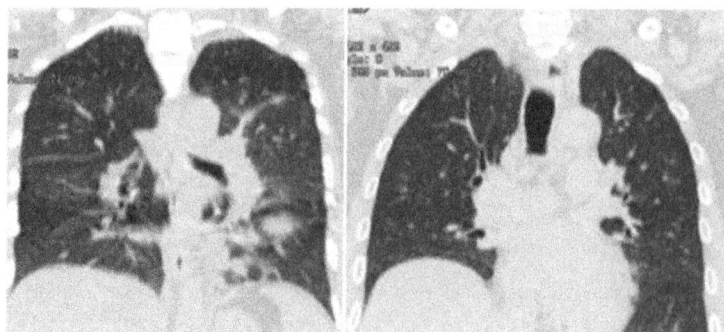

Fig. 1 Computed Tomographic Scans of the Chest of case A and case B

count 2.3×10^9/L) and thrombocytopenia (platelets count 28×10^9/L) had worsened.

Potential index case

The potential index case was a 72-year-old woman. She was the mother to cases A and B. Illness of potential index case began on May 21, 2016. She was sent to a local clinic by case A on the same day. Blood testing showed leukopenia (white blood cells count 3.83×10^9/L) and elevated blood sugar. She was treated for viral infection. On May 23, she had worse symptoms of fever (39 °C), bleeding gums, stomachache, diarrhea and malaise. Again, case A took her to a local community health center for treatment. Blood testing showed leucopenia (white blood cells count 2.38×10^9/L) and thrombocytopenia (platelets count 88×10^9/L). Dermal ecchymosis appeared on the index case's chest and upper lumber. On May 25, she felt nausea and vomited. She visited hospital D in Jiangsu province. Blood testing showed leukopenia (white blood cells count 1.83×10^9/L), thrombocytopenia (platelets count 32×10^9/L), elevated liver-associated enzyme levels (AST 805.4 U/L; ALT 220.0 U/L, coagulopathy (Prothrombin Time 13.7 s and APTT 64.1 s). Urine testing showed abnormal sugar (++), protein (++), occult blood (+++). Heteropathy was applied. However, she got worse and began convulsing. She died of multiple-organ failure on May 28. According to the guideline for prevention and treatment of SFTS [17], she was confirmed as a probable case of SFTS.

Epidemiological findings

The potential index patient was sick from May 21 and died on May 28. Case A took care of index patient during all the 8 days. Case B had visited index case on May

23 and 27. On May 27, both case A and B found bleeding from the mouth, nostrils, and ears of the potential index case. After the death of potential index case, case A and B had cleaned the body and directly touched the blood of the potential index case without any protection.

The potential index patient lived in a village near Tai Lake in Jiangsu Province, which is located to the southeast of China. The village is on a downhill, and she used to climb the hill every day as she had planted some vegetables on the hill. It is unclear whether the patient was bitten by ticks or not. However, investigation on the surroundings of the patient showed that ticks could be found in the village and in other places that the patient came into contact with on the hill. Both case A and case B had their own houses and denied history of tick bite or outdoor activities within 2 weeks before illness onset (Fig. 2).

Altogether, 19 ticks were caught through flagging from the hill and grassland. Eight rodents were caught on the hill, around the village or indoor around the residency of potential index case. Ticks could be found on the surface of rodents. Three out of ten dogs were found to be infected with ticks and tick index was 0.4.

Close contacts

A total of 32 close contacts including case C were identified in this family cluster. They were mostly relatives from the family. Three close contacts became ill. One was Case C, a 30-year-old female. She was daughter to case B and became ill on June 1, 2016 with the symptoms of coughing and a slight fever. She took some self-prescribed drugs but she could not remember the drug's name. On June 11, she accompanied her father (case B)

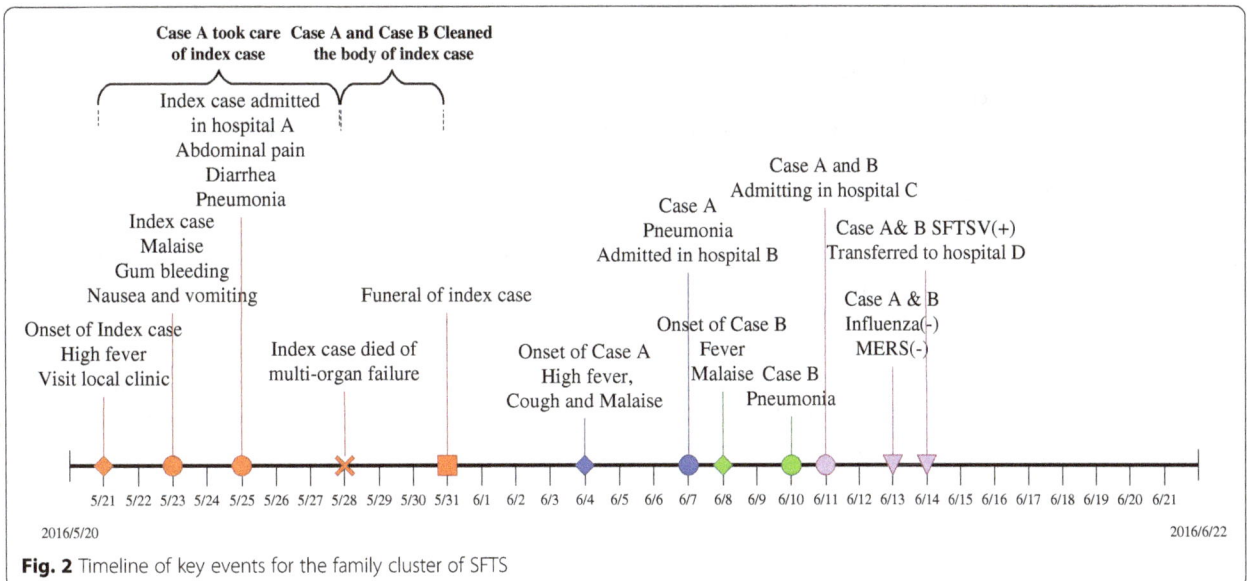

Fig. 2 Timeline of key events for the family cluster of SFTS

and her aunt (case A) to hospital C in Shanghai. She had a fever of 37.8 °C. Blood testing was normal at the time of admission. Rapid testing for influenza A was negative. She was admitted in hospital C and treated with antiviral medicine. She was discharged on June 14 when serum detection for SFTSV was negative. Another relative who became sick was the husband to potential index case's sister. He got fever on June 8, 2016 and recovered soon without any other symptoms. The third one who was an undertaker and had moved and cleaned the body of the potential index case. He had wiped the blood from the mouth of the potential index case. Other close contacts had no symptoms during the latent period after contact.

Laboratory testing

On June 13, serum samples were collected from case A and B. On June 14, C_t values of case A and B were 32 and 29 respectively in Real-Time PCR assay and both were positive to SFTSV. Sera of close contacts with fever or other symptoms were tested negative by Real Time RT-PCR including case C.

Discussion

We presented a family cluster of SFTSV imported from Jiangsu province herein. Three family members successively became ill. The potential index case died and two other proven SFTS cases developed a secondary infection following exposure to the potential index case. One secondary case had provided bedside care for potential index case and both the secondary cases had contact with blood from potential index case. As early as 2006, two clusters were suspected to be infected with a novel virus in Anhui province and patients from one cluster were confirmed to be SFTSV positive in 2012 [10]. Another family cluster was retrospectively identified in a hilly area about 110 km south of Nanjing in eastern China in 2007 [8]. In several family cluster reports of SFTSV in China and Korea, evidence of personal contact, especially blood contact was demonstrated [7–12, 18]. Most index patients reported in family cluster were infected through tick bites. Secondary patients in the family possibly became sick by contacting blood infected with SFTS. Genetic susceptibility was supposed to be one of the determinants for susceptibility of family members [19], which might explain why family members were more easily infected. However, person to person transmission was excluded in two family clusters reported in Zhejiang province [20]. In this family cluster, given the facts that two secondary cases had no history of tick bite or outdoor activities on the hill and case A and case B became sick 4 days and 7 days respectively, after the death of potential index case. Person to person transmission was suggested in this family cluster.

Lab-confirmed cases were reported in 16 provinces in China till 2014 [4]. More areas were verified as natural foci of SFTSV. Ticks could serve as a vector and reservoir of SFTSV and mice played a role in SFTSV transmission [21]. Ticks fed on SFTSV-infected mice could acquire the virus and transmit it to other developmental stages of ticks. SFTSV-infected ticks could transmit the virus to mice during feeding. SFTSV genomic RNAs were identified in *Apodemus agrarius* in Zhejiang province [22]. In this family cluster, the residence of index patient was located on a hilly area. Free ticks and mice were found in the surrounding environment and ticks were found feeding on mice. We inferred that SFTSV from ticks on the hill most likely caused the potential index case's infection though tick bite. However, more evidence will be needed to prove whether SFTSV was endemic in the region near Tai lake or not.

Secondary infection was person-to-person transmission. Two secondary cases had taken care of the potential index case and had close contact with the potential index case. First, two secondary cases had a history of coming into contact with potential index case's blood and handling or cleaning her corpse, which provided evidence of person-to-person transmission through blood contact. Second, in this family cluster, all three cases developed severe pneumonia at the early stage of infection, which was entirely different from most of other cases of SFTS. We proposed that aerosol person-to-person transmission probably existed in the family cluster. According to previous researches, typical clinical and laboratory manifestations of SFTS included fever, gastrointestinal symptoms, myalgia, chills, thrombocytopenia, and leukopenia [13, 14, 23, 24]. As a first group of serious symptoms, pneumonia was rarely observed in SFTSV infection. Confounded by influenza or avian influenza, it was difficult to be diagnosed. Atypical cases were easily ignored. However, researches had found that exposure to respiratory secretions led to nosocomial transmission of SFTSV among healthcare workers [25]. Positive results were detected in tracheal aspirate and gastric aspirate in an SFTS patient [26]. A cluster report in 2015 showed that SFTSV could be transmitted from person to person, by direct contact and/or aerosol transmission [27]. Our study gave more evidence for aerosol transmission in cluster. In addition, pneumonia may be an early onset symptom which should be explored in future research. One case of secondary-asymptomatic infection was found in a cluster in 2006 in Liaoning province and another asymptomatic case was reported in 2015 in Zhejiang province [28]. More integrated and sensitive clinical characters should be included in SFTS surveillance to identify possible SFTS cases.

Conclusion

A family cluster of SFTS was confirmed in Shanghai. Two family members were infected by SFTSV most possibly from one clinical SFTS case, who was potential index case for this family cluster. We should establish more surveillance system, within China and in the region, to identify more SFTS cases with atypical symptoms.

Abbreviations

ALT: Alanine aminotransferase; APTT: Activated partial thromboplastin time; AST: Aspartate aminotransferase; CT: Computerized tomography; pCO_2: Partial pressure of carbon dioxide; RT-PCR: Real-Time reverse transcription polymerase chain reaction; SFTS: Severe fever with thrombocytopenia syndrome; SFTSV: Severe fever with thrombocytopenia syndrome virus; TB: Tuberculosis; TCO_2: Total carbon dioxide

Acknowledgements

The authors thanks for Shanghai Huadong Hospital with data and sample collection and for Shanghai Jingan District Center for Disease Control and Prevention and Jiangsu Suzhou Center for Disease Control and Prevention for assistance in epidemiological investigation.

Funding

The study was sponsored by the 4th Round of Three-Year Public Health Action Plan of Shanghai, China (No. 15GWZK0101) and the 4th round of 3 years action plan on public health of Shanghai for overseas training plan for high-end talents (No. GWTD2015S02).

Authors' contributions

YYZ: epidemiological investigation, data collection, data analysis/interpretation, drafting of article, approval of article. HYW: concept/design, data collection, approval of article. JG: epidemiological investigation, data collection, approval of article. XZ: Laboratory detection, data analysis and interpretation, approval of article. RYZ: epidemiological investigation, data collection, approval of article. CZZ: epidemiological investigation, data collection, approval of article. HLB: epidemiological investigation, data collection, approval of article. ASA: critical revision of article, approval of article. HP: concept/design, data analysis/ interpretation, drafting article, critical revision of article, approval of article. All authors read and approved the final manuscript.

Consent for publication

Written informed consent was obtained from the patients for publication and any accompanying images.

Competing interests

The authors declare that they have no competing interests.

Author details

¹Shanghai Municipal Center for Disease Control and Prevention, Shanghai 200336, China. ²Shanghai Jingan Center for Disease Control and Prevention, Shanghai 200072, China. ³Global Health Program, Duke Kunshan University, Kunshan, Jiangsu Province 215347, China. ⁴Duke Global Health Institute, Duke University, Durham, NC 27710, USA. ⁵Department of General Internal Medicine, School of Medicine, Boston University Medical Center, Boston, MA 02118, USA.

References

1. Yu X, Liang M, Zhang S, Liu Y, Li J, Sun Y, et al. Fever with thrombocytopenia associated with a novel bunyavirus in China. The New Engl J of Med. 2011;364: 1523–32.
2. Tabara K, Fujita H, Hirata A, Hayasaka D. Investigation of Severe Fever with Thrombocytopenia Syndrome Virus Antibody among Domestic Bovines Transported to Slaughterhouse in Shimane Prefecture. Japan Jpn J Infect Dis. 2016;69(5):445–7.
3. Hwang J, Kang JG, Oh SS, Chae JB, Cho YK, Cho YS, Lee H, Chae JS. Molecular detection of severe fever with thrombocytopenia syndrome virus (SFTSV) in feral cats from Seoul. Korea Ticks Tick Borne Dis. 2017;8(1):9–12.
4. Li Y, Zhou H, Mu D, Yin W, Yu H. Epidemiological analysis on severe fever with thrombocytopenia syndrome under the national surveillance data from 2011 to 2014, China. Zhonghua liu xing bing xue za zhi. Zhonghua liuxingbingxue zazhi. 2015;36:598–602.
5. Zhan J, Wang Q, Cheng J, Hu B, Li J, Zhan F, Song Y, Guo D. Current status of severe fever with thrombocytopenia syndrome in China. Virol Sin. 2017; 32(1):51–62.
6. Pan H, Hu J, Liu S, Shen H, Zhu Y, Wu J, Zhang X, Zhou X, Wang C, Qu J, et al. A reported death case of a novel bunyavirus in Shanghai. China Virol J. 2013;10:187.
7. Tang X, Wu W, Wang H, Du Y, Liu L, Kang K, et al. Human-to-human transmission of severe fever with thrombocytopenia syndrome bunyavirus through contact with infectious blood. J Infect Dis. 2013;207:736–9.
8. Bao CJ, Guo XL, Qi X, Hu JL, Zhou MH, Varma JK, et al. A family cluster of infections by a newly recognized bunyavirus in eastern China, 2007: further evidence of person-to-person transmission. Clin Infect Dis. 2011;53(12):1208–14.
9. Wang Y, Deng B, Zhang J, Cui W, Yao W, Liu P. Person-to-person asymptomatic infection of severe fever with thrombocytopenia syndrome virus through blood contact. Intern Med. 2014;53(8):903–6.
10. Liu Y, Li Q, Hu W, Wu J, Wang Y, Mei L, et al. Person-to-person transmission of severe fever with thrombocytopenia syndrome virus. Vector Borne Zoonotic Dis. 2012;12(2):156–60.
11. Chen H, Hu K, Zou J, Xiao J. A cluster of cases of human-to-human transmission caused by severe fever with thrombocytopenia syndrome bunyavirus. Int J of Infect Dis. 2013;17(3):e206–8.
12. Yoo JR, Heo ST, Park D, Kim H, Fukuma A, Fukushi S, et al. Family Cluster Analysis of Severe Fever with Thrombocytopenia Syndrome Virus Infection in Korea. Am J Trop Med Hyg. 2016;95(6):1351–7.
13. Guo CT, Lu QB, Ding SJ, Hu CY, Hu JG, Wo Y, et al. Epidemiological and clinical characteristics of severe fever with thrombocytopenia syndrome (SFTS) in China: an integrated data analysis. Epidemiol Infect. 2016;144(6):1345–54.
14. Liu MM, Lei XY, Yu XJ. Meta-analysis of the clinical and laboratory parameters of SFTS patients in China. Virol J. 2016;13(1):198.
15. Ministry of Health, PRC. The key points of prevention and control of fever with thrombocytopenia syndrome by contact transmission. 2011. Available at: http://www.nhfpc.gov.cn/jkj/s3577/201108/90bfdcb5480c435b825d42c475be83fe.shtml. Accessed on: 29 Apr 2017.
16. Sun Y, Liang M, Qu J, Jin C, Zhang Q, Li J, et al. Early diagnosis of novel SFTS bunyavirus infection by quantitative real-time RT-PCR assay. J Clin Virol. 2012;53(1):48–53.
17. Ministry of Health, PRC. Guideline for prevention and treatment of severe fever with thrombocytopenia syndrome (2010 version). 2010. Available at: http://www.moh.gov.cn/mohwsyjbgs/s8348/201010/49272.shtml. Accessed on: 29 Apr 2017.
18. Gai Z, Liang M, Zhang Y, Zhang S, Jin C, Wang SW, et al. Person-to-person transmission of severe fever with thrombocytopenia syndrome bunyavirus through blood contact. Clin Infect Dis. 2012;54(2):249–52.
19. Sun J, Tang Y, Ling F, Chang Y, Ye X, Shi W, et al. Genetic susceptibility is one of the determinants for severe fever with thrombocytopenia syndrome virus infection and fatal outcome: An epidemiological investigation. PLoS One. 2015;10(7):e0132968.
20. Sun J, Chai C, Lv H, Lin J, Wang C, Chen E, et al. Epidemiological characteristics of severe fever with thrombocytopenia syndrome in Zhejiang Province. China Int J of Infect Dis. 2014;25(12):180–5.
21. Luo LM, Zhao L, Wen HL, Zhang ZT, Liu JW, Fang LZ, et al. Haemaphysalis longicornis ticks as reservoir and vector of severe fever with thrombocytopenia syndrome virus in China. Emerg Infect Dis. 2015;21:1770–6.
22. Ni H, Yang F, Li Y, Liu W, Jiao S, Li Z, et al. Apodemus agrarius is a potential natural host of severe fever with thrombocytopenia syndrome (SFTS)-causing novel bunyavirus. J Clin Virol. 2015;71:82–4.
23. Weng Y, Chen N, Han Y, Xing Y, Li J. Clinical and laboratory characteristics of severe fever with thrombocytopenia syndrome in Chinese patients. Braz J Infect Dis. 2014;18(1):88–91.
24. Wen HL, Zhao L, Zhai S, Chi Y, Cui F, Wang D, et al. Severe fever with thrombocytopenia syndrome, Shandong Province, China, 2011. Emerg Infect Dis. 2014;20:1 5.

25. Kim WY, Choi W, Park SW, Wang EB, Lee WJ, Jee Y, et al. Nosocomial transmission of severe fever with thrombocytopenia syndrome in Korea. Clin Infect Dis. 2015;60:1681–3.
26. Jeong EJ, Song JY, Lim CS, Lee I, Park MS, Choi MJ, et al. Viral shedding from diverse body fluids in a patient with severe fever with thrombocytopenia syndrome. J Clin Virol. 2016;80:33–5.
27. Gong Z, Gu S, Zhang Y, Sun J, Wu X, Ling F, et al. Probable aerosol transmission of severe fever with thrombocytopenia syndrome virus in southeastern China. Clin Microbiol and Infect. 2015;21:1115–20.
28. Ye L, Shang X, Wang Z, Hu F, Wang X, Xiao Y, et al. A case of severe fever with thrombocytopenia syndrome caused by a novel bunyavirus in Zhejiang. China Int J Infect Dis. 2015;33:199–201.

Permissions

List of Contributors

Cornelis H. van Werkhoven and Marie-Josee J. Mangen
Julius Center for Health Sciences and Primary Care, University Medical Center Utrecht, Utrecht, The Netherlands

Jan Jelrik Oosterheert
Department of Internal Medicine and Infectious Diseases, University Medical Center Utrecht, Heidelberglaan 100, 3584 CX Utrecht, The Netherlands

Douwe F. Postma
Julius Center for Health Sciences and Primary Care, University Medical Center Utrecht, Utrecht, The Netherlands
Department of Internal Medicine and Infectious Diseases, University Medical Center Utrecht, Heidelberglaan 100, 3584 CX Utrecht, The Netherlands
Department of Internal Medicine, Diakonessenhuis Utrecht, Utrecht, The Netherlands

Marc J. M. Bonten
Julius Center for Health Sciences and Primary Care, University Medical Center Utrecht, Utrecht, The Netherlands
Department of Medical Microbiology, University Medical Center Utrecht, Utrecht, The Netherlands

Yu jun Li
The First Affiliated Hospital of Jinan University, the West of Huangpu Street, Guangzhou, China
Department of Respiratory Medicine, Guangzhou First People's Hospital, Guangzhou Medical University, Panfu Road, Guangzhou, China

Zhu xiang Zhao and Zi wen Zhao
Department of Respiratory Medicine, Guangzhou First People's Hospital, Guangzhou Medical University, Panfu Road, Guangzhou, China

Chu zhi Pan
Department of Hepatobiliary Surgery, the Third Affiliated Hospital of Sun Yat-sen University, Tian He Road, Guangzhou, China

Chang quan Fang
Department of Respiratory Medicine, Guangzhou Red Cross Hospital, Tong Fu Zhong Road, Guangzhou, China

Hui ling Chen
Department of Clinic Laboratory, Guangzhou First People's Hospital, Guangzhou Medical University, Panfu Road, Guangzhou, China

Peng hao Guo
Department of Clinic Laboratory, the First Affiliated Hospital of Sun Yat-sen University, Zhong Shan Er Road, Guangzhou, China

Chengyi Ding, Jing Wang, Aoming Jin, Weiwei Wang, Ru Chen and Siyan Zhan
Department of Epidemiology and Biostatistics, School of Public Health, Peking University, 38 Xueyuan Road, Haidian District, Beijing 100191, People's Republic of China

Yuelun Zhang
Division of Epidemiology, The Jockey Club School of Public Health and Primary Care, The Chinese University of Hong Kong, Hong Kong, People's Republic of China

Zhirong Yang
Primary Care Unit, Department of Public Health and Primary Care, University of Cambridge, Cambridgeshire, UK

Le Wang, Zhishan Feng, Mengchuan Zhao, Shuo Yang, Xiaotong Yan, Weiwei Guo and Zhongren Shi
Institute of Pediatric Research, Children's Hospital of Hebei Province, 133 Zhonghua South Street, Shijiazhuang, Hebei Province 050031, China

Guixia Li
Institute of Pediatric Research, Children's Hospital of Hebei Province, 133 Zhonghua South Street, Shijiazhuang, Hebei Province 050031, China
Department of Laboratory Medicine, Children's Hospital of Hebei Province, Shijiazhuang 050031, China

Ching-Fen Shen
Department of Pediatrics, National Cheng Kung University Hospital, College of Medicine, National Cheng Kung University, 138, Sheng Li Road, North Dist., Tainan 70403, Taiwan

Tzong-Shiann Ho
Department of Emergency Medicine, National Cheng Kung University Hospital, College of Medicine, National Cheng Kung University, Tainan, Taiwan

Shih-Min Wang
Department of Emergency Medicine, National Cheng Kung University Hospital, College of Medicine, National Cheng Kung University, Tainan, Taiwan
Center of Infectious Disease and Signaling Research, National Cheng Kung University Hospital, College of Medicine, National Cheng Kung University, Tainan, Taiwan

Ching-Chuan Liu
Department of Pediatrics, National Cheng Kung University Hospital, College of Medicine, National Cheng Kung University, 138, Sheng Li Road, North Dist., Tainan 70403, Taiwan
Center of Infectious Disease and Signaling Research, National Cheng Kung University Hospital, College of Medicine, National Cheng Kung University, Tainan, Taiwan
Center for Infection Control, National Cheng Kung University Hospital, College of Medicine, National Cheng Kung University, Tainan, Taiwan

Nobuhiro Asai, Naoya Nishiyama, Yusuke Koizumi, Daisuke Sakanashi, Hideo Kato, Mao Hagihara, Hiroyuki Suematsu, Yuka Yamagishi and Hiroshige Mikamo
Department of Clinical Infectious Diseases, Aichi Medical University School of Medicine, 〒480-1195 1-1 Yazakokarimata, Nagakute, Aichi, Japan

Toyoharu Yokoi
Department of Pathology, Nagoya Ekisaikai Hospital, Nagoya, Aichi, Japan

Romaric Larcher and Erik Arnaud
Department of Internal Medicine, Caremeau University Hospital, 29 place du Professeur Debre, Nimes, France

Alix Pantel and Jean-Philippe Lavigne
Department of Microbiology, Caremeau University Hospital, 29 place du Professeur Debre, Nimes, France

Albert Sotto
Department of Infectious Diseases, Caremeau University Hospital, 29 place du Professeur Debre, Nimes, France

Marta Inês Cazentini Medeiros
Regional Laboratory Center of Instituto Adolfo Lutz - Ribeirão Preto and student at College of Nursing at University of São Paulo - Ribeirão Preto, São Paulo, Brazil

Samanta Cristine Grassi Almeida and Maria Luiza Leopoldo Silva Guerra
Bacteriologic Center of Instituto Adolfo Lutz Central–São Paulo, São Paulo, Brazil

Paulo da Silva and Ana Maria Machado Carneiro
Regional Laboratory Center of Instituto Adolfo Lutz - Ribeirão Preto, São Paulo, Brazil

Denise de Andrade
Ribeirão Preto College of Nursing at University of São Paulo - Ribeirão Preto, São Paulo, Brazil

Khalid Eljaaly, Samah Alshehri and Ahmed Aljabri
Department of Clinical Pharmacy, King Abdulaziz University, Jeddah Postal code 21589, Saudi Arabia
College of Pharmacy, University of Arizona, Drachman Hall – B306, 1295 N Martin Ave, Tucson, AZ, USA

Ivo Abraham
College of Pharmacy, University of Arizona, Drachman Hall – B306, 1295 N Martin Ave, Tucson, AZ, USA

David E. Nix
College of Pharmacy, University of Arizona, Drachman Hall – B306, 1295 N Martin Ave, Tucson, AZ, USA
Division of Infectious Diseases, Department of Medicine, University of Arizona, Tucson, AZ, USA

Mayar Al Mohajer
Division of Infectious Diseases, Department of Medicine, University of Arizona, Tucson, AZ, USA

Andre C. Kalil
Department of Internal Medicine, Division of Infectious Diseases, University of Nebraska Medical Center, Omaha, NE, USA

Claudia Fernanda de Lacerda Vidal
Tropical Medicine Health Sciences Center, Committee on Infection Control of Hospital das Clinicas, Universidade Federal de Pernambuco, Av. Professor Moraes Rego, 1235 Hospital das Clínicas - Cidade Universitária, Recife, Pernambuco 50670-901, Brazil

Aurora Karla de Lacerda Vidal
Department of Pathology, Institute of Biological Sciences, Universidade de Pernambuco, Hospital de Câncer de Pernambuco, Real Hospital Português de Beneficência em Pernambuco, Recife, Pernambuco, Brazil

José Gildo de Moura Monteiro Jr.
Cardiac Intensive Care Unit, Pronto-Socorro Cardiológico de Pernambuco, Universidade de Pernambuco, Recife, Pernambuco, Brazil

Aracele Cavalcanti
Committee on Infection Control, Pronto-Socorro Cardiológico de Pernambuco, Universidade de Pernambuco, Recife, Pernambuco, Brazil

Ana Paula da Costa Henriques
Committee on Infection Control, Real Hospital Português de Beneficência em Pernambuco, Recife, Pernambuco, Brazil

Márcia Oliveira
Intensive Care Unit, Hospital Agamenon Magalhães, Secretaria de Saúde de Pernambuco, Recife, Pernambuco, Brazil

Michele Godoy, Mirella Coutinho, Pollyanna Dutra Sobral, Claudia Ângela Vilela and Bárbara Gomes
Intensive Care Unit, Hospital das Clínicas, Universidade Federal de Pernambuco, Recife, Pernambuco, Brazil

Marta Amorim Leandro
Committee on Infection Control of Hospital das Clinicas, Universidade Federal de Pernambuco, Recife, Pernambuco, Brazil

Ulisses Montarroyos
Institute of Biological Sciences, Universidade de Pernambuco, Recife, Pernambuco, Brazil

Ricardo de Alencar Ximenes
Faculty of Medical Sciences, Tropical Medicine Health Sciences Center, Universidade Federal de Pernambuco, Recife, Pernambuco, Brazil

Heloísa Ramos Lacerda
Department of Infectious and Parasitic Diseases, Faculty of Medical Sciences, Tropical Medicine Health Sciences Center, Universidade Federal de Pernambuco, Recife, Pernambuco, Brazil

Jae-Uk Song
Division of Pulmonary and Critical Care Medicine, Department of Internal Medicine, Kangbuk Samsung Hospital, Sungkyunkwan University School of Medicine, Seoul, South Korea

Hye Kyeong Park and Hyung Koo Kang
Division of Pulmonary and Critical Care Medicine, Department of Internal Medicine, Ilsan Paik Hospital, Inje University College of Medicine, Goyang-si, South Korea

Jonghoo Lee
Department of Internal Medicine, Jeju National University Hospital, Jeju National University School of Medicine, Aran 13 gil 15, Jeju-si, Jeju Special Self-Governing Province 690-767, South Korea

In Ae Yoon, Ki Bae Hong and Ji Young Park
Department of Pediatrics, Seoul National University Children's Hospital, Seoul, South Korea

Hoan Jong Lee, Ki Wook Yun and Eun Hwa Choi
Department of Pediatrics, Seoul National University Children's Hospital, Seoul, South Korea
Department of Pediatrics, Seoul National University College of Medicine, Seoul, South Korea

Young Hoon Choi and Woo Sun Kim
Department of Radiology, Seoul National University Hospital, Seoul, South Korea

Hyunju Lee
Department of Pediatrics, Seoul National University College of Medicine, Seoul, South Korea
Department of Pediatrics, Seoul National University Bundang Hospital, Seongnam, South Korea

Byung Wook Eun and Young Min Ahn
Department of Pediatrics, Eulji Hospital, Seoul, South Korea

Eun Young Cho
Department of Pediatrics, Chungnam National University Hospital, Daejeon, South Korea

Hwa Jin Cho
Department of Pediatrics, Chonnam National University Hospital, Gwangju, South Korea

Marie-Josée J. Mangen and G. Ardine de Wit
Julius Center for Health Sciences and Primary Care, University Medical Center Utrecht, Heidelberglaan 100, 3584 CX Utrecht, The Netherlands

Susanne M. Huijts
Julius Center for Health Sciences and Primary Care, University Medical Center Utrecht, Heidelberglaan 100, 3584 CX Utrecht, The Netherlands
Department Respiratory Medicine, University Medical Center Utrecht, Utrecht, The Netherlands

Marc J. M. Bonten
Julius Center for Health Sciences and Primary Care, University Medical Center Utrecht, Heidelberglaan 100, 3584 CX Utrecht, The Netherlands
Department of Medical Microbiology, University Medical Center Utrecht, Utrecht, The Netherlands

Xingchun Chen
Department of Laboratory Medicine, People's Hospital of Guangxi Zhuang Autonomous Region, Nanning 530021, China

Lijun Wang
Department of Laboratory Medicine, Beijing Tsinghua Chang Gung Hospital, Tsinghua University, Beijing 102218, China

Jiali Zhou and Honglong Wu
BGI Tianjin, Tianjin 300308, China

Dong Li, Yanchao Cui and Binghuai Lu
Department of Laboratory Medicine, Civil Aviation General Hospital, Peking University Civil Aviation School of Clinical Medicine, No1. Gaojing Street, Chaoyang District, Beijing 100123, China

Vincent Yi-Fong Su
Department of Chest Medicine, Taipei Veterans General Hospital, No.201, Sec. 2, Shipai Rd., Beitou Dist., Taipei City 11217, Taiwan, Republic of China

Kang-Cheng Su
Department of Chest Medicine, Taipei Veterans General Hospital, No.201, Sec. 2, Shipai Rd., Beitou Dist., Taipei City 11217, Taiwan, Republic of China

Center of Sleep Medicine, Taipei Veterans General Hospital, No.201, Sec. 2, Shipai Rd., Beitou Dist., Taipei City 11217, Taiwan, Republic of China
Institute of Physiology, School of Medicine, National Yang-Ming University, No.155, Sec.2, Linong St., Beitou Dist., Taipei City 11221, Taiwan, Republic of China

Yi-Han Hsiao
Department of Chest Medicine, Taipei Veterans General Hospital, No.201, Sec. 2, Shipai Rd., Beitou Dist., Taipei City 11217, Taiwan, Republic of China
Institute of Physiology, School of Medicine, National Yang-Ming University, No.155, Sec.2, Linong St., Beitou Dist., Taipei City 11221, Taiwan, Republic of China

Kun-Ta Chou
Department of Chest Medicine, Taipei Veterans General Hospital, No.201, Sec. 2, Shipai Rd., Beitou Dist., Taipei City 11217, Taiwan, Republic of China
Center of Sleep Medicine, Taipei Veterans General Hospital, No.201, Sec. 2, Shipai Rd., Beitou Dist., Taipei City 11217, Taiwan, Republic of China

Yu Ru Kou
Institute of Physiology, School of Medicine, National Yang-Ming University, No.155, Sec.2, Linong St., Beitou Dist., Taipei City 11221, Taiwan, Republic of China

Ching-Min Tseng
Institute of Physiology, School of Medicine, National Yang-Ming University, No.155, Sec.2, Linong St., Beitou Dist., Taipei City 11221, Taiwan, Republic of China
Division of Thoracic Medicine, Department of Medicine, Cheng Hsin General Hospital, No.45, Cheng Hsin St., Beitou Dist., Taipei City 11220, Taiwan, Republic of China

Yu-Chin Lee
Sijhih Cathay General Hospital, No.2, Ln. 59, Jiancheng Rd., Xizhi Dist., New Taipei City 22174, Taiwan, Republic of China

Diahn-Warng Perng
Department of Chest Medicine, Taipei Veterans General Hospital, No.201, Sec. 2, Shipai Rd., Beitou Dist., Taipei City 11217, Taiwan, Republic of China
School of Medicine, National Yang-Ming University, No.155, Sec.2, Linong St., Beitou Dist., Taipei City 11221, Taiwan, Republic of China

Masahiro Aoshima
Department of Pulmonology, Kameda Medical Center, 929 Higashi-cho, Kamogawa, Chiba, Japan

Naoko Katsurada
Department of Pulmonology, Kameda Medical Center, 929 Higashi-cho, Kamogawa, Chiba, Japan Division of Respiratory Medicine, Department of Internal Medicine, Kobe University Graduate School of Medicine, 7-5-1 Kusunoki-cho, Chuo-ku, Kobe, Japan

Motoi Suzuki, Tomoko Ishifuji, Koya Ariyoshi and Konosuke Morimoto
Department of Clinical Medicine, Institute of Tropical Medicine, Nagasaki University, 1-12-4 Sakamoto, Nagasaki 852-8523, Japan

Makito Yaegashi
Department of General Internal Medicine, Kameda Medical Center, 929 Higashi-cho, Kamogawa, Chiba, Japan

Norichika Asoh
Department of Internal Medicine, Juzenkai Hospital, 7-18 Kagomachi, Nagasaki, Japan

Naohisa Hamashige
Department of Internal Medicine, Chikamori Hospital, 1-1-16 Okawasuji, Kochi, Japan

Masahiko Abe
Department of General Internal Medicine, Ebetsu City Hospital, 6 Wakakusacho, Ebetsu, Hokkaido, Japan

Andrea Gramegna, Marta Di Pasquale, Francesco Blasi and Stefano Aliberti
Department of Pathophysiology and Transplantation, University of Milan, Internal Medicine Department, Respiratory unit and Adult Cystic Fibrosis Center, Fondazione IRCCS Ca' Granda Ospedale Maggiore Policlinico, Via Francesco Sforza 35, 20122 Milan, Italy

Giovanni Sotgiu
Clinical Epidemiology and Medical Statistics Unit, Department of Clinical and Experimental Medicine, University of Sassari, Sassari, Italy

Dejan Radovanovic
Department of Biomedical and Clinical Sciences (DIBIC), University of Milan, Section of Respiratory Diseases, Ospedale L. Sacco, ASST Fatebenefratelli-Sacco, Milan, Italy

Silvia Terraneo
Respiratory Unit, San Paolo Hospital, Department of Medical Sciences, University of Milan, Milan, Italy

Luis F. Reyes and Marcos I. Restrepo
Division of Pulmonary Diseases and Critical Care Medicine, The University of Texas Health Science Center at San Antonio, San Antonio, TX, USA

Ester Vendrell
Intensive Care Unit, Hospital de Mataró, Consorci Sanitari del Maresme, Carretera de Cirera s/n, 08304 Mataró, Barcelona, Spain

Joao Neves
Internal Medicine Department, Centro Hospitalar do Porto, Porto, Portugal

Francesco Menzella
Department of Medical Specialties, Pneumology Unit, IRCCS Arcispedale Santa Maria Nuova, Azienda USL Reggio Emilia, Italy

Wujun Jiang, Min Wu, Jing Zhou, Yuqing Wang, Chuangli Hao, Wei Ji, Xinxing Zhang and Wenjing Gu
Department of Respiratory Medicine, Children's Hospital of Soochow University, Suzhou, China

Xuejun Shao
Department of Clinical Laboratory, Children's Hospital of Soochow University, Suzhou, China

Liping Zhu, Jie Bai and Di Xue
NHC Key Laboratory of Health Technology Assessment (Fudan University), Department of Hospital Management, School of Public Health, Fudan University, Shanghai, People's Republic of China

Yongcong Chen
School of Public Health, Lanzhou University, Lanzhou, People's Republic of China

Rongrong Zou, Kai Luo, Jing Yuan, Haixia Zheng, Lei Liu and Yingxia Liu
Shenzhen Key Laboratory of Pathogen and Immunity, State Key Discipline of Infectious Disease, Shenzhen Third People's Hospital, Shenzhen 518112, China

William J. Liu
Shenzhen Key Laboratory of Pathogen and Immunity, State Key Discipline of Infectious Disease, Shenzhen Third People's Hospital, Shenzhen 518112, China
NHC Key Laboratory of Medical Virology and Viral Diseases, National Institute for Viral Disease Control and Prevention, Chinese Center for Disease Control and Prevention, Beijing, China

Chuansong Quan, Dayan Wang and Guizhen Wu
NHC Key Laboratory of Medical Virology and Viral Diseases, National Institute for Viral Disease Control and Prevention, Chinese Center for Disease Control and Prevention, Beijing, China

George F. Gao
Shenzhen Key Laboratory of Pathogen and Immunity, State Key Discipline of Infectious Disease, Shenzhen Third People's Hospital, Shenzhen 518112, China
NHC Key Laboratory of Medical Virology and Viral Diseases, National Institute for Viral Disease Control and Prevention, Chinese Center for Disease Control and Prevention, Beijing, China
CAS Key Laboratory of Pathogenic Microbiology and Immunology, Institute of Microbiology, Chinese Academy of Sciences (CAS), Beijing, China
Center for Influenza Research and Early-Warning (CASCIRE), Chinese Academy of Sciences, Beijing, China

Yongfei Hu, Min Zhao, Jinghua Yan, Baoli Zhu and Shuguang Tan
CAS Key Laboratory of Pathogenic Microbiology and Immunology, Institute of Microbiology, Chinese Academy of Sciences (CAS), Beijing, China

Jue Liu and Min Liu
Department of Epidemiology and Biostatistics, School of Public Health, Peking University, Beijing, China

Kwok-Yung Yuen
State Key Laboratory for Emerging Infectious Diseases, The University of Hong Kong, Special Administration Region, Hong Kong, China

Yuhai Bi
Shenzhen Key Laboratory of Pathogen and Immunity, State Key Discipline of Infectious Disease, Shenzhen Third People's Hospital, Shenzhen 518112, China

CAS Key Laboratory of Pathogenic Microbiology and Immunology, Institute of Microbiology, Chinese Academy of Sciences (CAS), Beijing, China
Center for Influenza Research and Early-Warning (CASCIRE), Chinese Academy of Sciences, Beijing, China

Roni Nasser
Department of Internal Medicine "B", Ramabm Health Care Campus, HaAliya HaShniya St 8, 3109601 Haifa, Israel

Zaher S. Azzam
Department of Internal Medicine "B", Ramabm Health Care Campus, HaAliya HaShniya St 8, 3109601 Haifa, Israel
The Rappaport's Faculty of Medicine, The Technion Institute, Haifa, Israel

Mohammad E. Naffaa
Rheumatology unit, Galilee Medical Center, Nahariya, Israel

Tanya Mashiach
Epidemiology and Biostatistics Unit, Rambam Health Care Campus, Haifa, Israel

Eyal Braun
The Rappaport's Faculty of Medicine, The Technion Institute, Haifa, Israel
Department of Internal Medicine "H", Ramabm Health Care Campus, Haifa, Israel

Chimwemwe Tusekile Mula
Department of Clinical Nursing, Kamuzu College of Nursing, University of Malawi, Blantyre, Malawi

Lyn Middleton and Nicola Human
Department of Pharmacy, School of Health Sciences, University of KwaZulu-Natal, KwaZulu-Natal, South Africa

Christine Varga
Ohio State University Wexner Medical Center, Columbus, USA

Maria N. Chitasombat
Division of Infectious Disease, Department of Medicine, Faculty of Medicine, Ramathibodi Hospital, Mahidol University, 270 Rama VI Road, Ratchathewi District, Bangkok 10400, Thailand

Natta Ratchatanawin
Division of Dermatology, Faculty of Medicine Ramathibodi Hospital, Mahidol University, Bangkok, Thailand

Yingluck Visessiri
Department of Pathology, Faculty of Medicine Ramathibodi Hospital, Mahidol University, 270 Rama VI Road, Ratchathewi District, Bangkok, Thailand

Yiyi Zhu, Huanyu Wu, Xin Zhou, Renyi Zhu, Chunzhe Zhang, Hongling Bai and Hao Pan
Shanghai Municipal Center for Disease Control and Prevention, Shanghai 200336, China

Jie Gao
Shanghai Jingan Center for Disease Control and Prevention, Shanghai 200072, China

Abu S. Abdullah
Global Health Program, Duke Kunshan University, Kunshan, Jiangsu Province 215347, China
Duke Global Health Institute, Duke University, Durham, NC 27710, USA
Department of General Internal Medicine, School of Medicine, Boston University Medical Center, Boston, MA 02118, USA

Index

www.ingramcontent.com/pod-product-compliance
Lightning Source LLC
Chambersburg PA
CBHW082039190326
41458CB00010B/3406